Taking Care of Your Child

Important Addresses and Telephone Numbers

Please take a moment to put these numbers together here so that you can find them fast when you need them.

Emergency Room _____

_____

Poison Control Center _NATIONAL: 1-800-222-1222_____

_____LOCAL:_____

911/Ambulance _____

_____

Family Physician _____

_____

Pediatrician _____

_____

Specialist (specify) _____

_____

Dentist (office) _____

_____

Dentist Emergency Number _____

_____

Hospital (main number) _____

_____

Taking Care of Your Child

A Parent's Illustrated Guide to Complete Medical Care

EIGHTH EDITION

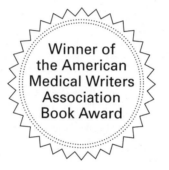

Winner of
the American
Medical Writers
Association
Book Award

Robert H. Pantell, M.D.
Donald M. Vickery, M.D.
James F. Fries, M.D.

Da Capo
LIFE
LONG

A Member of the Perseus Books Group

Dedication

To our parents, who first taught us about health

*To our mentors, Floyd Denny, M.D., and Helen Lamb, who first taught us
how to care for children*

*To innovators in child health, Evan Charney, Floyd Denny, Bob Haggerty,
Barbara Korsch, Clarence McIntyre, Terry Reilly, and Barbara Starfield,
who provide continuing inspiration*

To our children, patients, and their parents, who continue to teach us

Copyright © 2009 by Robert H. Pantell, James F. Fries, and Donald M. Vickery
Illustrations copyright © 2009 by Perseus Books Publishing, L.L.C.
Design and production by Eclipse Publishing Services
Set in 10-point New Baskerville

"Lights Turning Green" on pages 105–106 ©2001 Lenore Horowitz. Used with
permission of the author
M-CHAT on pages 502–503 ©1999 Diana Robins, Deborah Fein, and Marianne Barton

Cataloging-in-Publication Data is available from the Library of Congress
First Da Capo Press edition 2009
ISBN-13: 978-0-7382-1349-1

Published by Da Capo Press
A member of the Perseus Books Group
www.dacapopress.com

Da Capo Press books are available at special discounts for bulk purchases
in the U.S. by corporations, health plans, institutions, and other organizations.
For more information, please contact the Special Markets Department at
the Perseus Books Group, 2300 Chestnut Street, Suite 200, Philadelphia, PA 19103,
or call (800) 810-4145, or e-mail special.markets@perseusbooks.com.

10 9 8 7 6 5 4 3 2 1

A Note to Our Readers

This book is strong medicine. It can be of great help to you and your family. The medical advice is as sound as we can make it; many doctors have reviewed each section. But the advice will not always work. Like any sort of advice from your doctor, it won't always be right for you. This is our problem: If we don't give you direct advice, we can't help you. If we do, we'll sometimes be wrong. So here are some qualifications.

▲ If your child is under the care of a doctor and you receive advice contrary to this book, follow the doctor's advice; the individual characteristics of your child's problem can then be taken into account.

▲ If your child has an allergy or a suspected allergy to a recommended medication, check with your child's doctor, at least by phone.

▲ Read medicine label directions carefully; instructions vary from year to year, and you should follow the most recent.

▲ You know your child best; do not hesitate to follow your own judgment as to when to seek professional assistance.

▲ If your child's problem persists beyond a reasonable period, you should usually make an appointment to see the doctor.

BOOKS BY THESE AUTHORS

The Parent's Pharmacy
by Robert H. Pantell and David Bergman

The Common Symptom Guide
by John Wasson and Robert H. Pantell

Rudolph's Pediatrics: A Study Guide
by Robert H. Pantell, David Bergman,
and Maureen Shannon

Take Care of Yourself
by Donald M. Vickery and James F. Fries

Vitality and Aging
by James F. Fries and Lawrence M. Crapo

Taking Part: A Consumer's Guide to the Hospital
by Donald M. Vickery

Living Well
by James F. Fries

Arthritis: A Take-Care-of-Yourself Health Guide
by James F. Fries

The Arthritis Helpbook
by Kate Lorig and James F. Fries

*Lifeplan: Your Own Master Plan
for Maintaining Health and Preventing Illness*
by Donald M. Vickery

Contents

Chapter 9   Preventive Care   162

Acknowledgments

The following parents contributed to the development of this book, and their help was invaluable: Anne and Dave Bergman, Val Blanchette, Nora Blay, Jani Butler, Susan Charles, Libby and Milton Clapp, Linda Collins, David Curtis, Audrie Engbretson, Barbara and Joel Falk, Lee Hall, Mary Ann and Arthur Hanlon, Lenore and Larry Horowitz, Lois Kazmer, Michaline Krey, Shirley Lewis, Irmhild and Matthew Liang, Pit Lucking, Maria Maglio, Kay Neumann, Margaret Olebe, Suzanne Pennycook, Rosa Delgadillo Reilly, Kitty and Glenn Roberts, Marni Smith, Tom Stewart, Melissa Thornhill, Heather Van Nostrand, and Anne Wilkins. Many children also have contributed material: thanks to Loren and Matthew Loney, and Ciaran and Rylan Jacka, and Matthew, Gregory, and Megan Pantell.

We would also like to thank the following individuals for their assistance, support, and review: G. Robin Beck, M.D.; John Beck, M.D.; June Bernzweig, Ph.D.; Irene Cannon, M.D.; Mark Constantz; Doris Denney, R.Ph.; Larry Finberg, M.D.; June Fisher, M.D.; Susan Fisher-Owens, M.D., Victor Fuchs, Ph.D.; Judy Geisinger, M.S.W.; Dewleen Hayes; Halsted R. Holman, M.D.; Larry Horowitz, M.D.; Charles Irwin, M.D.; Al Jacobs, M.D.; Cynthia Kim, M.D., M.P.H.; Bev Kusler; Catherine Lewis, Ph.D.; Matthew Liang, M.D., M.P.H.; Tom McMeekin, M.D.; Carol Miller, M.D., Jane Morton, M.D.; Pat Moylan, R.N.; Kris Madsen, M.D.; Tom Newman, M.D., M.P.H., Margaret Olebe; Tom Plaut, M.D.; Shirley Rudd, R.N.; John Slane, R.Ph.; Tom Stewart, Ph.D.; Elihu Sussman, M.D.; Alan Uba, M.D.; John Wasson, M.D.; and Anne Wilkins.

We include special thanks for major conceptual guidance to David Bergman, M.D., and Marcia Pantell, M.S.W., M.P.H., Ph.D., and to Maureen Shannon, F.N.P., C.N.M., Ph.D. Maureen Shannon also contributed substantially to Chapters 1 and 2, and to Chapter 10, "Missing Children." Anne Bergman, M.S.W., Dr. P.H., contributed to Chapter 6, "Psychological Resources."

For continuing advice, review, and encouragement, we should like to acknowledge our wives, Maureen, Sarah, and Carol, and our children, Andrew, Elizabeth, Gregory, Gregory Michael, Matthew, Megan, and Meredith, and grandchildren Ryan, Connor, Kirsten, and Shane. Their daily input and effort make this as much their book as ours.

Finally, special insights for this edition were provided by the antics and challenges of Gregory and Megan, siblings who are $7\frac{1}{2}$ months apart in age, and the continuing adaptation and efforts at guidance of their older brother, Matthew. Inspiration for much of the new writing came from Maureen, who as a mother nurtured, refereed, dealt with earthquakes and hurricanes, earned a Ph.D., and did it all with style.

In Memoriam:
Donald M. Vickery, M.D.

Don Vickery died on November 22, 2008, at his home in Evergreen, Colorado, after a brief battle with a relentless cancer and is sorely missed by all of us who loved him. Don made major and legendary contributions to human health and improved millions of lives. He made a difference. He was the pioneering force behind "demand management" concepts and programs, showing that consumer-directed medical decision-making could improve health and reduce the need for medical care expenditures. He founded the Center for Consumer Health Education, now known as The Self-Care Institute, and Health Decisions International. He concentrated on wellness rather than illness, prevention more than cure, and the power of the patient over that of the doctor. Throughout, he worked successfully to establish new concepts of prevention through lifestyle changes and wise consumer decisions on a scientific evidence base. He authored and co-authored self-care books to bring wise decision-making to the public and also scientific articles for the health care professions. He was an original thinker, an extraordinary scholar, and a forceful advocate for better health for all.

Don trained at Harvard and Stanford Universities, was Board-certified in Internal Medicine, and was a Fellow of the American College of Physicians. He worked closely with Partnership for Prevention and the American College of Preventive Medicine, of which he was also a Fellow. He had an easy wit and a fine ironic sense of humor. He was easy to be with, motivating to talk with, and a pleasure to work with. This book, which we co-authored for over 33 years, has been a substantial part of his legacy. His contributions reflect his wisdom as a physician and father. We dedicate this edition, just completed at the time of his death, to his memory.

James F. Fries, M.D.
Robert H. Pantell, M.D.

Introduction

You can do more for your child's health than your doctor can.

This statement began the seven editions of *Taking Care of Your Child* and still rings true. Since the last edition, nearly 100 billion dollars has been spent by the National Institutes of Health directed to medical research. So it was shocking to learn that children born in 2008 are projected not to live as long as their parents. This unprecedented prediction was based, in part, on the deterioration of patterns and behaviors that parents can influence. Obesity is becoming one of the greatest threats to children's health, millions of teenagers are smoking, and problem behaviors such as drinking and substance abuse are taking increasing tolls. New medical technologies, such as fetal surgery, are more spectacular than the science fiction of the past. Advances in stem cell research hold a promise to dramatically alter the course of many chronic diseases, particularly since the resumption of funding by the federal government in 2009. New immunizations and strategies are available to protect children from serious infectious diseases. However, neither the diseases nor scientific breakthroughs that capture headlines are the principal determinants of whether your children remain healthy. Injuries still claim the lives of, or permanently disable, more young children than any other cause. As parents, you have it in your power to reduce injuries and save lives by securing your child in automobile safety restraints, insisting on the use of a bicycle helmet, and turning your water heater temperature down. You also have considerable control over your child's medical destiny by being informed about the availability of proven preventive measures, such as immunizations; by being aware of the risks and benefits of procedures for which there is no universally accepted policy, such as circumcision; and by modeling good health through eating sensibly and not smoking.

We are increasingly witnessing the consequences of family stress, school bullying, and neighborhood violence. Depression, drug abuse, and suicide are major concerns for children. It is no secret that families are under increasing stress. An important part of childhood is learning to cope with stress and adapt; however, children can become overwhelmed. Parents know their children best. Although parents cannot shield their children from today's family stresses and social pressures, parents have the responsibility to be alert to the signs of emerging difficulty and to enlist proper help.

We undertook this revision in response to the constantly changing forces affecting children's health and to keep current with medical advances available to children. Although most of the decision charts we developed have weathered well and required little or no revision, constant advances in our understanding of common problems have enabled us to make the charts more accurate. The increasing concern about autism, the ongoing national epidemic of obesity, the development of new technologies, and the change in approaching many symptoms also prompted an update. Some sections required expansion. Finally, we have included new material to update some of the major concerns of today's family, including recognizing autism, newborn jaundice, new approaches to managing common symptoms such as cough, and new vaccines against human papilloma virus and rotavirus.

Some things, however, have not changed. Your care and judgment are still the most important ingredients for fostering a lifetime of health for your child. A sound diet, a clean environment, and sensible living habits are the best way to reach this goal. However, illnesses and injuries are a part of growing up. Although some of these problems will require professional assistance, many can be handled at home. *The purpose of this book is to help you manage the common problems of childhood and to enable you to make better decisions about when to see a medical professional.*

Medical science encompasses a vast body of knowledge and an intricate technology. It is easy to become intimidated by the complexity of modern medicine and to feel uncomfortable making commonsense medical decisions. The most commonly encountered medical problems, however, are usually uncomplicated and inevitably get better by themselves. Each day you make sound decisions requiring good judgment in caring for your child. But there will always be a time when you are confronted with a new problem or an illness that is not typical. This book should help you in these times of uncertainty and improve your ability to judge how best to use your doctor.

There is an expression used by many medical educators: "When you hear hoofbeats, don't think of zebras." This has been our guiding principle. We have tried to focus in *Taking Care of Your Child* not on rare events that might happen, but on what probably will occur. Our own children have encountered a majority of the problems outlined in this book. Most of these problems can be successfully managed at home.

This book is divided into three sections. Parts I–III provide information helpful to understanding the several subject areas that we have found to be of greatest concern to parents. You will find discussions of pregnancy, birth, and physical development, as well as behavioral, school, and family problems and advice for staying healthy and for stocking the medicine cabinet. We have tried to give you both sides of issues such as home versus hospital birth, breast-feeding versus bottle-feeding, circumcision, and immunizations. Parts I–III provide background information for your role as parent and will assist you in developing a long-range strategy aimed at ensuring a healthy life for your child. In attempting to capture the complex feelings that develop between parent and child, we have relied on parents' statements of their experiences as well as some statements by children and adolescents throughout the book.

Part IV is the heart of this book; it provides specific guidance for more than 100 of the medical problems most likely to be encountered by infants, children, and adolescents. The charts in this section present step-by-step guidelines to help you decide on a program of home treatment or whether to make a telephone call or visit to your doctor. These charts are useful as an aid to your common sense and not as a substitute; you know your child best.

Part V provides a place to record growth, development, and medical information for each child.

As parents, we preside over the maturation of our children from complete dependence at birth to self determination less than two decades later. In gaining independence, a young adult needs to learn how to make personal and medical decisions with confidence. Teaching children to make independent decisions about their own health is one of the most important things a parent can do. The decision guidelines in this book can help you and your child with these important skills.

The typical child sees a doctor three to four times a year and has many more problems managed at home. Your family's experience with these scores of inevitable illnesses and injuries provides an opportunity for your children to learn, directly or by example, skills that will last a lifetime. The information presented in this book is intended to help you increase your confidence in the commonsense decisions you must make. In this process, you may save time and money, to be sure, but the real goal is to assist you in helping your child become a healthy adult.

Chapter One

A Child Is Coming

Pregnancy is as complex as any natural event in our lives. It is exciting, exhausting, fulfilling, fatiguing, happy, sad, simple, creative, and full of many more contradictions for both mother and father. In a few pages, we cannot do justice to a subject about which poets, parents, philosophers, and doctors have written extensively. Taking care of your child, however, begins with pregnancy. In this chapter, we will cover some of its most important aspects.

I'm Pregnant, We're Pregnant

There is no such thing as an unnatural feeling during pregnancy. Most parents experience a variety of emotions, from uncertainty and anxiety to satisfaction and exhilaration. To show the range of feelings, we quote from parents in this and the following chapters. But these are only a sampling of reactions. You will certainly experience emotions not found on these pages. Indeed, many people become concerned if they initially have no feelings about such an important occurrence. That, too, is a common experience, especially before parents can feel the first movements of the developing infant.

Many parents who have expressed tremendous anxiety about child raising during pregnancy find that the actual task is natural and rewarding. The advice of one mother is important to remember: "In having children and raising children, nobody is likely to experience something that hasn't happened to someone else. All of the emotions, from terrible fear to joy, have been shared by millions of others many times before."

Mother of Two   I hadn't given very much thought to what our lives would be like after the birth itself, which occupied most of my attention. If I thought at all about it, I guess I had a subconscious picture of myself in a Woman's Day *ad, one of those slightly out-of-focus pictures of a beautiful young mother in a pastel dressing gown nursing her baby in a pose of peaceful fulfillment. Was I surprised!*

Expectant Father   Libby kept asking me, "Aren't you excited about it?" She, of course, already was, and I had to admit, to her disappointment, that it was just hard to realize that we now had a baby on the way and

I really had no solid feelings or comprehensions about the child. She did come home wearing one of those tacky T-shirts with "baby" [in] bold across the front. My shy Libby did this. At first I wasn't too interested in being seen at the A&P with her and her new brazen shirt. But she was and still is proud of her tummy. I begrudgingly gave her my hand, which she pressed firmly on her tummy. I told her not to press too hard. I could hurt the baby. I still have a feeling of slight uneasiness when pressing on her tummy.

Expectant Father   *We're going into child raising with a lot of ignorance and a lot of trepidation. My cousins asked us to baby-sit for their four kids recently, and we realized for the first time we had very discordant philosophies about raising children. I always thought that I would naturally know how to raise kids—it never occurred to us we might have very different philosophies.*

Father of Two   *We had been trying for several months before Lenore got pregnant. When each month came and went with no pregnancy, we were filled with both relief and anxiety, and I think it is the mixture of the two emotions that is important. When Lenore did become pregnant, my first reaction was one of great exhilaration and excitement. But in a few days feelings of uneasiness surfaced. The exhilaration of starting a family was tempered by the uncertainty of not knowing what kind of change in our lives was to be forthcoming. Would we lose freedom? Would our new lifestyles be as comfortable as our present ones? Would the rewards justify the work? What was parenting all about anyway? We tended to try to cram many things into the nine-month pregnancy period. We had the feeling that each trip we took, each vacation, each special activity, each late-night dinner might be the last for a very long time. This ambivalence continued throughout the pregnancy, but as Lenore changed physically, I felt more sure that this was a very positive thing. The anxieties over the unknown were still present but somehow less important. Maybe they were replaced by the anxieties surrounding pregnancy and delivery. Would the baby be healthy? Would the delivery be easy? Would Lenore be well?*

Mother of Two   *I was totally unprepared for being almost solely responsible for her care. Why did I waste 9 months thinking about a birth that lasted only 20 hours instead of how to live with a dependent human being for another 20 years? I did not even see or hold a newborn in the time I was pregnant. I never saw breast milk or formula bottles.*

Mother of Two   *The one big thing that was taught in the Catholic Church was that in the event of a problem at birth, you were supposed to save the child. The doctors aren't allowed to make the decision, and they* *come out and ask the husband, and he's supposed to say, "Save the child." And I woke up upset and told David if that happened, I would really like a chance to try again.*

Taking Care of Yourself During Pregnancy

Taking care of your child begins prior to and during your pregnancy. Taking care of yourself during these periods is the same as living sensibly at other times, except that you are preparing (pre-pregnancy) or providing (if you are pregnant) for another individual. Your habits, such as smoking, drinking, or taking medications or drugs, may impact the success of conceiving and, when you are pregnant, will impact the developing baby. Most things that you did before becoming pregnant can continue without interruption. Some things in your life, however, will have to be altered. The "Additional Reading" at the end of this chapter provides information about preconception and pregnancy health care issues.

It is important for a woman to consider having a preconception health care evaluation by a qualified health care provider. This evaluation can assess for any situations that may require specific interventions to improve the possibility of experiencing a healthy pregnancy and birth.

Nutrition, vitamin supplementation, and medication administration both prior to and during pregnancy are factors that can influence pregnancy outcomes. Pre-existing conditions (e.g., diabetes mellitus, cardiac disease, HIV infection), risks of genetic diseases (e.g., Tay-Sachs disease, cystic fibrosis, hemophilia) or chromosomal abnormalities that you may or may not be aware of are important issues that ideally should be addressed prior to a pregnancy.

For example, if a woman who is planning a pregnancy is discovered not to have immunity to rubella (German measles) infection, she can receive a rubella immunization several months prior to pregnancy so that when she does conceive, her developing baby will be protected from birth defects associated with rubella infection. Women who are diabetic need to have very good control of their blood sugars prior to pregnancy to optimize both their attempts at conception and the progression of a normal pregnancy. Finally, something as simple as taking a small amount of folic acid (or folate) prior to and during the first 6 weeks of pregnancy has been shown to significantly reduce the possibility of giving birth to an infant with spina bifida.

Diet

A well-balanced diet is always advisable. Your nutritional status at the beginning of pregnancy is probably as important as what you eat during pregnancy. The exact amount that you'll need to eat during this time will vary according to your individual requirements, but common sense tells us that extremes are harmful.

Your total prenatal weight gain should be between 24 and 35 pounds (11 and 16 kg). Women who are underweight should gain 35 pounds, whereas obese women may need to gain as little as 20 pounds (9 kg). Gaining more than 35 pounds makes it harder to get back in shape after delivery. Most of the weight gained is for the infant, for the increased size of the uterus and breasts, and for more blood. Less than one-fourth of the weight is for increased stores of fat and protein. During pregnancy, you will need about 15% more calories and an additional 20 to 30 grams of protein on average each day.

Most women do not need to make elaborate dietary changes and write down their caloric intake during pregnancy. Common sense and a good diet will suffice. The increased nutritional requirements you will have throughout your pregnancy will increase during breast-feeding by another 200 calories per day.

These are the nutrients that are most important during pregnancy.

▲ Most of the extra calories you eat should come from increased **protein** (milk, meat, fish, poultry), the basic building blocks of fetal development.

▲ **Carbohydrates,** such as bread, potatoes, and cereals, also provide energy for the developing fetus. Restricting carbohydrates forces your body to rely on other sources of energy, such as fats. Too heavy a reliance on fats produces chemical by-products known as ketones, which alter your mood and are potentially harmful to both mother and fetus.

▲ **Fats** (butter, cheese, meat, whole milk) are also required for fetal development. They aid in the absorption of important vitamins.

▲ The requirements for **vitamins A and C** increase considerably during pregnancy, but an ordinary diet that includes fruits and vegetables will usually supply all your nutritional needs. Many doctors rely on vitamin supplements if they are uncertain of a woman's diet.

▲ Unlike regular vitamin supplements, prenatal vitamins provide more **folic acid,** a B vitamin found in milk and green vegetables. Folic acid is needed for the creation of blood. Adequate folic acid also reduces the risk of "neural tube defects," birth defects that result in problems with the infant's spinal cord. Therefore, taking supplemental folic acid six weeks before pregnancy and throughout the first several weeks of pregnancy is important for all women.

▲ The body requirement for **calcium,** important for maintaining sound bones and preventing muscle spasms, also increases considerably. Calcium is best supplemented with milk, cheese, or eggs. Broccoli and oranges are also rich in calcium, as are "bony" foods such as canned sardines.

▲ More **iron** is required for blood building. Foods rich in iron include meats, cereals, and many vegetables, such as peas, spinach, lima beans, and lentils.

The fetus's ability to obtain nutrition from the mother is remarkable. If a necessary nutrient is in short supply, the fetus will receive more of what is available. Improper nutrition first harms the mother, then the fetus.

Cravings

Many mothers report cravings for fruits and vegetables during pregnancy. These are undoubtedly your body's way of telling you what you need. Feel free to follow your cravings. Eat sensibly, and review your diet with a nutritionist or doctor should any questions arise.

Nausea

During the first three months of pregnancy, nausea and vomiting may interfere with your normal pattern of eating. Morning sickness occurs in many mothers, but others are most nauseated at supper time. Having frequent small meals is often the best way to obtain the nutrition you need. Many drugs used to treat nausea are potentially dangerous during pregnancy and should be avoided unless you have discussed the problem with your doctor and you both agree that medication is absolutely necessary.

Substances to Avoid

Since 1960, sassafras has been banned in foods because it was found to cause liver cancer in animals. Sassafras may still be available in some parts of the country as a tea. Avoid drinking it during pregnancy.

In 1977, the Food and Drug Administration (FDA) raised concern about artificial sweeteners. Although recent reviews are divided, we advise you to avoid them during pregnancy.

Because nearly all fish and shellfish contain small amounts of methylmercury, you should not consume more than 12 ounces weekly. Low-mercury fish include Alaska wild salmon, catfish, pollock, canned light tuna, and shrimp. Albacore (white) tuna is another common canned tuna that has more methylmercury than light tuna; weekly consumption should not exceed 6 ounces. Fish to avoid include shark, swordfish, king mackerel, and tilefish (see www.seafoodwatch.org and www.epa.gov/ost/fish).

Alcohol

Avoid alcohol. Drinking can cause the baby to suffer the birth defects and learning disorders classified as fetal alcohol syndrome.

Caffeine

Caffeine in coffee, cola, or medicines is safe in moderate amounts. Excess amounts can lead to difficulty becoming pregnant and poor weight gain of the fetus.

Tobacco

If you still smoke, this is the time to stop. Smoking interferes with the infant's normal growth and jeopardizes a successful pregnancy. Passive exposure to smoke is also dangerous and potentially interferes with brain development.

Exercise

Feel free to continue any physical exercise that you enjoyed before becoming pregnant. However, moderation is in order. This is not a good time to train for a marathon or begin an even moderately strenuous aerobics class. Skydiving and scuba diving are also not safe during pregnancy. In many parts of the country, there are now exercise classes especially designed for pregnant women.

Because of the fetus's ability to preferentially obtain an adequate blood supply, some of your physical reserves for strenuous exercise may be lost during pregnancy. Consequently, you may tire more quickly and feel faint, particularly at high altitudes. Basically, your body will tell you when to stop. You should also use your own judgment about certain types of physical exercise that involve the possibility of abdominal injury—for instance, skiing and hockey.

Traveling

With one exception, there are no traveling restrictions besides those dictated by common sense. As you approach the expected day of the birth, you should avoid trips that will place you out of striking distance of the site you have chosen for delivery. If you plan on flying in your ninth month, commercial airlines often request a letter in triplicate from your doctor, stating that he or she feels it is safe for you to fly.

Sex

Some women have decreased libido during pregnancy; for others the opposite is true. Both are normal. Intercourse is fine if everything is progressing normally. Women experiencing preterm labor or placenta previa (a placenta that is located over the cervical opening) should avoid both intercourse and orgasm because of the risk of increasing uterine contractions. In addition, vaginal bleeding, possible premature labor, or premature rupture of the amniotic fluid sac at any time during pregnancy are reasons to abstain.

After delivery, an episiotomy incision that is healing may make intercourse uncomfortable for several weeks.

Other than these situations, intercourse is possible whenever both partners are willing and able. If one of these problems arises, explore other forms of sexual pleasuring to maintain sexual intimacy.

Prenatal Testing

Some lab tests are done routinely on all pregnant women. These tests are important for mother and baby and are usually required by state law. They include blood tests for anemia and the mother's blood type, urine checks for infection and diabetes, and tests to check whether the mother has had certain infections, including rubella, syphilis, and hepatitis B.

Testing for the human immunodeficiency virus (HIV), the virus responsible for acquired immune deficiency syndrome (AIDS), is now recommended for all pregnant women. Many pregnant women who have HIV don't know that they are infected. Finding out if you are infected will enable you to obtain the important therapy you need. By taking anti-HIV medications during pregnancy, you can reduce the likelihood that your infant will become infected from 1 in 4 to less than 1 in 50. Most states now require that your doctor or nurse-midwife discuss this important testing option with you.

It is natural to worry about birth defects, which occur in 2 to 3% of infants at birth. Each year, there are newer and better ways to screen for some of the most serious defects. If one test indicates a cause for concern, doctors will often recommend a more advanced test to be sure that there is a problem.

Cystic Fibrosis

Cystic fibrosis is an inherited disease that can cause debilitating lung and gastrointestinal disease. Blood testing is now available and suggested for all couples planning a pregnancy or during pregnancy. If a mother tests negative, the baby cannot have cystic fibrosis, even if the father is a carrier. A father should be tested only if he wants to know whether he is a carrier.

Alpha-Fetoprotein Triple, Quadruple, and Multiple Marker Testing

An elevated level of a chemical called alpha-fetoprotein (AFP) in the blood can mean a number of things, including twins and inaccurate dating of the pregnancy. However, about 2 to 4% of women with elevated AFP are carrying an infant with *spina bifida* (an opening in the back revealing the spinal cord) or lacking a brain (*anencephaly*). Further counseling and diagnostic testing, including ultrasound and amniocentesis, are required if elevated AFP persists. In recent years this screening test has measured two additional pregnancy hormones (triple screen test) and inhibin-A (quadruple screen or multiple marker screen test). The test is now more accurate and can check for chromosome problems such as Down syndrome (Trisomy 21) or Trisomy 18. It is now recommended for all women at 15 to 18 weeks. Mothers older than 35 years should not rely on this test alone for Down syndrome but will probably also need amniocentesis.

Ultrasound (Sonogram)

Ultrasound is used in many fields of medicine. High-frequency, pulsating sound waves are bounced off an object and form an image on a screen. It is thus possible to determine the size, shape, and other important features of many parts of the body. For pregnant women, there are a number of important reasons to have a sonogram.

▲ An ultrasound is usually recommended after an abnormal screening test. For example, an ultrasound may determine whether a woman with an abnormal AFP test is carrying an infant with spina bifida or twins.

▲ Whenever there is the possibility of a pregnancy complication (for example, too much or too little amniotic fluid, slow or fast uterine growth) or of more than one baby, a sonogram should be done.

▲ Sonograms help to confirm the expected date of birth if the mother is unsure of her last menstrual period. Sometimes there is an important medical reason to be precise about the due date.

▲ Sonograms are also appropriate alongside amniocentesis, showing the doctor the location of the baby and placenta before and during the procedure.

▲ Ultrasound also can detect some of the physical characteristics that may indicate an increased risk for Down syndrome.

In some obstetrical practices, ultrasounds are routinely used to confirm or to date pregnancies. Some parents request sonograms because they want to have a "snapshot" of their baby in the uterus, to see the fetus move, or to know the sex of the baby. We do not think these uses are necessary. (In fact, sonograms are not very reliable on the question of the baby's sex.) The cost of the procedure is considerable: $100 to $200 per sonogram.

If ultrasound is recommended because you are at an increased risk of having a child with particular abnormalities, it is important that the test be performed by a radiologic group with expertise in pinpointing those abnormalities. Newer techniques with greater precision in detecting abnormalities include 3D fetal ultrasound, fetal MRI, and fetal echocardiogram. The risks of ultrasound appear to be exceedingly low. No documented complications have been reported for abdominal ultrasound. However, ultrasound should be reserved for medical reasons and not used for prenatal portraits.

Amniocentesis

Amniocentesis is a procedure in which amniotic fluid is removed from the uterus with a needle inserted through the abdominal wall. It is usually done at 16 weeks of pregnancy. (Later in pregnancy, if a premature cesarean delivery is planned, amniotic fluid may be tested to evaluate the infant's lung maturity.) The procedure is complex and expensive, requires a skilled doctor, and has complications. It is not for everyone.

Amniotic fluid reveals the following conditions.

▲ Genetic diseases such as Tay-Sachs disease, cystic fibrosis, sickle-cell disease, beta-thalassemia, and muscular dystrophy. In families with histories of metabolic disease, the risk of a child having the disease is usually 1 in 4 if both parents carry the gene for the disease.

▲ Chromosomal diseases such as Down syndrome, formerly known as mongolism. As women become older, the chances of having a child with Down syndrome increase. Only 1 in 1,250 women at age 25 will have an affected child, but 1 in 30 women at age 45 will. Advancing age is one reason to consider amniocentesis. Younger women who already have a child with Down syndrome may be concerned about having a second child with this condition. Although that seldom happens, many of these parents are interested in amniocentesis.

▲ A male fetus developing in a woman who carries the gene for hemophilia. Males can inherit this disease, but females cannot. Half of the males with carrier mothers will actually have hemophilia.

In the process of examining for abnormal or extra chromosomes, the sex of the child can be determined. You can ask your doctor not to reveal your child's sex if you so desire.

Amniocentesis is relatively safe, but there are risks. Spontaneous abortions and infant blood system problems (Rh sensitization) have occurred. When the procedure is performed by competent caregivers, however, the risk of a serious complication should be less than 1%. The risk of a spontaneous abortion after amniocentesis is less than 1 in 200.

Chorionic Villus Sampling

Like amniocentesis, chorionic villus sampling (CVS) provides information about the genetic and chromosomal characteristics of the developing fetus, but at an earlier stage of pregnancy (8 to 12 weeks). If a woman chooses an abortion because of information provided by this early test, the risks from the procedure are considerably diminished. However, CVS carries a slightly higher incidence of fetal death than amniocentesis. Again, it is essential to learn how risky the procedure is in the hands of your physician.

Percutaneous Umbilical Cord Blood Sampling

Percutaneous umbilical cord blood sampling (PUBS) is a relatively new procedure in which the fetus's blood is sampled directly. The advantage is that tests can be performed far more quickly, particularly chromosomal analyses. PUBS has risks and is not as widely used as amniocentesis or CVS. Ask your doctor about the risks.

All these diagnostic tests have ethical implications when coupled with the possibility of abortion, if you accept that practice. You need to decide which, if any, "disorders" warrant terminating the pregnancy. Also, a given inherited disease can affect one child much more seriously than another. What should be done with a fetus having a 50% chance of being born with a devastating disease? What do you do if you are looking for one problem and accidentally discover another?

If you are considering amniocentesis, CVS, or PUBS, discuss the test's implications at home and with your doctor. Doctors cannot tell you whether you should accept or reject a child with a given disorder. In the end, you should make a decision consistent with your own moral framework.

Medicine

All drugs are potentially harmful, and the risks associated with taking drugs increase during pregnancy because of potential harm to the fetus as well as the mother. Despite this, American women consume on the average 4.5 different drugs during pregnancy, and 80% of these medicines are not prescribed by doctors. Heavy medicine use is not surprising when one considers the number of drug messages we see and hear every day. Resist those messages!

As a rule, the majority of drugs that a mother takes will reach the fetus. The safety of most drugs now on the market has never been tested with respect to the fetus. Effects on infants are often discovered only after birth. Thalidomide, for example, was tested on rodents and did not produce the limb deformities that later resulted in human off-spring. Risks may be small—as low as 1 in 10,000 to 50,000 infants—but the consequences may be severe. There is no need to take even a small risk unless a medication is absolutely necessary.

Many medications change when stored over time and become harmful with age. Pregnancy is a good time to throw out all the medications on your shelf.

More than 200 drugs pose risks to a developing fetus. In some situations, however, these drugs may be needed for serious disease. In Table 1 (pages 13–14) we highlight a few common drugs that you should especially avoid, along with explanations of the problems they cause. Not all these associations are well documented. However, when considering infant safety, we feel that you should regard drugs as guilty until proven innocent. Before taking any medicine—even aspirin—while pregnant or nursing, consult your doctor. Other helpful information is available at www.nlm.nih.gov/medlineplus/druginformation.html and otispregnancy.org.

Aspirin

Some physicians recommend a low dose of aspirin to women who have experienced hypertension during previous pregnancies (preeclampsia) or to first-time mothers whose sisters or mothers have had that condition. Talk to your doctor about whether you should take one baby aspirin per day in the last half of your pregnancy to thin your blood and prevent blood clots in the placenta.

Immunizations

Avoid immunizations during pregnancy. This is especially true for rubella (German measles) immunizations. Women who receive rubella immunizations should avoid becoming pregnant for three months afterward. Although no birth defects have been reported in the few children born to women accidentally immunized with the rubella vaccine during pregnancy, the potential for problems remains. There does not seem to be any need to avoid contact with children who have recently been immunized.

Table 1: Drugs to Avoid During Pregnancy

Medication	Potential Problem in Infants
Alcohol—chronic abuse or high doses	Seizures, low blood sugar Growth retardation Birth defects
Amphetamines	Birth defects
Anticonvulsants Carbamazepine (Tegretol)	Facial defects Mental retardation
Phenobarbital	Congenital defects Bleeding at birth
Phenytoin (Dilantin)	Small size Facial defects
Valproic Acid (Depakote)	Brain and heart defects
Antidepressants Imipramine (Tofranil) Amitriptyline (Elavil, Etrafon) Lithium	Birth defects Birth defects Birth defects
Antihistamines Diphenhydramine—chronic use (Benadryl)	Seizures
Antihypertensive drugs (Captopril, Capoten)	Skull defects Small size Kidney problems
Antibiotics Sulfa Drugs	Jaundice
Tetracycline	Malformed teeth Suppressed bone growth Cataracts
Kanamycin	Hearing loss
Streptomycin	Hearing loss
Bronchial medications Potassium Iodide	Goiter
Caffeine—chronic heavy use	Growth retardation
Cocaine (illegal)	Brain damage Growth retardation Limb defects Kidney problems

Table 1: Drugs to Avoid During Pregnancy *(continued)*

Medication	Potential Problem in Infants
Diuretics Thiazides	Congenital defects (first trimester)
Ergotamine	Growth retardation
Hormones Estrogens (Diethylstilbestrol)	Vaginal cancer
Androgens	Masculinization of daughter
Progestins	Birth defects Growth retardation
Ibuprofen (Advil, Motrin—used late in pregnancy)	Lung problems
LSD (illegal)	Limb defects
Marijuana—chronic use (illegal in most states)	Unknown
Methotrexate	Spinal cord defects
Narcotics (illegal) (Heroin, Methadone)	Growth retardation Withdrawal symptoms
Nicotine (10 or more cigarettes daily)	Small size
Skin preparations Isotretinoin (Accutane) Acitretin (Soriatane) Etretinate (Tegison)	Birth defects
Tranquilizers Diazepam (Valium)	Decreased body temperature
Chlordiazepoxide (Librium)	Seizures
Barbiturates	Withdrawal symptoms Infant bleeding
Chlorpromazine (Thorazine)	Temperature regulation
Promethazine (Phenergan)	Bleeding
Vitamin excess C	Skin and intestinal problems
D	Heart valve problems
Vaginal preparations Metronidazole (Flagyl)	Cancer (in rats) Mutations (in bacteria)

Allergy Shots
Discontinue allergy desensitization treatments during pregnancy.

Pets

Some cats carry a disease called toxoplasmosis and can transmit it through their excrement. Like rubella, toxoplasmosis produces few symptoms in the mother (occasionally, fever or lymph gland swelling), but it is potentially harmful to the developing fetus. Toxoplasmosis is very common (30 to 40% of the population has had it). The more serious, relatively rare form of congenital toxoplasmosis appears in newborn children of women who became infected for the first time during early pregnancy.

If you have cats, your doctor can do a blood test that will reveal whether you have already had toxoplasmosis. If so, you need not concern yourself about this problem during pregnancy. If not, the commonsense approach is to avoid the cat's litter box and not to acquire a new cat. You can keep and love a cat that has been in the family for a while with relatively little risk.

Toxoplasmosis is also found in meat, but it is transmitted only in meat that has been undercooked.

Infections

It is impossible to avoid all infections during pregnancy. Immunizations before pregnancy can prevent some infections that are quite harmful to developing infants. Any exposure to an infection, particularly to illnesses that cause rashes, should be reported to your physician or nurse-midwife. Table 2 (page 16) lists the risks of certain infections, along with helpful measures regarding them.

Breast-Feeding or Bottle-Feeding?

Decide how you are going to feed your baby before the birth. Breast-feeding has many benefits for the baby and many think it is best for the mother too. It is considered the preferred feeding method by the American Academy of Pediatrics (www.aap.org/breastfeeding). If you do choose to bottle-feed, don't let this provoke feelings of guilt; 30% of women never attempt breast-feeding and only one third breast feed for more than a year. Bottle-feeding will not prevent you from providing your baby with intimacy and sound nutrition. Your baby will thrive when you make decisions that work for both you and your infant.

Table 2: Infections That May Occur During Pregnancy

Disease	Risk to Fetus	Suggestion
Chicken Pox	Disease that can cause fetal malformation in early pregnancy, severe newborn disease in late pregnancy	Avoid exposure; ask your doctor about immunoglobulin within three days of exposure
Fifth Disease (parvovirus B19)	Mild childhood disease that can cause a newborn to swell with fluid (hydrops)	Avoid children with characteristic rash (see page 432); consult your doctor
Hepatitis B	Infection	Have a hepatitis B screening during pregnancy, with treatment of infant at birth
Herpes	Genital infection that can lead to a brain infection in the newborn after delivery	Discuss with your doctor whether medication during pregnancy is needed
Human immunodeficiency virus (HIV)	Infection leading to AIDS	Have HIV screening during pregnancy, with appropriate treatment of mother and infant
Rubella (German Measles)	Infection in early pregnancy that can cause a variety of defects	Check immunization status before pregnancy
Toxoplasmosis	Disease that can cause fetal death or malformation	Check immunization status before pregnancy; avoid cat excrement and undercooked meat

Concerns about Breast-Feeding

Given the proper encouragement and assistance, nearly every mother can breast-feed. A few rare medical conditions, such as severe breast infections or infants with a cleft palate, may make breast-feeding more difficult.

Most drugs taken by the mother will be passed to the infant through breast milk. In general, therefore, never take any drug without consulting your doctor first. Some drugs that you should absolutely not take during breast-feeding are bromocriptine, captopril, cocaine, cyclophosphamide, cyclosporine, doxorubicin, ergotamine, lithium, methotrexate, phencyclidine, phenindione, and radioactive elements such as iodine. (See www.medlineplus.gov to check other medications.)

Infections can be transmitted through breast milk. This includes HIV, so HIV-infected mothers should not breast-feed unless there is no other source of infant nutrition. Similarly, mothers should not allow other women to breast-feed their infants because of the risk of HIV or other transmittable agents.

Many myths about breast-feeding make parents more anxious about this choice than they should be.

▲ Breast-feeding does **not** depend on your breast size. Large breasts contain mostly excess fatty tissue and in no way increase the ability to breast-feed.

▲ Inverted nipples are **not** an insurmountable problem.

▲ Breast-feeding does **not** interfere with poliovirus immunization.

▲ Breast-feeding does **not** cause more jaundice in newborns. In some instances, a baby may be taken off breast milk for several days to speed the resolution of the normal jaundice that occurs at birth. (See Jaundice, page 318.)

▲ Breast-feeding does **not** cause sagging breasts. However, for comfort it is important that you wear a brassiere that provides adequate support during your breast-feeding period.

▲ Although breast-feeding suppresses ovulation, it is **not** a reliable method of contraception.

Benefits of Breast-Feeding

▲ The baby receives nutrients in the proper proportion if the mother is eating a balanced diet. Only vitamin D supplementation is required.

▲ There is less chance of contaminating the milk than with bottle-feeding.

▲ Breast-feeding costs less than bottles, nipples, and baby formula, and it is in many ways more convenient. It does not require the paraphernalia of bottle-feeding. You don't have to run to the store in the middle of the night to buy formula. There is now widespread acceptance of mothers nursing in public.

▲ Breast-fed babies tend not to become fat as frequently as bottle-fed babies do. The composition, and therefore the taste, of breast milk changes during the course of a feeding. Thus infants will reject a breast after several minutes and move on to the other breast, even though the first breast still contains milk.

▲ The stools of breast-fed babies are lighter in color and looser than those of babies who are fed a formula. Because the stools are soft, breast-fed babies may have fewer irritations of the rectum, and they hardly ever become constipated. The more frequent stools will require more frequent changing of the infant. This looseness should not be interpreted as diarrhea. In fact, breast-fed babies have diarrhea less often. A strange bonus is that breast-fed babies' bowel movements smell better!

▲ For the mother, hormone release during breast-feeding causes rapid contraction of the uterus and encourages its return to normal after delivery.

▲ Breast-fed babies may have fewer ear infections.

Techniques of breast-feeding are discussed on pages 49–50. Nursing mothers associations and the La Leche League (www.llli.org) are always willing to help. The best place to get additional help is from a friend who has successfully breast-fed her baby or a lactation consultant (www.ilca.org).

Formula- or Bottle-Feeding

There are benefits to formula-feeding. The father can become involved in feeding very early. There is also somewhat more freedom of movement for the mother; a breast-feeding schedule may interfere with her ability to spend time away from the baby. (If parents choose breast-feeding, these problems can be reduced by using a breast pump to empty the breast when it becomes uncomfortable and having the father feed that milk to the baby with a bottle.)

Parents who choose bottle-feeding may be assured that today's commercial formulas are high quality. Great efforts have been made to produce formulas that are as close to breast milk as is feasible. Millions of Americans who were bottle-fed are a testimony to their overall safety.

Where tap water is safe for you to drink, it is safe for the baby. Sterilization is no longer necessary. Parents wishing to prepare several days' worth of feedings in advance should consider sterilizing, however, because bacteria can grow in the formula after it has been mixed.

Boil new nipples in water for a few minutes several times before using. This will remove the nitrosamides that some nipples have been found to contain. Also, use plastic bottles free of PCBs.

Infants suck naturally by squeezing their lower jaws and gums, using their tongues to push up on the nipple and keep it securely on the roof of the mouth. The usual bottle nipples permit milk flow more easily than the breast does. That causes infants to exercise their jaws less and to stick their tongues outward instead of upward to slow the rush of milk. Nuk nipples were the first type that allowed the infant to closely duplicate the sucking performed on the breast. Numerous nipples with this flattened shape are now available in latex and silicone.

Types of formula and techniques for bottle-feeding are discussed on pages 52–53.

Childbirth Preparation Classes

Preparing physically and psychologically is the key to a successful pregnancy for both parents. Learning to cope with some of the physical demands on mothers, such as eating to meet increased nutritional requirements, is usually pretty straightforward. Exercising to strengthen back and abdominal muscles is also important and readily achieved. (Standing in one place for a long time should be avoided during pregnancy.) But few exercises can prepare a woman for the demands on her perineal muscles. Similarly, the breathing best suited for labor is not something women have a chance to practice in daily life. Childbirth classes are useful for learning about these special physical demands of pregnancy.

The purpose of childbirth classes is to help the mother and father take an active part in the process of labor and birth. These classes attempt to focus the parents' energies during birth into productive psychological and physical activities, reducing their dependence on the doctor or midwife. Classes generally discuss in detail what occurs biologically during labor and delivery. They train women to use their bodies most efficiently to deliver a child. This includes physical and breathing exercises and demonstrations. In addition, classes teach the father or other partner how to help. Classes generally consist of six to ten two-hour sessions in the last three months of pregnancy. Many also include a tour and explanation of local delivery facilities.

Lamaze

The Lamaze method attempts to go beyond mere physical conditioning and elimination of fears. It is based on reconditioning, or changing the responses that the mother already has. The method aims to "convert delivery from the idea of pain to a series of understood processes in which uterine contraction is the leading phenomenon." By coupling a new breathing method with uterine contractions, Dr. Lamaze and his trainees hoped that the uterine contractions would stimulate breathing rather than pain.

It is unfortunate that Dr. Lamaze titled his original book *Painless Childbirth*. The purpose of prepared childbirth is to help the mother, father, and infant experience a safe, nontraumatic birth, but there is often still pain. Pain can be terrifying if misunderstood. It is not necessarily an evil force to be eliminated at all costs by drug or psychological anesthesia. The pain you may experience during swimming, running, or childbirth should not be hunted down and eliminated. In fact, very few natural childbirth classes have as their goal the creation of a "painless childbirth." Rather they strive for a childbirth in which the family is best prepared to deal with the event.

Parents should also realize that problems such as prolonged labor may occur despite the best preparation. Many problems have a physiological basis and are not the fault of the mother.

Other Types

Many parents dislike childbirth preparation classes that focus almost entirely on the physical aspects of delivery. They want more discussion of the emotional aspects. Several groups have developed childbirth preparation classes that focus on the feelings that parents experience during pregnancy, as well as on the reorganization of everyday life that the birth of a child brings about. The Bradley method has done much to bring fathers into the birth process.

We feel that all childbirth classes are helpful for most parents-to-be. Testimonials are the best evidence of their effectiveness. A recent study compared a group of women undergoing prepared childbirth with a group that had not taken any classes. There was no difference in the medical complications for mothers or infants in either group, but prepared mothers requested considerably fewer analgesics (pain medicines) and anesthetics. These drugs often make mothers and infants drowsy in the first few hours after delivery and diminish the quality of the interaction between them.

Sources

To find childbirth classes in your neighborhood, ask your friends, doctor, local hospital, or local nursing association. Many hospitals offer excellent classes on prepared childbirth, while others focus on how to understand hospital routines. Be sure you know the curriculum before you enroll.

If you are having difficulty locating childbirth classes, you may contact one of the following organizations.

▲ American Academy of Husband-Coached Childbirth
Bradley Method of Natural Childbirth
P.O. Box 5224
Sherman Oaks, CA 91413-5224
818-788-6662, 800-4A-BIRTH
www.Bradleybirth.com

▲ Lamaze International
2025 M Street, Suite 800
Washington, DC 20036-3309
202-367-1128, 800-368-4404
www.lamaze.org

▲ International Childbirth Education Association
  P.O. Box 20048
  Minneapolis, MN 55420
  952-854-8660, 800-624-4934 (book orders only)
  www.ICEA.org

Home Delivery, Hospital Delivery, or Something Else?

You have a choice of where your child is born and, in some areas, of which type of health care provider will attend your birth—doctor, certified nurse-midwife, or lay midwife. Paradoxically, people will spend hours doing comparative shopping for televisions and automobiles but automatically choose the local hospital for the birth of a child. The hospital can be an excellent place for your child to be born, or it can create problems.

Hospitals

How good is your local hospital? University affiliation does not necessarily ensure safety and quality. Each hospital must be judged on its own performance. How many deliveries are done there? Who attends these deliveries? Is a pediatrician available for emergencies? How often are cesarean deliveries performed? What indications does your hospital use for a cesarean delivery? There are no perfect guides to choosing the right hospital or for answering these difficult questions.

The hospital you choose should treat the entire family with respect. It should be supportive of your wishes for your childbirth. Most hospitals allow fathers in the delivery room. If you plan on having the father present, be sure to ask beforehand. Ask about the hospital's "routine" choices for medication and anesthesia. You want care consistent with your wishes, not "routine" care. If you feel uncomfortable with certain procedures, negotiate before your delivery or look elsewhere.

At Home

We occasionally get questions about home delivery. In many countries, delivery of children at home is the rule. The experience with home deliveries in countries such as England and Holland has been excellent. Women are carefully followed throughout their pregnancies, and those who have no complications are delivered at home by people with training and experience. In some countries, even first deliveries are performed at home. Other countries have a policy of doing home deliveries only for the second and later pregnancies.

The fact that home deliveries are safe in many countries does not mean that they are safe in your community or right for you. If you find someone offering to assist with your child's birth at home, ask about his or her qualifications. Is he or she a lay midwife, a nurse-midwife, or a doctor trained in obstetrics? How many deliveries has the person done? Is he or she prepared to deal with an emergency? What backup facilities are available? Does the person have admitting privileges at a hospital? In general, we discourage home deliveries, especially given some of the alternatives now available at medical facilities.

Other Options

In most communities, hospitals have set up comfortable, "homey" rooms for childbirth. These rooms are often called "alternative birthing rooms." In the event of an emergency, the mother is wheeled down the hall to the conventionally equipped delivery room.

In several areas of the country, more structured "out-of-hospital birthing centers" exist. Many of these centers are staffed by both certified nurse-midwives and doctors, and they have excellent hospitals nearby should the mother or baby require more extensive care.

Most communities have several options for delivery of your child, and you should find out about them. We feel that rather than beginning with a categorical decision ("I want a home birth" or "I want a hospital birth"), you should begin with the question, "What is the best method of delivery for me and my child in my community?"

Additional Reading

Planning for Pregnancy, Birth, and Beyond, 2nd rev. ed., American College of Obstetricians and Gynecologists Staff (New York: NAL, 1997).

Husband-Coached Childbirth, 5th ed., Robert A. Bradley (New York: Bantam, 2008).

Essential Exercises for the Childbearing Year, 4th rev. ed., Elizabeth Noble (Harwich, Mass.: New Life Images, 2003).

While Waiting: A Prenatal Guidebook, 3rd rev. ed., George Verrilli and Anne Mueser (New York: St. Martin's Press, 2002).

Chapter Two

The Big Event

Just as in pregnancy, the big event, birth, is full of complex emotions for both mother and father. Here are some of the feelings that parents have shared with us.

Mother of Six   *Great joy sweeps over you, but not on schedule. They placed my newborn son on the bed beside me. I looked at the child, and I did not recognize him. It's odd when you have felt his every move from the moment he started to move . . . when he has been a physical part of you for so long. Even though you don't even know the sex of the child, you still expect to recognize him . . . and you look at this total stranger. . . . You find out what his face looks like . . . a new and totally unknown face, a whole new and different person you have to get to know, . . . and with the knowing comes the loving.*

Mother of Two   *Although I had excellent prenatal care and access to the most enlightened and modern practices, the emotion I felt strongest after Mary's birth was anger and resentment toward myself and members of the medical professions. Why specifically—too much time was spent on reading, exercising, and talking about giving birth. I got sucked in by the movie star syndrome of the big event. How I would have natural childbirth, breathing, learning about my body, the muscles and how they worked, learning about pain, about control, learning my script, being undrugged and awake so I could experience birth, so I could see another baby coming out of my body. Hey, for 9 months I read about it, talked about [it], drove everyone nuts—and I loved every minute of it. After laboring 19 hours at home, I finally was driven, screaming and contorted with pain, to the hospital, where I expected to die. After being quickly gassed, but not soon enough to feel a mid-forceps delivery, I passed out and missed Mary's birth.*

But I loved her intensely the moment I saw her; she was really special. I could spot her the minute I walked into the nursery; she was so fair and bald and her head so lumpy. I was so proud of her and myself.

Mother of Three   *It is almost impossible to have any kind of relationship with the unborn baby. When I saw Peter for the very first time, he was lying in a plastic bassinet and had stopped crying very soon with his eyes wide-open, seemingly looking around. I thought he was so* *beautiful! . . . After this initial feeling of joy, it was a matter of getting used to this little warm, cuddly, and sleepy living thing. I didn't sense any immediate attachment; it was an adjustment to something very new. The feeling of wanting to protect this new presence, nurse it, and take care of it was very strong—I guess this is what they meant by "motherly instinct."*

Mother of Four   My husband couldn't care less if it was a girl or a boy—he was so frightened something would happen to me—he only wanted to know, "Are you all right?"

Mother of Two   I had a lot of depression because it didn't go according to the book. I read all the books and did all the exercises and learned how to blow, but nobody prepared me for any of the things that might happen. And I felt that because I was healthy and was not 4-foot-10, people looked at me funny when I told them I had a C-section. They seemed to be saying, "What's wrong with you? You seem to be big enough to have a baby." You need to know that it's not your fault. I felt guilty for 6 months because I thought if I had only breathed right, I would not have had 60 hours of labor.

Father of Two   The labor and delivery process ended with a feeling of great exhilaration, an indescribable feeling, unmatched by anything else I have ever known. Somehow everything was right with the world, and nothing could be wrong.

Stages of Labor

Most women begin labor in the fortieth week of pregnancy, but 10 to 15% have premature labor. Many premature labors do not proceed to delivery, ending after a short time. For many days before delivery, the mother may experience contractions known as Braxton Hicks contractions. The contractions are thought to prepare the uterus (womb) for delivery and to thin and widen the mouth of the uterus. This process is known as effacement and dilation.

The first stage of labor begins when contractions in the uterus become more regular and intense. It is often difficult to tell precisely when this stage begins, and there are frequent false starts. Often a small amount of bloody mucus may appear several days before labor. Contractions may come regularly, strongly, and at short intervals, and then suddenly cease. True labor has generally begun when contractions are 10 minutes apart. These contractions may be felt in the lower abdomen or the lower back.

During the first stage of labor, the mouth of the uterus (cervix) proceeds to open (dilate) more and more. Generally, this first stage becomes shorter with each pregnancy. It often lasts for 6 to 18 hours in the first pregnancy but only 2 to 5 hours in the second pregnancy. The end of the first stage of labor is known as transition and is often the most tiring period. In transition, the cervix dilates 8 to 10 cm (3 to 4 inches), the size required for the infant's head to pass through the birth canal. It is for this stage that childbirth class preparation is often the most helpful, because relaxation is important.

The second stage of labor is usually much shorter than the first. It usually lasts about 1 to 2 hours for the first child and 15 to 30 minutes for subsequent births. The second stage starts when the cervix is fully dilated and ends when the child is delivered. During the early phases of the second stage, some pain medications or anesthesia are usually administered.

The third stage is usually the shortest and lasts from several minutes to half an hour. During the third stage of labor, the placenta (afterbirth) is delivered. The doctor or midwife examines the placenta carefully to ensure that no parts still remain in the uterus. Any parts of the placenta remaining in the uterus must be removed because they can become a serious cause of bleeding later on.

Rupture of the Membranes

Throughout pregnancy, the developing infant rests in a pool of fluid enveloped by the amniotic sac. During the first stage of labor, this fluid cushions the child's head. The amniotic sac generally bursts by itself at the end of the first stage of labor. Frequently, the amniotic sac will begin to leak fluid or rupture even before labor has begun. This will usually bring about the beginning of labor. The absence of fluid does not directly interfere with labor, but an amniotic sac that has been ruptured for more than 24 hours increases the chances of infection. If labor has not begun and a large rush of fluid indicates that the amniotic sac has ruptured, contact your doctor.

The amniotic sac is often ruptured artificially at the end of the first stage of labor to facilitate the delivery. This is a painless procedure.

Medications Used During Labor

All medications that are given to the mother reach the child. No medications should be used automatically. For certain conditions, however, medications can be used with relative safety after careful deliberation by the doctor.

Sleep Medications

Sleep medications are sometimes used for women who are having false labor or who have been in and out of labor for several days and may have had little or no sleep. The mother's fatigue may carry a greater risk to both mother and child than a mild sleeping medication does. Barbiturates such as Seconal, Nembutal, and Luminal are frequently used as sedatives.

Pain Medications

Most childbirth classes equip mothers to cope with some of the pain of labor. However, as one obstetrician notes, "There is a reason they call it *labor* and not brunch!" Labor can be uncomfortable, and analgesics (pain relievers) should be made available when other techniques fail. Such medications reduce the pain of labor but do not completely eliminate it. Strong narcotic pain relievers and tranquilizers such as Demerol and Nisentil may be used on occasion. These medications enter the infant's bloodstream and have temporary depressing effects on him or her. However, pain can interfere with the progress of labor and also affect the infant.

Anesthesia

Anesthesia involves the complete elimination of pain by blocking the nerve impulses at either the local, spinal, or brain level. Several kinds of anesthesia are used in childbirth. Discuss them with your doctor before labor begins.

General anesthesia is rarely used in the United States today, although it is sometimes used after the first stage of labor is complete. With general anesthesia, the mother has no awareness of either pain or the birth of her child. We do not believe that general anesthesia has any place in routine deliveries. It may be used in complicated deliveries, where extreme relaxation of the mother's uterus and birth canal is necessary to perform a complicated obstetrical maneuver such as rotation of the infant. General anesthesia may also be used when a cesarean delivery must be performed.

Spinal anesthesia is administered at the end of the first stage of labor and results in complete absence of pain from the mother's waist down. This procedure was popular several years ago, but it is being used less and less today. Complications are possible in both mother and child, and postpartum headaches often trouble the mother. Again, this is an acceptable procedure for complicated deliveries or when the mother is experiencing moderate pain.

Epidural anesthesia (lumbar epidural block) is similar to spinal anesthesia, but it can block the pain fibers more specifically than spinal anesthesia. (For example, it can cause pain elimination specifically in the lower abdomen, perineum, and vagina.) It is administered during the second half of the first stage of labor. The possible complications associated with this type of anesthesia include slowing the woman's labor and lowering the mother's blood pressure.

Caudal anesthesia is given in the second half of the first stage of labor. It is generally administered lower in the spine than spinal anesthesia. It can be given continuously by a small tube inserted into the lower portion of the back. Caudal anesthesia has many of the same problems as spinal anesthesia, including the possibility of lowering the mother's blood pressure and causing postpartum headaches.

Pudendal block anesthesia eliminates pain in the woman's external genitalia. This provides partial anesthesia during the second stage of labor and during repair of spontaneous or surgical cuts of the birth canal (episiotomy). Some episiotomy repairs require an additional local injection of Xylocaine.

Pitocin and "Induced Births"

Oxytocin is a natural hormone that causes contractions of the uterus. The body produces it during labor to intensify contractions. The body also produces it after labor to make the uterus contract and to decrease uterine bleeding. An infant sucking on the mother's breasts stimulates the production of oxytocin and hence uterine contractions.

Pitocin is synthetic oxytocin. It should not be used routinely to augment natural contractions or to induce delivery of a child at a convenient time. It may be of great assistance to women who are more than two weeks past the due date or in cases where the infant is in distress. Pitocin may also help during prolonged labor or to aid uterine contractions after labor. It is administered intravenously. Too much Pitocin can cause such painful or excessively strong uterine contractions that depressant drugs must be used to counteract the force. Whenever Pitocin is being used, physicians able to perform cesarean sections should be present just in case a C-section is required.

Fetal Heart Monitoring

Fetal heart monitoring has long been accomplished by listening to an infant's heartbeat through a stethoscope. A strong, regular heartbeat is a sign that an infant is doing well during labor. A significant, prolonged drop in heart rate or in the intensity of the heartbeat is a sign of distress that may necessitate a cesarean delivery to prevent damage to the infant.

Electronic monitors have replaced the stethoscope for keeping track of an infant's heartbeat. In some cases, external monitors are used to keep track of both uterine contractions and fetal heartbeat by means of electrodes strapped to the mother's abdomen. In other cases, internal fetal monitors are used. Electrodes are inserted during the first stage of labor and are placed directly on the infant's head. This requires rupture of the amniotic sac, if it has not already ruptured. Some of these monitors are capable of measuring the acidity (pH) of the infant's blood as well as the infant's heartbeat. The mother's uterine contractions are also measured.

The theoretical advantage of fetal monitors is that they help detect early infant distress. Many women object to them on the grounds that they interfere with mobility during labor. There is, however, a more significant disadvantage to fetal monitors. With the use of fetal monitors at certain hospitals, the rate of cesarean deliveries has doubled. Yet the rate of newborn complications in hospitals not using fetal monitors appears no different from the rate of complications at hospitals using monitors and having a higher number of cesarean deliveries.

Because all the risks and benefits of fetal monitors have yet to be clarified, they should not be used routinely. For low-risk pregnancies, professional organizations have recommended either listening for the infant heart rate every 15 minutes in the first stage of labor and at least every 5 minutes in the second stage or using electronic monitors at the same intervals. We do feel, however, that fetal monitors can be important in high-risk or complicated pregnancies, or when the mother or baby develops a problem during labor.

Delivery Room Procedures

Episiotomy

An episiotomy is an incision made in the skin between the lower end of the vagina and the anus to enlarge the vaginal opening and ease the birth. Many obstetricians feel that an episiotomy minimizes damage to both infant and mother. They argue that these straight incisions heal better and hurt less than the irregular tearing that might otherwise occur.

Although the American College of Obstetricians and Gynecologists believes that episiotomy is useful in some situations, the organization states, "The routine use of episiotomy is not necessary and leads to a delay in the patient's resumption of sexual activity." Discuss episiotomy with your doctor or midwife beforehand so that you will know what to expect.

Breech Deliveries

Breech deliveries are not really "feet first"; they are actually "hips first." Although about 3% of births are breech, most of these occur in premature or multiple (twins or triplets) births. It is difficult to assess them precisely, but breech births are more complicated and carry greater risks to the fetus. Cesarean deliveries are often performed to deliver babies from the breech position.

Cesareans

A cesarean delivery (C-section) is a surgical procedure performed under general anesthesia to remove the infant from the uterus through the abdominal wall. C-sections are performed in about 20% of births. Because they are so common, parents should understand the procedure in the event that it must be performed. Discuss this possibility fully with your obstetrician.

There are many reasons for doing a C-section. Sometimes the infant's head is larger than the mother's pelvis can accommodate. Or labor may suddenly stop; this often occurs spontaneously, and sometimes because of drugs. Prolonged labor usually is a physiological problem and not caused by the mother's actions. Less common reasons for performing a C-section include a placenta implanted in front of the cervical opening, complications of diabetes or other illnesses, signs of significant fetal distress, or other serious problems of the developing infant.

C-sections are relatively safe, although they carry a higher complication rate than vaginal deliveries. Because more sensitive methods for detecting fetal distress (such as fetal monitors) are now available, minimum distress is being discovered more often. That has led to a higher number of C-sections. The benefits of basing C-section decisions on these new monitoring techniques have not yet been proved.

Having one C-section does not mean that you cannot have a vaginal delivery in subsequent births. Nearly three-quarters of women who have had C-sections are able to have future vaginal deliveries.

Premature Labor and Births

Between 5 and 10% of all infants are born more than two weeks before the due date. A number of factors account for these premature births. Some are caused by an error in calculating dates, and some are due to premature inducement of labor or cesarean section. Infections, long-standing illnesses, poor nutrition, and complications of pregnancy also can lead to premature labor. However, the majority of premature births are unexplained. Often a mother who has had a good diet, exercised regularly, avoided drugs, and received proper medical care will begin labor early.

Many women experience premature labor contractions because of the nature of the uterus. Considerable progress has been made in managing premature labor so as to prevent premature births. Contact your doctor or midwife immediately if labor begins early.

Because labor contractions are extraordinarily fatiguing if they go on for more than a few days, bed rest is usually recommended when they arrive early. This can be particularly frustrating if friends and relatives react by envying you for being "catered to." In reality, lying down for a long time can produce sore and weakening muscles. In addition, the mother is often plagued by questions such as "Did I do something wrong?" and "Is my baby going to be all right?" Some of your strongest support may come from mothers who have had the same experiences.

It is quite common for women experiencing premature labor to be prescribed medicines to reduce uterine contractions. Although many medicines are now being used for this purpose, including magnesium sulfate, nifedipine, indomethacin, and ritodrine, only ritodrine has been approved for premature labor by the Food and Drug Administration (FDA). A combination of bed rest and ritodrine is often a successful regimen, but many women still deliver prematurely.

Fortunately, the chances of a premature infant surviving and developing normally are excellent. Often survival rates are better in centers with considerable experience in premature infant care—be sure your hospital is ready for your baby. Many premature infants are faced with temporary respiratory problems because of immature lungs (hyaline membrane disease or respiratory distress syndrome). Other premature infants have problems with infections. Competent medical care can do much to help infants with these problems. Recent work suggests that corticosteroid hormones given to mothers who go into labor before 34 weeks can prevent some respiratory problems in infants.

Parents are often surprised by the appearance of premature infants. They are certainly not as big and cuddly as many parents expect. They appear quite frail and are often connected to a variety of monitoring and other devices. It may be difficult to locate the child among the machines. Nevertheless, you are just as important to your premature child as to your full-term child. Holding and cuddling the infant are important and are encouraged in many nurseries. Premature infants who have significant human contact grow stronger faster than those who do not.

Newborn Procedures

Delivery room procedures should encourage the unity of the family while ensuring the safety of the infant. More and more infants are given to their mothers immediately after birth, and often breast-feeding starts in the delivery room. There are many reasons why we approve of this process. Stimulation of the mother's nipples encourages uterine contractions and thus decreases bleeding. Holding the baby and looking at him or her gives parents an early opportunity to experience the presence of their child and to explore their feelings about this new addition to their family. We encourage both parents to hold the infant. Although we agree with recent advocates that bathing infants in warm water immediately after birth is soothing, we feel that giving parents the opportunity to hold their new child is more important and gratifying for all.

Child development experts have placed a tremendous emphasis on the first few minutes of life. These first minutes are important, but so are the first days, weeks, months, and years. If the delivery doesn't go as planned and you miss out on your child's first few minutes, don't worry; there will be many more shared experiences to come.

Hospitals vary in their newborn routines, so you may want to spend some time becoming familiar with your local hospital's procedures before your delivery. Following is a list of the most common routines. All of them are designed to improve the safety of your infant's hospital stay.

▲ Deliveries should be attended by an individual responsible for caring for the infant as soon as he or she is delivered. This caregiver need not be a pediatrician. Most delivery room nurses can manage the common problems of the first few minutes of life. Complicated pregnancies or complicated deliveries, such as breech births, should be attended by a pediatrician or another doctor who will care for the baby immediately after birth.

▲ We have never seen an infant held up by the feet at birth and smacked so that he or she will begin crying. That is for the movies. Most infants breathe and cry spontaneously at birth. When the infant's chest moves through the mother's narrow birth canal, most of the fluid is forced from the infant's lungs. Most infants have their mouths and upper respiratory passages suctioned to remove that considerable amount of fluid. This facilitates breathing.

▲ The delivery room should be equipped with infant warmers, or the infant should be wrapped snugly in a blanket. It takes a while for a baby's internal temperature regulation to begin performing smoothly. One of the worst things that can happen to an infant is a rapid drop in body temperature. This can occur if a wet infant is left exposed at normal room temperature.

▲ Babies should be examined promptly after birth for any signs of distress. The initial assessment should include evaluation of color, tone, activity, respiratory rate, and heart rate. Often this initial evaluation is expressed as a number from 1 to 10, known as the **Apgar score.** This score is not a predictor of the child's intelligence or health. A more thorough examination is usually performed within the first few hours of life.

▲ All infants should have prophylactic eye medication administered. In most states, this is a legal requirement. The purpose of the eye medication is to stop infections from the gonococcus bacterium (gonorrhea). Gonococcal conjunctivitis is a major threat to the infant and is a common cause of blindness. Although most mothers are certain that they do not have and never have had gonorrhea, this disease can remain hidden for many years. The most common eye medications are erythromycin and silver nitrate, which may cause several days of tearing in the newborn. Erythromycin is also effective against another, more common infection known as chlamydia.

▲ New babies should have a vitamin K injection. A newborn's immature liver is often unable to produce this vitamin, which is necessary for making one of the components of blood that prevents hemorrhaging. Before the administration of vitamin K became routine, hemorrhaging was common in newborns.

▲ While in the hospital, an infant should be examined daily by a doctor, and daily conferences should be held with the parents to discuss any questions or concerns they may have.

Newborn Blood Screening

Father of Four   When I look at my grandchildren I am so grateful that my daughter was one of the first infants in the country to have PKU detected and treated.

Upon discharge from the hospital, all babies have blood tests for inherited diseases. Blood is usually obtained from the infant's heel.

Screening for rare but treatable diseases is a major scientific success story. At the time of our first edition in 1976, newborns were only tested for PKU (phenylketonuria, a disease that leads to mental retardation but that can be treated with an appropriate diet). Now there are nearly 30 tests available to identify conditions for which there are effective treatments. In addition to testing for PKU, all states screen for hypothyroidism (a disorder of the thyroid gland that affects growth and causes mental retardation), galactosemia (an inability to digest lactose due to a missing enzyme, which leads to brain damage or death if untreated), and sickle cell disease (a blood disorder accompanied by problems of blood clotting and inability to fight certain infections).

State policies vary on testing for other inherited disorders; virtually all states require 4, others as many as 30. If a disease runs in your family, ask your doctor if a newborn screen is available. Information on state screening is available at www.genes-r-us.uthscsa.edu and www.marchofdimes.com.

Human immunodeficiency virus (HIV) testing is recommended for all pregnant women. If the mother was not tested during pregnancy, it is recommended for newborns. If a newborn's test is positive, it signifies infection in the mother but not necessarily in the baby. Infants who test positive immediately begin receiving medicines to reduce the likelihood that they will become infected. Most do not. Mothers also have the opportunity to begin their own HIV care and to learn how to avoid transmitting the virus to their baby (such as not breast-feeding).

Hearing Screening

New technologies have provided us with the ability to test hearing in newborns. Along with the American Academy of Pediatrics (AAP) we believe every newborn should be screened. Several types of tests now measure newborn hearing more accurately than the response-to-hand-clapping techniques of the past. One type of test (otoacoustic emissions) detects problems with the inner and middle ear while another (auditory brainstem response) checks the nerve and brain functions needed for hearing. Both are simple and noninvasive. The tests are not perfect. If an infant tests abnormal, more extensive evaluation should be performed by an audiologist and physician within three months. Even if normal, some infants should be rechecked. These include infants who have had serious infections, high bilirubin levels at birth, facial anomalies, head trauma, or fluid in the middle ear for three months. If someone in your family has had hearing loss or you are concerned about your infant's hearing, request a test.

Circumcision

Both parents should carefully consider before the birth whether to have a son circumcised. Circumcision involves the surgical removal of the foreskin of the penis. There are several commonly used techniques to perform circumcision. In one technique the child is sometimes sent home with a small plastic ring still in place around the penis. The ring will eventually fall off. We mention this because doctors occasionally forget to tell the parents, and the plastic ring can cause considerable anxiety.

Circumcision has its historical roots in both ritual and health. It does prevent *balanitis,* an infection beneath the foreskin, and *phimosis,* the inability to retract the foreskin. These problems can cause swelling of the foreskin and even obstruction of the urinary stream. Infants who are uncircumcised are also more likely to develop urinary tract infections. When uncircumcised boys have fevers in infancy, they should be tested for urinary infections. However, the overwhelming majority of uncircumcised boys never develop medical problems.

Less than 5% of newborn boys have retractable foreskins. By three years old, 90% of boys have retractable foreskins. It is difficult and unnecessary to retract the foreskin in a newborn infant. Retraction usually becomes easy after several months. Phimosis is frequently seen in children who are beginning to take responsibility for their own bathing but who do not retract the foreskin and wash the glans of the penis carefully. Phimosis does not occur with proper hygiene.

In some children, the end of the penis has not completely developed, and the child is unable to produce a forceful stream of urine. This problem, termed *hypospadias,* is not a dangerous medical problem, but it can create difficulties if the boy cannot use a urinal like other males. It can also be a cause of infertility. One of the surgical procedures to correct this problem requires that the foreskin be intact. Unfortunately, this procedure cannot be used if the foreskin was removed by circumcision.

Complications from circumcision are rare, but they do include damage to the penis itself.

Other arguments for and against circumcision have been made with varying degrees of scientific support. Cancer of the penis has been said to be more common in uncircumcised males, and cancer of the cervix may be more common in the sexual partners of uncircumcised males. Uncircumcised males also are more likely to contract sexually transmitted infections when engaging in unprotected sexual intercourse. Some people believe that a man's sexual pleasure is enhanced by the presence of the foreskin, but others believe that it is diminished. Neither argument has been substantiated.

Finally, there are those who worry, "Will he be like everyone else?" or "Will he be like his father?" Circumcision is an optional procedure, and there will no doubt be plenty of circumcised and uncircumcised boys around. We feel that medical procedures should be done for medical reasons and not to make boys look like somebody else. The AAP agrees and at this time does not believe scientific data are sufficient to recommend routine neonatal circumcision.

Taking Your Child Home

The joy of taking your child home can be offset by many challenges. In the past, to minimize costs, health insurance companies began limiting the hospital stay for new infants and mothers to less than 24 hours. Although studies have differed in their findings on how these "drive-through deliveries" affect patient health, legislation has been passed making 48 hours the standard stay for vaginal deliveries; mothers who have C-sections usually stay longer. Most hospitals have developed sensible criteria for discharge. Criteria for the baby include full-term healthy baby, normal exams, normal lab values, good feeding, and success in urinating and having a bowel movement—and for the parent, sufficient parent skills and confidence to care for the infant.

While early discharge unquestionably causes problems for some infants, and is frustrating for many parents, it remains an option. If you feel that you would like to leave early, discuss this with your physician. Although there are certainly better places to be than a hospital, the surveillance and support provided by maternity and neonatal care nurses continue to be valuable services.

If you leave the hospital early, inquire about home nursing visits. Many hospitals and health plans offer such visits. They save money for you and your health plan while providing valuable services.

Following are some of the things you should prepare for when leaving the hospital.

Hospital Routine

There are usually quite a few people coming in and out of the hospital room: nurses and doctors assessing mother and baby; administrators with paperwork; hospital staff with food; etc. Hospital paperwork must be completed. Generally, the father can attend to this, although many hospitals now have someone from the financial office drop by the room so that the mother can complete the paperwork herself.

Most hospitals permit unlimited visiting by fathers; young children may be screened for illness before being allowed entry to the maternity ward. A young child may be anxious about the mother's return and overjoyed to see her come out of the ward, only to be restrained from embracing her by hospital rules. The mother usually is provided with a wheelchair when leaving the ward (like it or not) and generally is not allowed to have contact with her older children. Although there are many compelling arguments against these rules, your hospital may enforce them, and you should be prepared to deal with their effects on your other children.

Product Samples

Many hospitals provide a package of goodies for the parents to take home for their new child. These goodies are supplied by the companies making the products and not by the hospital or your doctor. They are advertising samples. Some of them may be useful, but many are not. Although they are free, they can cost you money in the long run and get you started on some bad habits.

A typical package will include the following:

▲ **Infant formula.** This is very often a prepared liquid or liquid concentrate and is fine if you are going to bottle-feed your child. The samples are handy to have and have a long shelf life. If you do choose to use infant formula, however, remember that powdered formulas are more economical than liquid. Check at your local supermarket to see which is most cost-efficient. There are no clinically significant differences between the major commercial products now on the market.

▲ **Lotions, creams, and ointments.** Use these on yourself if you wish, but most infants do not need such preparations. We do not recommend the routine use of any skin preparation for children. For management of diaper rash, see page 374.

▲ **Powders.** Baby powders have been used for centuries to keep babies dry, but the best way to dry a baby's bottom is to dry the baby's bottom. As soon as the child urinates, the effect of the powder is gone. If you choose to powder your child, place the powder in your hand and then place it on the child's bottom. Shaking powder from a distance will spread a cloud of dust, and the infant can inhale it.

▲ **Cotton-tipped swabs.** Swabs can be used to clean a newborn's umbilical cord stump with alcohol, but they should never be used to clean the inside of children's ears. Wax is produced within the ear canal for a purpose. It usually becomes a problem only when it is pushed into the ear canal with a swab. We tell parents never to put anything smaller than their elbows in a child's ear.

▲ **Vitamins.** All infant formulas are supplemented with the vitamins needed for your child's proper growth and development. Infants who are breast-fed need only vitamin D supplements (see page 49).

The Drive Home

The number one killer of children in this country is injuries. The leading accidental killer is the automobile. The risk to your child from the automobile is greater than the risk from childhood infectious diseases and cancer combined. Always be careful with kids and cars.

You may want to hold your baby in your arms on your way home from the hospital, but this is not in anyone's best interest. The driver will probably be excited about bringing the baby home and will be less attentive to road conditions than usual. We have heard of tragic injuries in this setting. Have an **infant car seat** ready to use on the way home. Some hospitals may not let you leave with the infant unless you have a car seat.

Remember that children should *never* sit in the front seat. The backseat is safer, whether or not your car is equipped with air bags, which are potentially deadly to children. Children should always wear seat belts—as should parents. A discussion of infant car seats can be found on pages 192–193.

Arriving Home

Upon arriving home, you need time and attention for yourself, your new infant, and your other children, who probably are anxious to see that you still love them. These are the most important items on your agenda. Contact with friends and relatives is secondary. If a friend or a relative will be staying with you, we advise that he or she help with the household chores and free you for time with your children. Well-meaning relatives too often come between older children and their mother. Older children need reassurance from their mother, as well as their grandmother, that their mother still loves them.

Mothers who have no relative or no husband to help at home can seek help from neighbors, friends, social agencies, and employment agencies.

Chapter Three

Your First Concerns

Is there life after birth? Becoming a new family is a major physical and emotional adjustment for everyone. Here are some thoughts on this new experience from parents we know.

The First Child

Father of Two   *The first several weeks made it very clear that our lives had changed fundamentally and unalterably, partially for the better, partially not. We were tied to the breast-feeding schedule. Our freedom of movement was over. Our nights were continually interrupted. There were times I resented the change—resented the baby for bringing them about and felt guilty because it seemed unconscionable to hold such feelings toward such a small, adorable, helpless infant.*

Father of Three   *During the early months, I don't remember feeling as close physically or emotionally to the baby as I do now. Was it because my wife had everything so under control and was breast-feeding? Or was it because I was still working? I don't know. The first time I held the baby, even though I had held others before, was a fairly nervous time. He seemed very small and fragile, and I was afraid of letting his neck fall down for fear of causing some whiplash injury.*

Mother of Four   *You take a diaper off the top of the pile, and your husband says, "That one is dusty." With the first baby you waste a lot of unnecessary time on things like that.*

Mother of Six   *We take on a 24-hour-a-day job with a pathetic lack of skills with which to cope. And for the mother and father who have been accustomed to being effective and successful at their own work, the feeling of gross incompetence leads to a great resentment.*

Mother of One   *After four years of peaceful dinners enjoyed after hectic days, my husband and I resented the interruption. I felt an obligation toward the baby but also sympathy for my husband. We felt guilty that we were being selfish. After discussions with friends, we decided that our feelings were shared by many couples adjusting to a new member in their family.*

Father of Two   Other couples talked about it, but we never had the experience of feeling restricted by our new addition. In fact, it was pretty nice to have an excuse to stay home.

Mother of Six   The responsibility lasts for 24 hours each day, and the decisions are all yours. You can't put the problem aside or pass it on. I believe this is the essence of the trapped feeling so common in new parents, much more than the fact that they can't go to the party because there is no sitter available tonight.

Mother of Two   This is the first time in my life that any individual had the right—not the privilege—to call on me 24 hours a day any-place, and I had the obligation to go. Nobody had ever done that to me before. I was a schoolteacher, and my husband used to say, "Ha! This one doesn't go home at 4:30."

Mother of Two   Coming from a large family, I knew the mechanics of caring for babies, but somehow I didn't remember babies as so small and weak. I had a feeling of nervous anxiety, not depression. Sue's breathing was so irregular I found myself checking her constantly, really expecting to find her dead from crib death or suffocation from not being able to lift her head up high enough.

Mother of Two   I nursed Tally for six months and once again felt anger at those women who had full breasts at the right time instead of the three months of engorgement, leaking, pain. Pain? Maybe I was the only one. Maybe I wasn't relaxed enough, not in tune with my body. Something must be wrong with me. Only after talking with other mothers—some successful, some not—did I discover that the "letdown reflex" is often painful.

Mother of Four   With my first baby, we were living abroad and even had two maids, but I still had no time to make even Jell-O for dessert. I asked myself, what was I doing? It seemed that I had no time for a bath. Now that I have four, everything is organized, and there's plenty of time.

The Second Time Around

Mother of Six   I guess the second time around it is all more real. . . . You know about the new person arriving . . . and the joy is easier. And then you discover they never both sleep at the same time.

Mother of Two   *This is what the days were like.*
  6:00 A.M. Feed/change Jeremy
  8:00 A.M. Dress Mirah; breakfast/clean up
 10:00 A.M. Feed/bathe Jeremy; change Mirah
 12:00 P.M. Change Mirah; lunch/clean up
  2:00 P.M. Feed/change Jeremy; change Mirah for nap
  3:00 P.M. End of Mirah's nap
  4:00 P.M. Change Mirah
  6:00 P.M. Feed/change Jeremy; dinner for Mirah
  6:30 P.M. Larry burps Jeremy; I fix dinner
  7:00 P.M. Dinner/clean up
  8:00 P.M. Bath for Mirah; dress for bed
  8:30 P.M. Ice cream for Mirah
  9:00 P.M. Bed for Mirah
 10:30 P.M. Feed/change Jeremy; pray he sleeps through the night
 11:30 P.M. Fall exhausted into bed

Mother of Two   *The first night home, I put Rick down and went to bed. I woke up a short while later because I realized I had not checked on Alan and tucked him in again—something I always did. I forgot Alan was in the house. That made me feel strange and also sad. About three nights after Rick was born, I was playing with Alan when Rick started crying. I had to leave Alan to feed Rick, and I felt myself resenting Rick because he had broken in on a special time.*

Mother of Four   *After the first baby, I never cried once, and I thought there was no such thing as the postpartum blues. When Emily was born, I brought her home, and I woke up one morning and burst into tears. David was still in bed, and he put his arms around me and said, "What's wrong?" I said, "I'm very unhappy about that baby." And he said, "I know." And we both decided, wrongly, that since we had had another little girl, we were very disappointed.*

Mother of Two   *I felt guilty because Sarah was so jealous of her sister, and I was hard-pressed to devote an "hour," as my pediatrician had recommended, to her exclusively. I also felt badly that I was not so involved in the new baby's personality as I was in Sarah's. The little things, like rolling over, that Sarah did that thrilled Will and me seemed less exciting the second time around.*

Mother of Two   *I have almost unconsciously learned to use my left hand while the baby is cuddled and nursing on the right. It's amazing how I can now manage to eat my dinner—not quickly, it is true— during two-year-old tantrums and three-month-old cranky crying, talking to one and holding the other. I sometimes think that hardening of the eardrums must be estrogen related.*

Father of Two   *The second baby was a very different experience. The peaks of exhilaration were lower, although present. The valleys of anxiety were not nearly as deep, although they too were present. My God, what an added increment of work! Two sets of diapers. Two car seats. Two feeding schedules. Two sleeping schedules. But not that much more restriction. We were able to accommodate to it. We resumed our other lives more easily.*

Mother of Two   *We found that we were spending most of our time with people who had children. They understood the constant interruption and irrational and seemingly destructive behavior of our children.*

Mother of Five   *It is more important for the child to feel loved than for the house to look good. The three-year-old will remember you sitting down and drawing silly faces for him with a warm glow. He won't feel the same about you mopping the floor and his not being allowed in until it is dry. I remember the Montreal taxi driver who said it always worried him if he came home to a tidy house. It made him wonder if his kids had had any fun at all that day.*

In the first few days at home, new parents often spend a great deal of time checking their new baby. Perfectly normal infants often appear strange in some way, causing concern to new parents. The purpose of this section is to describe the sometimes surprising features found in normal newborns.

There are undoubtedly things that you will notice about your newborn that are not covered in this discussion. Most doctors are more than willing to sit down and explain the concerns that parents have over their babies. Very often, however, parents forget to ask about a small item because of the excitement of having their child and because of the chaos of the hospital ward. We suggest that you write down any questions about your baby and make sure you get a satisfactory answer to each one.

Activity

Infants spend much of their time sleeping. The newborn may spend 18 or even 20 hours sleeping, the 6-month-old 16 to 18 hours, and the 1-year-old 14 to 15 hours. For more on sleep, see pages 80–81. You may observe several types of sleep states. In one state, the child will be motionless and have regular breathing. In another, the baby's breathing will be irregular, the eyes will flutter, and the hands will move.

Infants also exhibit different stages of being awake, the least satisfying of which is crying. This is the infant's most obvious way of communicating needs, frustrations, and discomforts, but there are other subtle ways of communicating that parents can learn to recognize.

Infants spend much of their quiet time looking and watching. In this stage, the infant is exploring the world with his or her eyes. He or she will stare intently into the parents' faces and follow them across the room. Babies have certain likes and dislikes in shapes, patterns, and even colors. These preferences have been demonstrated even in the first few hours after birth. In the "active alert" state, the infant is looking around actively, as well as moving the arms and legs.

Newborn babies are often disappointing to parents who expect laughing, gurgling infants. The image of babies most of us have is actually when they are four to eight months old. Newborns are exciting, but it will be months before they laugh and gurgle.

Breathing

Infant breathing patterns are often irregular. An infant may pause for 5 to 10 seconds between breaths. This is known as periodic breathing. This breathing pattern, characteristic of a certain state of sleep, is normal for newborns, and infants normally outgrow this pattern within the first few months of life. It should not be of concern to parents unless it persists for a number of months. A longer pause—20 seconds, or if a baby turns blue—is known as an apneic spell. Apneic spells require that you contact your physician immediately.

Sudden Infant Death Syndrome (SIDS)

Many parents fear that their infants will stop breathing and become victims of SIDS. Although SIDS is the leading cause of death beyond the newborn period, it is important to remember that the risk is less than 1 in 1,000 before age one and declines rapidly after six months. The risk of this syndrome is higher for children whose siblings had the problem and for premature infants.

Do not panic if your child's breathing is erratic, with the child not taking a breath for 10 to 15 seconds. Discuss pauses longer than that with your doctor. There are a number of ways to diagnose and manage erratic breathing, including monitors and medications. Parents who have experienced a previous loss of a child should discuss the benefits and risks of an apnea monitor with their physicians.

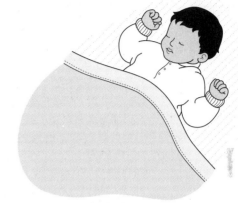

Sleeping position for infants. Studies have shown that healthy infants who sleep on their back or side are less vulnerable to sudden infant death syndrome (SIDS). Some infants with respiratory or intestinal problems may be better off sleeping on their stomach, however. Consult your doctor.

Parents can reduce the risk of SIDS by following these rules.

▲ It is essential for the mother not to smoke during her pregnancy or after birth. Infants who die from SIDS are two to three times more likely to have mothers who smoke.

▲ The American Academy of Pediatrics recommends that healthy infants sleep on their backs. There is convincing evidence that infants who sleep on their stomachs are more vulnerable to SIDS. Since the American Academy of Pediatrics recommended in 1992 that infants sleep on their back, SIDS has decreased more than 40%. Premature infants and those with respiratory or intestinal problems may do better sleeping on their stomachs. In those circumstances, you should rely on your doctor's judgment.

▲ As a general rule, babies should not sleep on pillows or soft surfaces. Infant cushions have even been banned because of the risk of suffocation.

▲ Maternal smoking during pregnancy and overheating have also been implicated in SIDS.

Parts of the Body

The Skin

At birth, most infants are covered by a thick white material known as the **vernix caseosa.** This covering is generally washed off within the first day, but often some of the material is missed. Do not be disturbed to find white, sticky material behind your child's ears and in the ear folds.

The baby's skin will frequently peel in the first week or two of life. This is another normal occurrence during the newborn period. There are a number of other rashes that are extremely common in the newborn and are not serious. (See Baby Rashes, page 372.)

Birthmarks

About 50% of American babies are born with a birthmark. While **salmon patches** are seen in lighter skinned babies, slate gray spots are common in babies of color. A salmon patch, when located in the center of the forehead or on the eyelids, is also known as an "angel's kiss." If it is located on the back of the neck, it is called a "stork bite." Virtually all salmon patches will disappear in the first few months, although occasionally a stork bite will remain.

Many babies have a slate gray discoloration around their buttocks. This is found in about 95% of African-American babies, 80% of Asian-American babies, 70% of Hispanic babies, and 10% of white babies. It also will disappear by age 6 or 7 years.

Strawberry marks are often barely visible at birth. If they can be seen, they are red and white. They gradually grow, achieving their biggest size at about 6 months of age. Occasionally they are quite large. Strawberry marks are gone in 50% of children by age 5 and in 70% of children by age 7. In extremely rare cases, these strawberry marks trap some of the blood cells (platelets) that assist in preventing bleeding problems. For platelet problems, doctors will administer medicines (steroids). Virtually all strawberry marks will disappear if left alone. Large persistent ones can be surgically removed after the child is older than 6 years.

Port-wine stains are large purple marks that occur in about 3 in 1,000 babies. They are a cosmetic problem if they appear on the face. There are currently no good methods for removing these stains. X rays are harmful and must be avoided. Cosmetics may be used to cover these spots. If a port-wine stain covers an entire eyelid, there may be an associated problem of seizures, which will require medical help.

Finally, infants may have brown or black hairy or nonhairy **moles.** More than 2% of white babies and 20% of black babies have these moles. They do not disappear. Because there is a risk of large moles developing into cancer, many doctors recommend their removal soon after birth. You should discuss the problem with your doctor.

The Head

The head is the largest part of the infant's body at birth. As such, it frequently shows signs of its tight passage through the birth canal by being misshapen **(molding)** or by having a circular swelling on the back. This swelling, known as a **caput succedaneum,** results from the child's head pushing against the mother's pelvis during labor. It generally disappears within two to three days. Another type of swelling that may appear in the same area is a **cephalohematoma,** caused by bleeding under the scalp. This swelling can be distinguished from the caput succedaneum in that it is generally found only on one side of the scalp. Cephalohematomas usually take longer to disappear than caputs but are of no concern unless they are so large that there may have been significant blood loss.

In addition, the head may have marks from the pressure of forceps, if they were used in the delivery. These marks are very common and should resolve within a few days.

The two soft spots on the infant's head are called fontanels. The size may vary greatly. Normal fontanels range in size from 1 to 3 inches (3 to 8 cm). When the infant is asleep, they will ordinarily be flat. When the infant is crying, the fontanels will bulge upward. They also will rise and fall regularly with the infant's heart rate. The front fontanel, on top of the head, will close at about 12 months of age. The smaller, back one will close before 6 months.

The Eyes

Infants can see quite well from birth, although they do have some difficulty focusing for the first few months of life. One of the most frequently asked questions is what color the child's eyes will be. Most newborns have the same eye color—bluish gray. Eye color generally cannot be determined accurately until sometime after the third month.

Yellowness of the "whites" of the eyes, also known as **jaundice,** is usual in newborns. The newborn liver is not as capable of handling the normal breakdown products of human red blood cells as is the adult liver. This causes a certain amount of jaundice for the first few days of life. An extremely high level of jaundice can be a problem. If you are concerned about jaundice after you go home from the hospital, call your doctor promptly. Sunlight is beneficial in reducing the amount of jaundice in newborns, but use caution because infant skin is extremely sensitive to the sun. A special type of lighting (phototherapy) can be used to reduce the level of jaundice.

Occasionally, the eyelids may be swollen because of pressure placed on them in the birth canal. This swelling usually resolves by three days of age.

Tears are absorbed by tear ducts located in the inner aspect of the eyes. Excess tearing in only one eye may signal a blocked tear duct.

The doctor will usually examine the newborn's eyes carefully at birth, including giving the baby a test for vision. Frequently, however, the doctor will arrive on the scene when the infant is sleeping or cry-ing, and the test is not adequate under these conditions. Thus, it is usu-ally the mother who confirms that her infant has good vision by checking whether the child follows her face and eyes as she moves from side to side. The doctor also will examine the lenses of an infant's eyes to make sure there are no cataracts. In addition, the doctor will use an ophthalmoscope to examine the backs of the eyes, known as the retinas for any blackening, which would indicate the presence of a retinoblastoma, an extremely rare but treatable tumor of the eye in newborns.

Crossed eyes are common in newborn babies. (See Vision Prob-lems, page 330.)

The Nose

Most textbooks tell us that infants must breathe through their noses. Therefore, doctors and parents pay a lot of attention to clearing the nostrils of excess mucus and debris. Seldom does mucus completely block the nostrils, however, and we have found that infants adapt quickly to mouth breathing, so parents need not worry too much about clearing the nose.

Babies also have protective reflexes that enable them to turn away from potentially suffocating situations. In putting infants down to sleep, it is important to lay them on their backs, and not on a soft pil-low, to reduce the risk of suffocation or SIDS.

Newborns sneeze a lot. This sneezing is not an indication of a respiratory infection or an allergy; it is a normal reflex.

The Mouth

Often parents will notice little white spots on the roof of an infant's mouth, directly in the midline. These are known as **Epstein's pearls** and are normal in newborns.

Years ago, many parents worried about their infants being tongue-tied. Literally, this means that the frenulum, the piece of tissue on the bottom of the tongue that attaches to the floor of the mouth, is short. A short frenulum will not interfere with the child's speech. However, it will interfere with the child's ability to stick his or her tongue out as far as other children can, with the ability to catch M&Ms thrown in the air, and occasionally with the ability to lick an ice cream cone quickly down to nothing. The inability to perform these acts can be troublesome to a child, so the frenulum can be cut if you wish. This is a simple proce-dure, but it should not be carried out until the child is much older and actually experiences some disability.

The Face

The newborn's face is subjected to a considerable amount of pressure as it comes through the birth canal. This pressure may rupture very tiny blood vessels and cause a purple rash known as **petechiae.** This rash will generally resolve within two weeks.

In addition, infants often develop white dots with red bases all over their faces. This is known as **newborn acne.**

If your child has a widespread rash, your doctor may tell you that he or she has *erythema toxicum neonatorum.* Again, this is a harmless rash of the newborn period. (For more information, see Baby Rashes, page 372.)

The Hands

Infants ordinarily keep their fists clenched. You may notice that your baby has long fingernails. An infant's fingernails are generally soft but can scratch his or her skin. If the fingernails look long or scratch marks seem to be appearing on the infant (or on you when you hold the baby close), you may cut the nails. Almost any nail-clipping instrument, or even your teeth, will do, as long as you are careful.

The Chest

Many parents are surprised to find that their infants, boys as well as girls, have swollen breasts. This is a response to the mother's hormones, which have crossed the placenta and are found in the fetal blood. Swelling of the breasts usually disappears within the first month of life, but it may last for two to three months. Occasionally, a breast discharge may occur.

The Abdomen

The **umbilical cord** is of frequent concern to parents. This cord consists of a gelatinous white material through which run two arteries and one vein. The cord will dry up in 1–2 weeks. During that process there may be a smell caused by bacteria on the cord. A little alcohol applied to the cord will destroy the bacteria but does not need to be used routinely. In one to three weeks, the cord will get smaller, develop a brownish color, and fall off, often with a slight amount of bleeding. If an area of redness develops on the skin surrounding the cord, consult your doctor.

Swelling or hernias of the navel are very common in African-American babies, far less common in white babies. Almost all of these hernias disappear by themselves. For more information, see page 160.

The Genitalia

The genitalia of both boys and girls are swollen in the newborn period because of the presence of maternal hormones. Boys have swollen, enlarged scrota, and girls have enlarged genital lips and clitorides. The swelling should subside within several weeks. Vaginal discharges and bleeding occur frequently (see pages 476 and 478). The foreskin in most newborn boys cannot be retracted (see page 480).

The Feet

An infant's feet assume many unusual positions. It is easy to understand why if you think of the cramped quarters in which he or she has recently been living. Most babies have feet that are turned in, with the soles facing each other. They will assume a more normal position within a few months. Parents can check the normality of the feet by wiggling them about. It should be possible to wiggle an infant's foot into all the positions that your own foot can assume.

Feeding

The feeding of infants and children is more than just satisfying the hunger urge. There are, in fact, three goals of feeding.

1. To meet the nutritional requirements of children so that they can grow.
2. To help children develop muscle and coordination skills. As infants become older, they learn to feed themselves. This requires complicated skills, such as reaching the tongue around a spoon, grasping the spoon, and eventually inserting the spoon into the mouth.
3. To assist infants and children in developing social skills. Eating is a social activity that involves interaction with other family members.

Breast-Feeding

With proper guidance and encouragement, most mothers can master the technique of breast-feeding. Nevertheless, some mothers, through no fault of their own, will be unable to breast-feed. Many doctors are supportive, but few have the experience to be truly helpful. Often the maternity nurses at the hospital are helpful in providing early instructions. Many hospitals, health systems, and communities now have professional lactation services. Another source of help in breast-feeding is a friend or neighbor who has successfully breast-fed her baby. The La Leche League (www.llli.org) or a local lactation consultant (www.ilca.org) are also good sources for advice on breast-feeding techniques.

Do not let anyone undermine your desire to breast-feed. Also, while current guidelines strongly recommend breast-feeding for 6 months, do not let anyone push you into nursing longer than you are able. Work and living situations always impact our choices. Rely on your own judgment after you have listened to expert advice. Judge for yourself how long you want to breast-feed. Two weeks, two months, and two years are all acceptable choices.

Preparation

Recommendations vary widely about the proper preparation of the breast for breast-feeding. By and large, we do not feel that very much preparation before birth is necessary. We suggest a commonsense approach. During the last few months, wash the breast with a damp washcloth and no soap. Avoid most creams and lotions, although using lanolin on the areola (the dark area around the nipple) is acceptable. Exposing the nipples to air or massaging them several months before birth sometimes helps. The purchase of several supportive nursing bras is a good investment for most mothers.

Milk Content

An infant can be put to the breast within minutes after birth. For the first several feedings, the breasts produce a material known as **colostrum.** Colostrum is rich in antibodies that protect the child against infections. There is no need to worry about the number of calories in your milk during the first several days because infants are born with extra weight that will tide them over until the high-calorie milk comes in. Between the third and fifth day after birth, milk begins to come in abundantly.

Although you may have heard that the iron content in breast milk is low, the baby's intestines absorb the iron so well that supplemental iron drops are seldom necessary. Vitamin D is the only supplement breast-feeding babies need; it should be started shortly after birth in dosages of 200 IU daily.

Remember that you are no longer eating just for yourself but also for your infant. Drink whenever you're thirsty. Be sure to drink 2 quarts (2 L) of liquids a day: 1 quart (1 L) of milk and 1 quart of any other favorite nonalcoholic drink. Limit coffee and colas to a cup a day.

Techniques

You can nurse lying on your side or sitting up. Leaning forward a little in the sitting position helps.

Placing the nipple near the baby's mouth stimulates the **rooting reflex,** which will help the baby find the nipple. Don't nudge the child with your finger, or he or she will root toward the finger. You may need to use your finger to hold the top part of your breast away from the infant's nose to allow him or her to breathe. Babies will let you know if they are having trouble breathing by pushing off the breast or opening their mouths and crying.

Besides the rooting reflex, infants have a **sucking reflex** that forms the basis for their feeding. After an infant has been sucking for a while, a vacuum is created, and a tight seal is formed by the mouth around the nipple. You can avoid irritation to the nipple by breaking that vacuum before removing the infant from your breast. Just insert your finger between the infant's gums to break the seal.

The mother also has reflexes that assist her in breast-feeding. Seeing or hearing her child, or even hearing another child's cry, will begin the flow of milk.

Feeding a small, premature baby can present special problems, but they can often be overcome. Indeed, many nurseries feel that breast milk is more important for premature infants than for full-term babies. Special bottles with "premature" nipples are available. Until the premature child is strong enough to suck and control the flow of milk, you can use a breast pump and bottle-feed with these small nipples.

Timing

Newborns require feeding every two to three hours. (Every four hours is unusual.) Frequent, prolonged feedings promote initial milk production. Once the milk is in, the feedings may help prevent engorgement. You should begin by allowing the child to suck for several minutes on each breast, gradually building up to about 15 minutes on each breast by the third day of life. The infant will reject a partially full breast because the taste of the milk changes somewhat during feeding. The child should be allowed to reject one breast and move to the other one. If your breast is so full that the infant is having difficulty grasping the nipple, press out some milk by using your thumb and index finger to squeeze the breast at the areola.

Many mothers who breast-feed find that the father can begin giving a supplemental bottle within the first two months. The father should usually give the supplemental bottle at the same time each day, although this is not a rigid rule. To prevent breast engorgement, mothers may pump their breasts while the father gives the supplemental bottle. Some parents prefer to have the mother pump her breasts and have the father bottle-feed the breast milk. Other women find that their breasts adjust within a short period of time to the uneven schedule that is created by the father's feeding.

You might experience some soreness during the first few days of breast-feeding, but if any pain or discomfort persists after a few days:

1. Check your baby's positioning. In a cradle hold, your baby's body should be parallel to you: chest to chest, tummy to tummy.

2. Make sure your baby is latched on to your areola, with his or her lips curled out.

3. If your breast becomes engorged, breast-feed more frequently. Apply a warm compress before breast-feeding. Express some milk manually by massaging your breast to soften your breast. A softer areola will help your baby latch on better.

Call your doctor if pain persists after you have taken these steps.

Babies have their own style of eating. Some are ravenous eaters, others are picky, and still others seem to fall asleep shortly after they begin nursing. They all feed differently, but all thrive beautifully. Your baby will let you know his or her style early.

Your baby should be getting enough milk if:

1. He or she nurses 8 to 10 times per day for at least 10 to 15 minutes on each side.

2. He or she stools at least 2 times per day and has at least 4 wet diapers per day. Many babies will stool after each feeding in the first month of life. Most babies will have 6 to 8 wet diapers per day.

3. You can hear your baby swallowing.

4. You can see breast-milk in his or her mouth.

5. Your breast feels fuller prior to breast-feeding (especially after a longer interval) and softer after breast-feeding.

Medications that should be avoided/given with caution when breast-feeding include:

▲ Acebutolol
▲ Atenolol
▲ Bromocriptine
▲ Cyclophosphamide
▲ Cyclosporin
▲ Doxorubicin
▲ Ergotamine
▲ Lithium

▲ Methotrexate
▲ Phencyclidine
▲ Phenindione
▲ Phenobarbital

Drugs of abuse—amphetamines, cocaine, heroin and, phencyclidine—have all been associated with adverse effects in nursing infants.

In addition, if it is medically necessary for diagnostic testing for a mother to receive a radioactive substance, breastfeeding should be suspended according to the time frame specified by the professional familiar with the radioactive substance.

The following helpful hints are from mothers who have breast-fed.

Mother of One   *The more relaxed you are about it, the easier it is. In the early weeks, there is bound to be some tension, but it can be minimized, and with it the process becomes natural and easy. Try to find a comfortable place in the house where you will have the things you need close by and won't have to get up to interrupt the feeding. Either having the telephone within reach or turning it off is helpful.*

Mother of Two   *Set the feeding time aside for you and the baby to relax together. Keep interruptions and distractions to a minimum. This may be hard if you have other children. It is a good time to listen to music, watch TV, or read. It may be your only chance to sit and do these things.*

Mother of Two   *Wear loose clothing, especially things you can pull up from the bottom, which will give you more privacy in public than things that button and zip up in front. You can also take along a small blanket or shawl to shield you and the baby.*

Mother of Two   *By hand-expressing a little milk or putting the baby to [the] breast, you can relieve some of the pressure of engorgement. If it really becomes bad, hot compresses work. But take heart; generally it will occur only the first month or two, until you and the baby are synchronized.*

Bottle-Feeding

All commercial formulas are safe and provide excellent nutrition for your infant. Three companies provide the majority of infant formulas, while some store chains now offer their own brand names. Ross Laboratories' main formula is Similac, Mead Johnson produces Enfamil, while Nestlé Carnation provides Good Start. Each of these companies is continually striving to improve its product to more closely resemble breast milk.

The basic Similac with Iron that has been sold for years has removed linoleic acid and is available as Similac Advance with Iron. Two important ingredients found in breast milk, DHA and ARA, have been added to formulas to produce Enfamil LIPIL, Similac Advance, and Nestlé Carnation Good Start Supreme DHA & ARA. We recommend (as does the American Academy of Pediatrics) formulas fortified with iron (not "low iron").

A large variety of formulas are available for special situations. For infants allergic to cow's milk protein (lactose intolerant), soy-based formulas are available (Similac Isomil, Enfamil ProSobee, and Nestlé Good Start Supreme Soy). Hydrolysated formulas break down the cow's milk protein to be more easily digestible. Hydrolyzed formulas include Similac Alimentum Advance, Enfamil Nutramigen Lipil, Enfamil Pregestimil (also helps with problems absorbing fat), and Nestlé Carnation Good Start Supreme. The latter has a whey hydrolysate that, in one study, was found to be helpful to infants with colic. Hydrolyzed formulas used in the first four to six months may benefit some infants at high risk to develop allergic problems.

Take care to mix the formula according to the instructions; using too little water can cause serious problems for the infant. The temperature of the formula need not be higher than body temperature; room temperature is fine. Do *not* use the microwave oven to heat formula. Uneven heating can result in the infant swallowing a patch of liquid that is too hot.

Children who are bottle-fed need an iron supplement. Most commercial formulas are available with or without supplemental iron. We recommend iron-fortified formula until one year of age. By then, iron intake from other foods should be adequate, and milk or formula should account for only one-third of the child's calories. We do not recommend cow's milk until one year of age. Also, young children should get whole milk. After age two, 2% milk can be given. The fat percentage can drop further after school entry.

How Much Milk or Formula?

A newborn needs about 50 calories for each pound of weight (or 110 calories per kg) daily. By age one, that requirement drops to about 45 calories per pound (100 calories per kg). Formula and breast milk provide 20 calories per ounce (30 g). Thus, a newborn weighing 7 pounds (3 kg) needs about 350 calories, or 17½ ounces (500 g) of milk or formula, each day. Such calculations are seldom necessary, however. Infants will let you know when they are hungry or full.

Most newborns will not take more than 3 ounces (90 g) of milk or formula at one time, and hence they require about six feedings a day. Don't be surprised if feedings are as frequent as every two hours or if the time interval varies daily. As infants become older, they can eat more and be fed less often. Middle-of-the-night feedings often usually fall by the wayside when the infant starts sleeping through the night around the fourth month. By six to nine months, the infant should be getting about one-third of his or her calories from sources other than milk or formula. By one year of age, most infants will be satisfied with three meals and an occasional snack.

Solid Foods

Recommendations by experts about when to begin solid foods change about once a decade. Almost all infants are capable of digesting solid foods at birth, but their tongues are not coordinated enough to feed them these foods easily. Most experts feel that there is no need to begin solids until six months of age. Many parents, however, claim that children sleep through the night better if they receive a solid feeding late in the evening. Children with a strong family tendency toward allergic disorders may do better if they don't receive solid foods until six months of age. If such a baby doesn't seem satisfied with formula alone, it is possible to add rice cereal to the formula to thicken it. Rice cereal is highly unlikely to cause an allergic reaction.

Infants between four and six months of age generally do well on most packaged strained foods or baby foods. These foods tend to be expensive, and generally have a fair amount of added water, however, so some parents prefer to prepare their own baby foods at home. There are a number of books about making baby foods that will be acceptable to your child, as well as several types of machines to prepare them.

Between 6 and 9 months of age, some children are given "junior" foods, which are baby foods with more texture. Finally, between 9 and 12 months of age, most children are capable of eating finger foods or table foods.

The best guideline for feeding your child after the first year is to feed him or her small portions of everything you eat. Make sure to include foods from all the basic food groups.

▲ Milk and cheese
▲ Meat, fish, and chicken, or their protein equivalent in eggs, cheese, or beans

▲ Fruit
▲ Yellow and green vegetables
▲ Bread, potatoes, and cereal

Feeding Ability

Most children have a vigorous sucking ability at birth, although many do not perfect this skill until they are four weeks old. At four months, the infant will begin to show signs of waiting for food. For instance, the child's arm will often move at the sight of food. The infant will develop more tongue control, sticking out his or her tongue for the spoon. Place the food well back on the child's tongue; he or she still cannot remove the food from the spoon with the tongue. At this age, the infant will swallow a fair amount of air and need periodic burping.

Between five and six months, infants develop lip control and can bring their lips to a cup. The hands also are developing at this age, and the child will be able to grab a bottle with both hands. Soon the baby will bring the hands to the mouth and begin to develop the ability to grasp a spoon with the hand.

Between 6 and 9 months of age, the child will learn to remove food from the spoon and might be able to drink from a cup. The child also will learn to eat a cracker without any assistance. Between 9 and 12 months of age, the infant will achieve better finger control and be able to use the fingers to obtain small pieces of food. He or she will try to use a spoon alone, but the spoon is more often a toy than a feeding instrument. The child will be able to hold a cup but often will spill its contents. At this age, the child will begin to become choosy about foods. Although infant taste buds are quite developed, infants may be more sensitive to food texture than to taste and are likely to reject foods because of texture.

The period between 12 and 15 months is one of the more trying times for parents. Children begin throwing food and utensils and become more assertive in rejecting certain foods. Between 15 and 18 months, their muscle skills become more sophisticated, and they can handle a cup full of liquid without spilling. Between 18 months and 24 months, children can handle a cup well and drink through a straw. The social aspects of feeding will become more evident at this age, as the child will begin to say "eat," to name certain foods, and to know when food is "all gone." At least three of a child's first six words are usually related to food. At this age, children also begin feeding their favorite stuffed animals or dolls. By 3 years of age, a child should not be spilling very much and should be able to coordinate talking and eating.

Nutrition Facts

Serving size: 3/4 cup (27 grams)
► Servings per container: about 12

Amount per serving

	Cereal alone	With 1/2 cup Vitamin A & D fortified skim milk
Calories	90	130
Calories from fat	10	10

		% Daily Value
Total Fat 1g	2%	2%
Saturated Fat 0g	0%	0%
Polyunsaturated Fat 0.5g		
Monounsaturated Fat 0.5g		
Trans Fat 0g		
Cholesterol 0g	0%	0%
Sodium 190mg	8%	11%
Potassium 85mg	2%	2%
Total Carbohydrate 23g	8%	10%
Dietary Fiber 5g	20%	20%
Sugars 5g		
Protein 2g		
Vitamin A	0%	4%
Vitamin C	10%	15%
Calcium	0%	15%
Iron	2%	2%
Vitamin E	2%	2%

Sugar and other ingredients. The nutrition label found on many foods provides helpful information about many substances in addition to sugar (highlighted). Fats, sodium (salt), vitamins, and minerals are among the items listed. On cereal labels such as this one, the figure for sugar content sometimes reflects the presence of fruits, which naturally contain sugar and raise the cereal's overall sugar content. Also check the number of servings per container. Too often a container with 6 servings is consumed in 1 or 2 snacks.

Social Eating

Feeding is an integral part of a child's social development. During mealtime, children learn how to interact with the family and choose their foods. Parents should not take the socializing power of appetite too far, however. We are not fond of using foods, such as desserts, to reward children and feel that a child should not be forced to eat a disliked food as a punishment.

Feeding time can become a battleground between parents and offspring. Some of these battles may be avoided if parents realize that children naturally tend to fulfill their nutritional needs. Although it may seem unbelievable to many parents, studies have shown that nine-month-old children will select a nutritionally balanced meal when presented with a wide variety of foods. These children do not become overweight or underweight. Often a child's tastes differ from day to day. A food rejected one day may make an entire meal the next, and the resulting diet is well-balanced.

A child's nutritional requirements change dramatically in the first year of life. After a year of age, growth slows down. Infants gain about 2 pounds (900 g) a month in the first six months of life, about 1 pound (450 g) a month in the next six months. Between 1 and 6 years of age children gain only 4 to 5 pounds (2 kg) a *year*. Children won't leave the table hungry; their appetite is a good guide. We hope this knowledge makes it easier to tolerate a child's pickiness.

As children become older, the dinner hour is often the one time when all family members are assembled in one spot. This is an important social time. Watching television or reading during dinner is wasting time that could be better spent with the family. Good communication during dinner is an important means of promoting mental as well as nutritional health.

Overeating

Overeating and obesity have turned into a national childhood epidemic of disastrous proportion. Unlike a broken bone or a strep throat, being overweight poses a substantial risk for the early onset of diabetes and heart disease and chronically robs children of self esteem. When our first edition appeared in the 1970s only 4% of school-age children were overweight compared with over 17% today. One state reports 40% of children are overweight and 25% are obese. The obesity rate has doubled for preschoolers and teens. More than 30% of children are currently at risk for diabetes or heart disease.

The causes are clear:

▲ High calorie foods of limited nutritional value barrage our children in ads as well as school lunchrooms and vending machines.
▲ Food portion sizes have exploded, with standard sizes for fast food drinks and burgers doubling or tripling since the 1970s.
▲ Many schools have eliminated or cut back on physical education programs.
▲ Kids typically watch more than four hours of television daily (with additional time spent on electronic games or computers).
▲ Children increasingly are driven or bussed to school and other organized activities.

Teaching children to eat the right foods in the right amount is one of the most important jobs of a parent. For children, knowing what to do is necessary but not enough to prevent obesity. Parents need to be role models for their children. A parent who would never allow smoking in the house should be as vigilant in keeping the wrong foods in the wrong amounts off the dinner table.

Here are a few practical suggestions.

Top 10 things to help children achieve healthy weight

1. No more than 1 hour of screen time (TV and video game) per day

2. Play (be active) for at least 1 hour per day

3. No soda! (or other sugared beverages)

4. No juice; eat fruit instead

5. Eat 5 fruits or vegetables each day

6. Eat smaller portions and wait 20 minutes before second helpings

7. Help children set health goals and provide a nonfood reward when kids make their goals

8. Provide a safe food environment at home; if it's not in the house, they're less likely to eat it and you're less likely to argue

9. Limit the amount of white fluffies you eat (white fluffies are simple carbohydrates without fiber, like white rice, white bread, pasta, etc.)

10. Exercise with your children; walk together, bike together, go to the park—be active together

Remember, parents with weight issues can attend a variety of helpful programs such as WeightWatchers. Lessons learned will help with all at home.

Additional information can be found on the following websites:

www.cdc.gov/healthyweight/children

www.aap.org/obesity

Food Additives

There are more than 2,700 known **additives** in the foods we consume. Two-thirds of these have no known nutritional benefit. They include food colorings and artificial flavorings. The harm caused by useless additives is unknown but potentially unlimited. Some food additives, such as preservatives, are necessary, but most are not. Any foreign substance can cause an allergic response in a sensitive individual, so these additives undoubtedly cause many allergic reactions. Research is currently under way to determine whether food additives are responsible for behavioral problems as well as allergy problems. Evidence suggests that food additives may affect behavior in some children, but it is not conclusive.

Additional Reading

The Premature Baby Book, Helen Harrison and Ann Kositsky (New York: St. Martin's Press, 1983).

Your Amazing Newborn, Marshall H. Klaus, M.D., and Phyllis H. Klaus (Cambridge, Mass.: Da Capo Press, 2000).

Raising Healthy Eaters, Henry Legere, M.D. (Cambridge, Mass.: Da Capo Press, 2004).

The Premature Baby Book: Everything You Need To Know About Your Premature Baby From Birth to Age One, James Sears, Martha Sears, Robert Sears, William Sears (New York: Little, Brown, 2004).

The Breastfeeding Book: Everything You Need to Know About Nursing Your Child from Birth through Weaning, Martha Sears and William Sears (New York: Little, Brown, 2000).

New Mother's Guide to Breastfeeding, Joan Younger Meek, editor (Elk Grove, Ill.: American Academy of Pediatrics, 2002).

Chapter Four

Growth and Development

One of the greatest rewards of being a parent is watching your children grow. The excitement of witnessing your child's first steps or hearing your child's first words is difficult to exaggerate. As the years roll by, scrapbooks become as important to parents as the writings of their favorite authors. Home movies are more entertaining than this year's Academy Award winners.

Parents with no interest in history suddenly become meticulous historians of their child's life. The precise timing of the first step, the first word, the first birthday party, and the first date is remembered after the date of the Magna Carta has long been forgotten. As other historians do, parents remember battles—the battle of the bottle, the battle of the toilet. Momentous pacts and treaties also have their day.

Parents also grow. They learn to deal with the trauma of beheaded toy bears, bogeymen in the dark, departing friends, and illnesses in brothers, sisters, and pets. In just a few years, parents watch their children grow from complete dependence to total independence.

Watching children grow is fun, but sometimes it can be worrisome. Parents are easily and naturally concerned that their children are not developing properly, and sometimes parents worry unnecessarily. As a society, we often seem preoccupied with predicting the future success of our offspring. A child throwing a ball at an early age should prompt excitement but not necessarily anticipation of a career in sports. And children who read at an early age may be destined for mechanical or artistic interests rather than a scholarly life.

In this chapter, we discuss patterns of growth and development, as well as some of the tools used to measure and predict this process.

What Does Normal Mean?

Is my child normal? Why is Johnny so short? Why does George still wet the bed—he's almost eight? Why didn't my second child start to walk as early as my first? The spirit of competitiveness lives in all of us. We worry unnecessarily about things such as whether Suzie will walk before the little girl across the street does.

Although children are constantly developing in all areas, certain areas can develop more rapidly because of the individual needs of the child. For example, consider a child growing up in a large family.

Whereas most of us have dinner with many people only at Thanksgiving or other holidays, the youngest child in a large family may experience these fun, chaotic events every night. To survive, that child may well develop quick hands at an early age. But later in childhood, a child from a smaller family will catch up.

The opposite seems to occur in the development of walking ability. With many heavier bodies running about, a small child in a large family is likely to be knocked over frequently. It is common to see late walking in these children, but they often develop other means of locomotion. Some are clever enough to get their older brothers and sisters to carry, push, or pull them about. Others develop the skill of rapid creeping or scooting. Children are constantly developing and adapting to their environments. They are adapting in the way that is best for them and not according to schedules printed in textbooks.

Variability

Another important consideration in interpreting the limits of "normal" is the concept of **variability.** Variability describes the outside limits of the age at which a given skill should develop. For example, most children begin to smile by about three to four weeks of age, but some children begin on the first day of life, and other children don't begin until they are seven to eight weeks of age. We say that the average child smiles at one month, but the variability is either a month earlier or a month later.

As tasks become more and more complicated, the variability increases. Most children sit at about 6 months, but the variability is between 4 and 8 months. Most children walk at 12 months, but some begin as early as 9 months, and others may not walk until 16 months or even later. Verbal ability has even greater variability. Some children say three words (other than mama and dada) before 12 months of age; others may be almost 24 months before this is accomplished. Beethoven was said to be composing and playing music at the age of 3 years, but adults 10 times that age have difficulties with these tasks. Variability limits are far more meaningful than single "normal" values in interpreting whether a given milestone has occurred on schedule. In other words, a child who does not walk at the average age of 12 months is still normal if he or she is walking at 16 months. However, that child will be considered abnormal if he or she is not walking by the age of 3 years.

Normality in one area of development does not guarantee normality in all others, and abnormality in one area does not signify abnormality in others. Consider a child who, for whatever reason, has acquired an injury that affects muscle (motor) development. This child may lag considerably in sitting, walking, and the more sophisticated locomotion skills but still acquire language, social, and other skills at the appropriate ages.

Intelligence

A common misconception is that a child's intelligence can be predicted by observing how rapidly he or she develops in the first year of life. Except for rare cases of severe retardation, development rates offer very little help in predicting ultimate intelligence, let alone whether that person will use his or her intelligence creatively, productively, or not at all.

Experts can put only a fuzzy border around what is normal and what is abnormal. Nobody can say what your child will be like in the future. A child who is developing slowly at first may develop rapidly later on. Other children may develop very rapidly initially and then slow down. Most usual are periods of alternating rapid, slow, and average development in response to changes in season, changes in family composition, and other changes not yet determined.

It is natural to worry about your child's development. No two children are alike and all have different strengths and weaknesses. Minor differences between your child and your neighbor's are expected. While Jason had a vocabulary of 4 words at a year and Jasmine only 1, she was able to count at 3 while he could not until he was 4. Some children do have developmental problems, however. Don't be shy about sharing your concern with your child's physician during regular checkups. Most problems with children's development are detected first by parents, not doctors! A good resource for learning about your child's developmental progress is http://brightfutures.aap.org/web/. The "Ages and Stages Questionnaire" is used by many professionals to help identify children who may have developmental issues worth further investigation.

Autism

Considerable attention has been paid in recent years to an increase in autism, and many parents worry about this problem. One thing you need not worry about is a link between thimerasol in immunizations and autism. A number of scientific groups have scrutinized this issue and were unable to find any evidence linking the two. In addition, vaccines are now thimerasol free except for some flu vaccines. Nevertheless, about 1 in 1,000 children will have a form of autism, a genetically based condition of brain development. About 5% of children with autism have a sibling with a similar condition. There is a broad spectrum for autism (autism spectrum disorder) with some individuals being severely disabled while others are famous authors. Autistic children have difficulties with language, social interactions (such as making eye contact), and behavior. The following should prompt an evaluation for autism:

▲ No babbling, pointing or other gestures by 12 months
▲ No single words by 16 months
▲ No two-word phrases by 24 months
▲ Doesn't respond to name

The diagnosis of autism first appeared in the diagnostic manual established by the American Psychiatric Association in 1980 and autistic disorder (AD) in 1987. For autistic disorder, six criteria must be met from a list of more than a dozen items addressing a child's social interactions, communication skills, and repetitive behaviors. As the diagnosis of AD has increased, along with educational services available through the 1990 Individuals with Disabilities Education Act, other diagnoses of children with developmental problems have decreased. In other words, there is not necessarily an influx of this problem but a re-classification of the many developmental challenges that children and parents have always experienced. Today, many children with a wide variety of developmental issues surrounding social interaction difficulties are now being considered as potentially having an autism *spectrum* disorder (ASD).

While ASD is a new label, the general approach to detecting developmental issues in children has remained constant. As a parent you should always be vigilant and bring concerns about development and behavior to your child's health care provider. In the first year of life you can pay particular attention to your child's social skills, particularly interacting in a playful and reciprocal manner. Verbalization is also important starting with cooing and moving towards the formation of words. There are numerous developmental screening tools. Your child's health care provider may ask you to fill one out at home or in the waiting room. *Ages and Stages* is now used in many offices (www.agesandstages.com). For ASD screening many clinical offices now rely on the Modified Checklist for Autism in Toddlers (M-CHAT) that can be found in the Appendix.

An evaluation will typically include hearing tests, potential lead screening, and other formal diagnostic tests. For more information see www.aap.org/advocacy/archives/mayautism.htm.

Growth

Your Child's Weight

The physical growth of infants is remarkable. They usually double their weight in the first four to five months of life and triple their weight by the time they are one year of age. The average baby's height increases by a full 50% by the end of the first year. At birth, a child's head size is already nearly 60% of its adult size. By age three, the head will be nearly 90% of its adult size. As the previous section explains, however, these are *average* gains. There are wide variations that are normal. Except in cases of rare diseases, physical growth is determined by two factors: proper nutrition and heredity.

Proper nutrition begins during pregnancy and continues throughout infancy, childhood, and adult life. The measure of growth that is most sensitive to nutrition is, of course, weight. Children largely make up their own minds about when and what to eat. There are periods when children will refuse to eat a great deal of food. Remember that if your child will not eat carrots or spinach for a day or so, it will have no effect on his or her weight, and certainly it will have no effect on height or brain growth. Prolonged periods of not eating will eventually affect weight, height, and ultimately brain growth, but malnutrition of this severity is extremely uncommon in the United States.

Most parents are concerned by their children's eating habits. Indeed, in discussing problems with parents, we have found that *all* children at some point seem to eat too much or too little and not enough of the right kinds of foods. It is hard for children *really* to eat too little if presented with food. Hunger cravings are biological, and the survival instinct is strong. Normal children always eat enough.

More often, the problem is that children eat too much. A child in the first year who eats too much gets chubby and undergoes several invisible changes. An excess number of fat cells may develop within his or her body. According to one theory, once these fat cells have multiplied, they send out messages that help determine appetite cravings. Although losing weight in the future will decrease the size of these fat cells, their number will remain the same. Excessive eating also can stretch the size of the stomach. Because hunger pains occur when the walls of the stomach contract against one another, stretched stomachs require more food to decrease that empty feeling. Other factors appear to determine eating patterns. For example, thin people seem to be able to tell precisely when they have had enough food and will not eat anymore. Recent studies have documented that some obesity is due to a gene that is responsible for continued eating even beyond the point when hunger is satisfied.

Children learn eating patterns from their parents, and proper weight is partly culturally determined. In some countries, being heavy is considered a sign of prosperity, and the same holds true for some subcultures in the United States. A wide range of weights must be considered normal.

Your Child's Height

Genetic factors are important to physical growth. Tall parents tend to have tall children, and short parents tend to have short children; it is as simple as that. However, an interesting phenomenon called "regression toward the mean" has been observed. Tall parents have children who are taller than average but shorter than their parents. Short parents have children who are shorter than average but taller than their parents.

Children grow upward, but not steadily. For long periods, children may not grow at all. At other times, they may exhibit rapid growth spurts. Your doctor will record the growth of your child on a growth chart similar to those shown on pages 496–501. After recording a series of heights and weights at different ages, you can visualize the growth of your child. If growth is extremely fast or stops for a long period, it will show up on the graph much more clearly than through the traditional marks on the closet wall. Don't worry too much about how your child compares to the "normal" lines on these charts. At some time during growth and development, most children will be high or low in something. Usually, the growth rate is roughly parallel to the lines on the growth chart and does not deviate more than two or three lines from the original. A prolonged period of delayed growth requires investigation. The charts will also help you with the problems of being **overweight** (page 302) and **underweight** (page 304).

Hormone Treatments

Height has always seemed a trivial characteristic by which to judge any person. Unfortunately, our culture has traditionally placed values on various heights. Being tall has been seen as an asset for boys but may be a problem for girls. Some parents are concerned that their children will be handicapped by being too tall or too short, and they seek out ways to change growth patterns.

Many tall women can remember being teased because of their height when they were younger; parents wish to protect their daughters from such experiences. A few parents have also been concerned that their daughters may grow too tall for a ballet career. Hormones that will prematurely stop bone growth are available, but they are dangerous and have numerous side effects. To be effective, these hormones are best given before puberty—too early for most girls to make serious career decisions about ballet. Once these drugs stop growth, it cannot be restarted. Except for very unusual circumstances, we do not recommend the use of these hormones. Furthermore, as we see in the attention being paid to basketball players and fashion models, tall women are now viewed with respect.

Other parents have heard about **growth hormone** for increasing height. Growth hormone is produced naturally by the pituitary gland and is effective in children who have a deficiency of the substance in their bodies. Growth hormone has recently been found to be effective in children with extreme growth problems. Some doctors and pharmaceutical companies have been promoting this drug for children whose height is below average but who are not extremely short. Because of potential side effects, use of this hormone should be restricted to severe growth retardation.

Growth at Puberty

Initially, growth is controlled by two hormones: growth hormone and thyroid hormone. During puberty, additional hormones kick in. These hormones are also responsible for the development of sexual characteristics in boys and girls. However, they play only a minor role in human sexual *behavior,* which is far more directed by psychological factors.

As an adolescent reaches puberty, the pituitary gland increases the secretion of a hormone called follicle-stimulating hormone (FSH). FSH in women stimulates the ovaries to produce estrogen (female hormone) and in men stimulates the development of sperm. In males, another pituitary hormone stimulates the increase in testosterone (male hormone) from the testicles. Testosterone can also be produced by the adrenal glands in men and women.

Boys

For boys, no single dramatic event makes clear that puberty is on its way. There is a typical sequence of changes, however. These changes may not be immediately obvious, because they tend to occur over a fairly long period. They usually begin between the ages of 9 ½ and 14, but some of the changes are so subtle that they may not be noticed until later.

In most boys, enlargement of the testicles begins at about age 11 and continues until about age 18. Penis enlargement usually begins about a year later and continues until about age 16. Pubic hair generally does not begin to appear until about age 13 ½, although some 11-year-old boys show signs of early pubic hair. If there are signs of pubic hair development before age 10, a call to the doctor is in order.

Testosterone—which is responsible for the enlargement of the penis, testicles, and growth of pubic hair—is responsible for the development of axillary and facial hair, voice changes, adult body odor, acne, and increasing muscle mass at about age 15.

Half of all boys will experience some enlargement of one or both breasts. Commonly, there may be a lump or tenderness under one or both nipples. This can be easily explained on the basis of hormonal changes, but it is often very embarrassing. Your son will need your help and support without having undue attention drawn to this condition. Obesity may accentuate this problem by giving the appearance of very large breasts, while at the same time making the penis and testes appear small. Occasionally, breast enlargement may be so great and so prolonged that you and your son may wish to discuss the possibility of cosmetic surgery with your doctor. Usually, however, the condition resolves itself within a year.

Girls

The process of sexual maturation in girls usually starts about two years before the first menstrual period. The first sign of puberty typically occurs at age 9½ for white girls and age 8 for African American girls. For many girls, development starts earlier and is still normal. Signs of puberty before the age of 6½ require an evaluation by your doctor. Although the age at which changes occur can vary widely, the sequence of these changes is pretty much the same in all girls. Breast development begins first and is followed shortly by the appearance of pubic hair. Hair under the arms begins to increase about a year later. Between ages 11 and 13, a growth spurt results in a noticeable gain in height. Menstrual periods begin around age 11½. Over this entire period, there is some change in the way fat is distributed over the body, particularly in the hips and buttocks. Widening of the hips, as well as development of the uterus, vagina, and external genital organs, also occurs. Problems associated with vaginal discharge and menstrual problems are discussed on pages 476 and 478.

Variation in breast development is often a cause for concern. Breasts usually begin to develop one to two years before the first period, but they may not develop until up to two years after the onset of menstruation. Often one breast develops more rapidly than the other. This may be embarrassing, but most breasts reach nearly equal size by age 18. Sometimes girls worry that the areola (the dark area surrounding the nipple) may be elevated too much or not enough. The areola is elevated in about 75% of women and not elevated in the remainder. Both patterns are normal. Inverted nipples are not a problem and need no treatment other than reassurance.

The size of the breasts also concerns many girls. We are happy to note a decline in the emphasis on huge breasts as the ultimate sign of sex appeal. Still, most girls worry about being flat-chested, even though virtually none of them will be. The problem is usually one of timing. Remember that the breasts may not begin to develop until two years after menstruation starts and may not be fully developed until age 19 or 20. It is perfectly possible for one 13- or 14-year-old to have undergone very little or no breast development, while most of her friends will be well into the process. Your reassurance is an important factor in easing your daughter's anxiety. Efforts at stimulating breast development artificially have no place in the developing child or mature woman. Oral or topical estrogens are potent drugs that should not be used to promote cosmetic changes.

Excessively large breasts also cause concern. Emotional support from parents, as well as physical support from a good brassiere is important during adolescence. Surgical procedures for breast reduction may be considered by older adolescents and their parents.

Development

New Skills

Watching your child grow in size is only part of the fun of being a parent. Development of coordination is even more exciting, and infants quickly acquire a variety of skills. They develop muscle abilities, which give them mobility and allow them to explore. They develop extremely fine motor abilities, which enable them to accomplish complex tasks such as playing a musical instrument. They develop the ability to convey anger, disappointment, or love through facial expressions. Language develops so that they can express their needs. Gradually, language abilities become more sophisticated until children are able to use words to express feelings.

Social skills provide early rewards for children. Smiling begins very early, often in the delivery room. Soon this smiling becomes more specific, as infants are able to recognize their parents and acknowledge that their parents are exhibiting warm feelings toward them. Gradually, children learn how to play games with others. Soon afterward, they learn how to share things, and ultimately they develop the capacity to love. Learning is one of the more complicated skills, progressing from primitive basic memory to abstraction, moral judgment, and creativity.

How Babies Learn

There has been a tremendous amount of research in the past decade focusing on how babies learn. Scientists are now proving what millions of mothers (and fathers) suspected all along: Babies are phenomenal learning machines and this learning begins moments after birth. There has been extraordinary progress in understanding the biologic processes of the brain as well as how parents and the world shape an infant's mind. What distinguishes the current generation of researchers in the field of cognitive psychology is the creative use of experiments to understand what babies know and how babies learn. The experiments often rely on techniques such as observing eye movements or recording heart rates to decide whether babies prefer one sight or sound or smell to another. We now know that at birth babies prefer human faces and voices and can soon distinguish familiar from unfamiliar faces and sounds.

Babies are really the world's most sophisticated learning machines, and their learning incorporates billions of inputs from parents and their surroundings. Today's cognitive scientists have taught us that infants are also scientists performing ever more complex experiments as their brains mature. Alison Gopnik, Ph.D., and her colleagues describe many of these experiments in *The Scientist in the Crib*. They describe babies' minds as analogous to special computers made of neurons instead of silicon chips. But the programming is so extraordinarily powerful that "Bill Gates's little daughter has already solved problems that Bill, with all his billions, is still unsuccessfully trying to crack." The White House Conference on Early Childhood Learning provides us with an excellent summary of knowledge about infant learning (www.ed.gov/pubs/How_Children/foreword.html). Practical information can be found at www.ed.gov/parents.

The message is clear. Babies learn at an amazing pace by interacting with parents and their environment. Wonderful changes occur when a mother sings to an infant or a father smiles and shakes his head. There is little or no evidence that spending hundreds of dollars on special programs designed to build better babies will do anything. Leonardo DaVinci, Thomas Jefferson, and Wolfgang Mozart achieved moderate success despite lacking the benefit of video- or computer-based learning programs.

Sequence of Skills

Skills develop in an orderly, rather than a haphazard, fashion. Much pediatric and psychological research has focused on this sequence and has helped to establish the expected order of events and the limits of "normal." Attempts to correlate the age at which something happens with future capabilities have not been very successful, however.

As an example of the logical building of increasingly complicated skills, let us look at the sequence of development required for a child to use a pencil. The first stage in the sequence is reflex control. All infants have what is known as a **grasp reflex.** They will grab and hold on to any object placed in their palms, such as a finger or a pencil. Doctors may demonstrate the strength of an infant by allowing him or her to clasp each of the doctor's index fingers and then lifting the child off the table. The infant will demonstrate his or her strength admirably, but this is not a sophisticated use of the hand. There is no control over this reflex, and the child will clutch anything placed in the palm. Indeed, you may notice how your infant keeps his or her hands clasped in a fist for most of the first few months of life.

As the nervous system develops, the child overcomes the grasp reflex, usually by about three months. The infant is now ready to use the hands in a different fashion. By about four months, infants can keep their hands open and hold on to objects placed in them. Although their vision is good, their coordination is not sophisticated enough to reach for an object and retrieve it. Infants will usually overshoot the object.

At five months, infants' retrieval abilities get better. The process known as raking begins, as children bring objects closer by using the entire hand. At nine months or so, infants achieve control of the thumb and forefinger and can bring them together to pick up tiny objects such as raisins, pennies, and pills. Soon your infant will be picking up these objects, examining them, and ultimately placing them in his or her greatest exploratorium, the mouth. Development of this finger-to-thumb pinching motion is unique to humans. Unfortunately, this ability also places infants at risk for stuffing the nose, mouth, and ears full of "goodies" and "baddies."

By now, infants are able to let go of items voluntarily. The ability to release items in a projectile fashion—better known as throwing food on the floor—begins around a child's first birthday.

After a year, things progress rapidly. Hands that learned to release toys voluntarily only a few months earlier are now gentle enough to release one block precisely on top of another. By age two, your budding engineer can create a tower six stories (or blocks) high. Like any engineer pleased with his or her work, the child will feel the need to leave records of his or her successes, and the ability to draw develops. At first the child will draw with crayon in fist, but before the third year begins, the child will hold the crayon as an adult does. Pencils are somewhat trickier than crayons, but the child will soon master the skill of holding a pencil as well.

Finally, the apprentice needs help from the master craftsman. A child cannot develop artistic skills without paintbrush and paper. But necessary as these raw materials and practice time are, the child also needs encouragement. Children are social beings; a smile or kind word lets your child know that you are pleased with his or her progress.

This evolutionary sequence illustrates most other processes in child development, such as walking. The general rules are as follows:

▲ The child must overcome involuntary reflexes to attain voluntary control.

▲ There is a logical progression; cruder movements always precede finer movements.

▲ The child must coordinate several senses. For example, to build a tower of blocks, the child relies on sight, depth perception, and balance.

▲ A skill can develop only when the nervous system is mature enough. Building a tower of blocks is impossible for a six-month-old, no matter how much exposure to blocks the child has had.

Individuality

The growth of every individual is unique; this is the most important point of this chapter. Even identical twins brought up in a similar fashion will grow differently and ultimately do different things with their lives. Children will demonstrate their unique tastes, even for music, at an early age.

Furthermore, an infant is an active participant in creating his or her environment. A baby will quickly learn how to manipulate his or her parents. For example, the child will learn that jabbering will, as if by magic, produce parents. Parents sometimes substitute a favorite teddy bear when a child cries or jabbers, rather than spend time with the child. Or a parent may comfort a child vocally when physically occupied with other tasks. The infant quickly decides whether these responses are enough. They may suffice for a time, but then the game begins again as the infant discovers a new way of drawing attention. Quieter infants may use smiling or eye contact, rather than voice, to make their demands known. In some way, however, your infant will actively influence your behavior. This is part of how you develop as a family.

Toilet Training

Toilet training is an important developmental milestone for toddlers and their parents. The skills required for bowel and bladder control are similar. Because these skills are acquired at slightly different ages, we will discuss them separately. Both are the culmination of a long series of accomplishments, and parents play an important role by recognizing, reacting to, and rewarding each accomplishment.

Bowel Control

Young infants have a reflex known as the **gastrocolic reflex.** About 20 minutes after eating, an infant will have a reflex bowel movement. This reflex, like other early reflexes, will gradually diminish, usually by 12 to 15 months of age. Willful control of bowel elimination can develop only after the child has overcome this reflex.

Many parents recognize this happening and begin toilet training by capitalizing on the reflex. We have all heard stories of children being toilet trained by the age of 6 months. These children are, of course, not really toilet trained, but instead are passing stools in a regular pattern determined by the gastrocolic reflex. Some parents have confused the natural disappearance of this reflex with a conscious decision by their 12-month-old to be uncooperative. This is far from the truth; a 12-month-old is still much too young to toilet train. Other skills must develop and mature first.

The child must be able to sense that a bowel movement is occurring. Most children acquire this knowledge after one year of age. (Parents can often recognize that their child is producing stool by facial expressions or other gestures.) Initiation of bowel control is often begun at this time, most often unconsciously. You will often mention "BM" or some other term when the child is having a bowel movement. The association between act and language will have begun, but the final act of this complex learning task will not be accomplished for another year or two.

After the child is able to detect the sensation of a bowel movement, he or she becomes able to sense the presence of fecal material in the rectum before it passes. Following this, the child begins to achieve some muscular control over the passage of the stool. Newborn infants have no anal control. This muscular coordination develops at different ages in different children. Some children develop it early in the second year of life, others not until the end of the third year. The rare child with a neurological condition may develop this control much later or not at all.

The length of time that a child can use muscular control to withhold the stool gradually increases. In the middle of the second year, the child may be able to tell you that a bowel movement is on the way, but the movement probably will have occurred before you reach the toilet.

Children should not be rushed to the toilet. Frantic activity can be a frightening experience for children, who might associate normal body functions with dirt and disgrace. Of course, many households have such a high level of activity that rushing may be normal. In short, the speed with which you take your child to the toilet should be similar to the speed with which you do other things with your child.

The Potty
Once your child begins to inform you of an impending bowel movement, you can begin taking the child to the toilet ("potty"). Most children will be able to do this when they are two to three years old. Introducing your child to the toilet should be a relaxed affair. Initially, there is no need even to remove the child's pants. Consider that the child's potty is often on the floor, where it tends to be colder than elsewhere in the room. Sitting on a cold seat can be a shocker for anyone, especially a two-year-old. Merely associating the bowel movement with the potty is enough at first. Staying there too long should be avoided. (The energy level of a two-year-old is such that the child will not wish to remain on the potty too long anyway.)

A potty that sits on the floor generally seems more secure than a toilet seat placed way up high on that big toilet. It is also easier to push with the feet on the ground. A portable potty also can be easily taken on trips, and it becomes the individual possession of the child. Initially, when the child produces a stool, it should be allowed to remain in the potty for a while. The child will be pleased with the product and may be disappointed when it is taken away. One friend, confronted with a shocked two-year-old noticing her missing stool, invented the "BM birdie" who needed the stools. His daughter was satisfied with the explanation and loved to talk about the birdie. Remember also that the roar of the toilet can be frightening to a child. Seeing this roaring monster consume a stool can upset a two-year-old, though it may thrill a three-year-old.

A major accomplishment during the long process of development is the ability to put things off, or delay pleasure. Learning to postpone urges can take months or years. (Indeed, many adults have trouble postponing some urges.) Having a bowel movement is a biologically pleasurable experience. A child learns to delay this pleasure in order to receive something equally pleasurable—a parent's reward. The child is beginning to make decisions about the pleasures that social behavior can bring. A two-year-old appreciates the social interaction with Mom and Dad. Smiles and praise, not overdone, should accompany potty sitting.

Praise can be more laudatory when a bowel movement is produced, but it should also accompany nonproductive sittings. You should not keep your child sitting on the potty until he or she produces a bowel movement. Children take time to learn, and there will be many dry runs. Persisting will frustrate both you and your child. When your child is tired of sitting, the time is up.

Generally, a child's second year is a period of negativism. He or she will frequently say no. This negativism is an important developmental milestone, for the child is developing an individual personality that is not a part of Mother or Father. The drive toward independence will eventually motivate a two-and-one-half-year-old or three-year-old to control bowel movements. However, the early part of this struggle for independence may mean a struggle over who will make the decisions about bowel movements. It does not pay to engage in battles over this issue. Reward or disengagement is the key. Punishment will only intensify the child's opposition and prolong the struggle.

Bladder Training

Bladder control in children follows the same developmental sequence as bowel control, lagging behind bowel control in most children. At birth, infants urinate by reflex when their bladder is stretched to a certain point. As they get older, they can hold larger and larger amounts of urine.

By 18 months, children can sense when they are urinating. The muscular ability to hold urine in the bladder is usually acquired between the ages of two and one-half and three and one-half years. Usually by the age of two and one-half, the child is well on the way to learning bowel control, and bladder control often follows soon after. Many toddlers are very concerned about being in control and learn quickly to hold on to their urine. They are training themselves by holding their urine longer so that they may spend more time at play or gain the social rewards offered by their parents.

Because calling Mom or Dad for assistance in going to the potty is a handy way of getting attention, parents can expect some dry runs. Accidents should also be expected, because a child at this age can easily become preoccupied or forget the urge to urinate.

Daytime bladder control is achieved by age three in 85% of children and by age four in more than 95% of children. Occasional accidents will occur. Often older children with the "giggles" will have accidents even in school. Children will usually learn bladder control quicker when their older brothers or sisters are around to help demonstrate.

Bed-Wetting

Nighttime dryness takes longer to achieve. Nearly 20% of five-year-olds and more than 10% of six-year-olds are still subject to frequent nighttime wettings. By contrast, some three-year-olds, if taken for a late-night trip to the bathroom, will make it through the night just fine. Expect an occasional accident, but avoid any sort of punishment. Children should not be kept in overnight diapers until they are 100% dry. These diapers do not encourage the child to develop his or her control. (See Bed-Wetting, page 298.)

If bed-wetting remains a problem after age 6, consult your doctor during a regular checkup. Because bladder control, like bowel control, is the culmination of a sequence of sensory, muscular, learning, and social development, a competent medical professional will investigate all these areas. Most therapy focuses on the social aspects of changing this behavior. Medication may occasionally be necessary. Surgery is virtually never needed. Frequently, improvement occurs when the child makes the decision that a dry bed is important, such as when visiting a friend or relative.

Relying on a drug to increase urinary retention through increased muscular control or to decrease urine production or on an alarm to modify behavior through negative reinforcement is a narrow approach to a complex phenomenon. These methods have a role, but only as part of a therapeutic process involving coordination of efforts with child, parents, and professionals. Don't buy the devices advertised in the back pages of many magazines.

Additional Reading

Infants and Mothers: Differences in Development, rev. ed., T. Berry Brazelton, M.D. (New York: Dell, 1983).

Toddlers and Parents: A Declaration of Independence, rev. ed., T. Berry Brazelton, M.D. (New York: Dell, 1989).

Touchpoints: Your Child's Emotional and Behavioral Development, T. Berry Brazelton, M.D. (Cambridge, Mass.: Perseus Books, 2000).

The Magic Years, Selma H. Fraiberg (New York: Scribner's Reference, 1996).

The Scientist in the Crib: What Early Learning Tells Us About the Mind, Alison Gopnik, Andrew N. Meltzoff, and Patricia K. Kuhl (New York: Harper Paperbacks, 2000).

Your Baby and Child: From Birth to Age Five, 3rd rev. ed. Penelope Leach (New York: Knopf, 1997).

Chapter Five

Personality and Behavior

The complexity of human personality development cannot be discussed in a single volume, let alone in a single chapter. Freud, Piaget, Erikson, Sears, Maccoby, and hundreds of other scientists have devoted their entire lives and thousands of volumes to expanding our knowledge in this area. In this chapter, we provide a framework for personality development that can help you understand some of the common behavioral problems you may encounter.

Infancy: Birth to One Year

Each infant is born with an individual temperament. Theories that a child's personality depends entirely on environmental factors are now felt to be untrue; infants are individuals from the very start. Some come out active and screaming and remain at a high level of activity throughout life. Others are very mellow at birth and continue with this personality trait.

We now know that infants exert a strong influence over their parents' behavior toward them. An active child will quickly learn how to attract his or her parents' attention. These active children, with their many demands, will force parents to interact with them more often and will often encourage parents to provide them with more play objects. Quieter children may show the greatest pleasure while being held or merely looking at a parent. Quiet activity pleases this type of child the most, and parents, sensing this pleasure, respond with the level of activity that the child enjoys most. Often a child will interact differently with each parent.

When infants have quiet times, they are listening, learning smells, judging distances, and developing intellectually. During active times, they are moving and discovering limbs, exercising muscles, and developing coordination.

The newborn quickly learns how to obtain food. Babies are born with reflexes that enable them to suck vigorously and locate the nipple on the breast by rooting, but they must learn how to make the milk appear. Crying most often serves this function. Parents influence the baby's behavior by modifying feeding schedules to their own preferences. Infants quickly develop an interest in their environments. They soon learn that toys can be manipulated by kicking and reaching; hence they begin to control their surroundings.

Infants can be troublesome before the terrible twos. A majority of the mothers in a study by Emily Szymowski and Robert Chamberlin describe their one-year-olds as *attention-seeking, stubborn, clingy, temperamental, restless, noisy,* and *fidgety.* The three most common descriptions, however, were *cheerful, curious,* and *friendly.*

Within the first few weeks of life, children are already becoming social and beginning to smile. Smiling is clearly an expression of joy. From birth to six months, infants will often smile at anything and all people who please them. By six months, many children can recognize the faces of their principal caregivers. Faces other than those may bring anxiety, terror, and screaming. Children raised in households with many people may not experience as much anxiety.

Crying

Crying is a normal activity of all infants and serves many functions. In a newborn, crying helps the lungs adjust from the fluid-filled amniotic sac to an air-filled world. Infants cry in response to their needs when they are hungry, wet, cold, or, on occasion, in pain. This crying is a way of communicating with their parents and is effective because it usually produces the necessary response—a parent to alleviate the need. Parents quickly become adept at distinguishing different types of cries: those signaling hunger, pain, boredom, or anger.

Some crying is not due to a specific need of the infant, however. Neither hunger, wetness, nor pain is responsible. The infant is merely fussy. Holding and rocking does not always relieve this type of crying, but parents need not be concerned about this fussiness.

More than forty-five years ago, T. Berry Brazelton did a study of healthy infants that revealed that two to three hours of fussiness per day in the first few months of life was to be expected. Some infants were fussy for as much as four hours a day. Fussy crying increased gradually, becoming most prolonged by six weeks of age, and declined thereafter. By three to four months, most infants were fussy less than one-and-one-half hours daily. Most of the crying seemed to occur between the hours of 6:00 P.M. and 10:00 P.M. Unfortunately, this crying occurs at a time of day when parents are tired and becoming more irritable themselves. (For further discussion, see Colic, page 462.)

Crying may also occur as a result of the child's being frightened by a loud noise or a sudden movement. Some infants cry in response to lights going on or off.

As an infant grows older, crying becomes less frequent. Children can delay their need for gratification longer and longer. Older infants, however, begin to miss their parents and will cry when they are lonely. By six months of age, a child has come to recognize his or her parents and consequently recognizes their absence. Some people recommend holding an infant if he or she is crying because of loneliness. Others warn that cuddling children after crying will spoil them. We believe in a commonsense approach. A few whimpers when a child wakes up at night and is lonely need not be attended to. Frequently, playthings in the crib will serve to comfort the child. If the whimpering persists, often the voice of the parent is enough to quiet the child. If crying becomes intense and prolonged, hold and comfort your child.

Beyond one year of age, crying is often a product of the child's frustration at not being able to control his or her surroundings. This is, of course, a healthy sign of personality development, but it can disrupt the family. You can tolerate this crying better if you understand it.

As children become older, crying can be triggered by emotions. It is helpful for parents to teach a child to say that he or she is angry or frustrated rather than to demonstrate these feelings by crying. Sadness and separation are also frequently accompanied by crying.

Crying can be a sign of pain, especially in a young child who cannot verbalize the presence of a headache, stomachache, earache, or sore throat. If illness is causing the pain, other symptoms will usually be present as well.

Sleeping

An infant's typical sleeping patterns can be extraordinarily fatiguing for parents. A parent may feel frustrated if he or she hears that a friend's infant always sleeps from 8:00 P.M. to 8:00 A.M. or reads an article claiming that by three, four, or six months, your child should be sleeping through the night.

Individual sleep patterns and requirements vary tremendously. The average infant sleeps approximately 16 hours a day, with some infants sleeping as few as 10 hours and others sleeping as many as 22 or even 23 hours. As children get older, their sleep requirements gradually decline. By one year of age, children sleep only about 14 hours. By four years of age, they sleep an average of 12 hours, and by age 8, they sleep an average of 9 hours, but as few as 6 and as many as 13 hours.

Newborn infants have as many as five or six sleep cycles throughout the day. By one year of age, most children have just two sleep cycles—an afternoon nap and evening sleep. Most children outgrow their need for an afternoon nap by the time they are five years of age, but even many adults choose to take an afternoon nap whenever possible.

The length of a child's sleep cycles will increase markedly in the first year, but a substantial number of children wake up in the middle of the night throughout the first two years. One study that recorded the sleep of nine-month-olds revealed that although two-thirds of them woke up during the night, only 22% of their parents reported the night waking. Thus, in a sense, "sleeping through the night" is a phenomenon that involves *both* children's sleep and parents' sleep. It really means "letting Mommy and Daddy sleep through the night."

Although night waking can exhaust parents, you may find some solace in knowing that this pattern is normal for infants. As they become older, you should not encourage them to stay awake with food, holding, or other forms of attention, but merely attend to the child's immediate comfort and safety. As infants enter their second year, following a regular bedtime ritual can decrease their anxiety over separation and facilitate their going to sleep.

Using a bottle to get children to sleep has some drawbacks. It makes children subject to increased numbers of dental problems and earaches. You can give your child a bottle before putting him or her to bed, but the child should drink the milk sitting upright, and you should not let the milk remain in contact with the child's teeth for a long period of time. (In other words, babies should not routinely go to sleep "teething" on a bottle.) It is far better to give a child a "transitional object" such as a teddy bear than to give a bottle to provide comfort when getting to sleep.

Eventually, it is important for children to learn to fall asleep on their own. Most children awake several times during the night. If they are used to falling asleep in a parent's arms, they will expect these arms at 3:00 A.M. Develop a pleasant ritual and then place your child in the crib—awake. Do this either at naptime or evening bedtime. If your infant protests, listen to the protest for about 3 minutes (use a watch, or you'll be back in 20 seconds). Then return, comfort your child with your voice or a touch, as appropriate, and leave shortly thereafter. You can now leave for up to 4 minutes. Repeat this process gradually increasing the time away. This approach is preferable to deciding one night to let your baby "cry it out" and has been popularized by Richard Ferber. Most infants learn how to put themselves to sleep within a week using this technique. Relapses will occur, and you must alter the routines to accommodate illness and other events.

Toddlers

Toddlers are moving from being totally dependent on their parents to trying to control themselves and their universe. They begin to discover their individuality and try to determine how much power they have as individuals. Toddlers are at an age of daring exploration. They will climb ladders far too high, run much too far away, and try to eat dangerous things. Parents of children in this age group must set limits without overprotecting a child. The child must learn what is too high, what is too hot, what is too sharp.

Children are very negative during this period. Because of the child's extreme inquisitiveness, parents find themselves saying no often. The child, however, is driven by a burning desire to explore and to control anyone who tries to interfere with those explorations. The constant "no, no, no" of the child is meant to ensure his or her autonomy. Toddlers will often say no when in fact they have every intention of doing what their parents ask. Again, this is their way of telling you who is in charge. Their "no" really means, "No, I'm not going to do it because you want me to do it, but I will do it because I feel like it and because I am in charge here." Parents would do well to employ some diplomacy. Every diplomat knows how important it is for the opponent to save face. Parents can let the child say no while at the same time making sure that he or she does what is expected.

Like the "no" syndrome, temper tantrums in toddlers are often a reaction to a world they cannot control. It is their way of dealing with parents whom they perceive as interfering with their autonomy. The tantrums are a sign of toddlers' frustration, not only with parents and the world but also at their inability to communicate that frustration. As children become more verbal and are more able to express their anger, temper tantrums become far less frequent. A parent can be most helpful by encouraging children to communicate their feelings directly rather than using tantrums or other aggressive acts. Try not to let tantrums become a successful tactic for your child to obtain a goal.

Despite the first steps toward independence, the toddler still requires a tremendous amount of holding and touching. These interactions are important for children in this age group to develop their personalities.

It is not easy being a parent of a two-year-old. For that matter, it's not easy being a two-year-old. This period often creates the greatest amount of anxiety for parents and has been dubbed the "terrible twos." The terrible twos may not seem so terrible if the parents realize what is going on. Their task is to aid the toddler in becoming independent. This requires not only tremendous affection and more patience than at any other stage of development but also a thorough understanding of what the child is going through.

Sleeping

Many of the sleep problems of childhood are based on the fact that children's sleep patterns are different from those of adults. Many parents would prefer that their children go to bed at 7:30 or 8:00 in the evening and awaken shortly after the parents arise. These wishes do not correspond to the needs of all children. We feel that some sleep problems can be avoided by careful planning. Children get to sleep most easily when there is an established, predictable routine. If children are wound up because of exercise or vigorous play, it will be difficult for them to go to bed; ordering a child into bed at such a time is futile. A good wind-down routine consists of a nighttime bath, toothbrushing, and a story in bed. These activities calm children and provide a time for parents and children to enjoy each other.

Young children often do best with night-lights in their rooms. You can expect your toddler to spend some time talking or playing after you have left the room. There is no need to interrupt this activity. Some children may begin whimpering after the parents leave the room. Common sense, as well as the age of the child, should dictate your response. (For more information, see the section on crying on pages 79–80.)

It is common for children to wake up between 5:00 and 6:00 A.M. Younger infants may prefer to spend time in bed babbling and playing with toys. Toddlers generally rush off to their parents' rooms upon awakening. Depending on the hour, some parents prefer to bring the toddler in bed with them so that they can get an extra hour of sleep. This approach is entirely a matter of parental choice. Sometimes three- and four-year-olds go through periods of trying to sleep in their parents' beds. Although there is no harm in permitting this activity occasionally, we do not encourage parents to allow children to sleep with them for prolonged periods.

Fears

Fear of the dark and nightmares are so common that we should probably not even consider them problems. The best approach to fear of the dark is to use a night-light. Nightmares occur commonly in children of preschool age, and generally you can handle them with a few minutes of cuddling and reassurance. Rarely, children experience something called night terrors, which are quite distinct from nightmares. Night terrors occur in a different stage of sleep, and the child is generally hysterical and cannot be comforted. Persistent night terrors require medical help.

A frequent cause of sleep disturbances is the use of medications. This is particularly true with antihistamines and decongestants, which can interfere with the child's normal sleep patterns. If your child is having trouble sleeping and is simultaneously taking a medication, consult your doctor about the problem.

Thumb Sucking and Pacifiers

All infants are born with a sucking reflex. Because of this reflex, they will suck on a fist, finger, nipple, or anything else that comes in contact with their mouths. The sucking is, of course, necessary for feeding. Hence, an infant soon associates sucking with a feeling of satisfaction and security. As the child grows older, it is normal to suck on fingers, pacifiers, or favorite objects. Often the child will hold a favorite object in one hand and suck the thumb of the other, or the child will suck a thumb and insert a corner of a blanket or teddy bear's ear in the mouth as well.

Sucking on objects, as well as thumb sucking, occurs most frequently between the ages of one and two and one-half. Sucking increases when the child is anxious, tired, hungry, or stressed. There is no need for concern about these activities. They are perfectly normal and demonstrate resourcefulness in finding a way to deal with stress and anxiety.

Several words of caution: **Pacifiers** should not be sweetened, because this can encourage the development of cavities in the teeth. Pacifiers should be of hard rubber and should have a "skirt" larger than 1½ inches (4 cm) in diameter to protect the infant from suffocating. Several deaths have been reported from pacifiers with a small skirt lodging inside infants' mouths. Some liquid-filled pacifiers have been found to be contaminated with bacteria. Remove any strings attached to pacifiers to lower the risk of strangulation.

Children will generally outgrow **thumb sucking** by the age of five. Parents should not make an issue over thumb sucking, because this will heighten the child's anxiety and hence increase his or her need for a pacifying object. Persistent thumb sucking beyond age five should be discussed during a regular medical visit.

Temper Tantrums

Temper tantrums are common in children between 15 months and 4 years of age, and tantrums almost invariably arise when there is conflict between parent and child. The pattern of the tantrums is familiar to many parents of toddlers. A child is asked to do something—put down a toy, come in for a nap—and returns a few "nos" in response. When the child realizes that he or she is not going to be indulged, an outburst begins. There may be kicking, crying, shouting, rolling on the floor, fist banging, and spitting. As often as not, these displays are put on in public. You will probably feel embarrassed and want to beat a hasty retreat with your child. Even at home, you will be tempted to take evasive action.

A good approach to temper tantrums is to ignore them as much as is humanly possible. It is important that your child not get his or her own way after a tantrum. Punishing the child briefly and then indulging him or her ensures repetition of the tantrum. You are then essentially teaching your child that temper tantrums are effective in getting what is desired. Giving in even occasionally will prolong the persistence of these outbursts.

The best approach to temper tantrums is to try to prevent them. Understand the development of a child's personality, be consistent in discipline, and take a commonsense approach as to what demands and restrictions are reasonable for your child. As children grow older, parents should teach them to verbalize, rather than demonstrate, their feelings. It is better for a child to say "That makes me mad" or "I'm frustrated" than to display anger through physical acts of violence. It also is easier for parents to deal rationally with verbal, rather than physical, protests.

Breath-Holding Spells

The same factors that may precipitate a temper tantrum—conflict, frustration, anger, a contest of wills—cue some children into breath-holding spells. Breath-holding spells can also occur as a result of pain. Such spells are most common around the first year of life but occur anywhere from a few months to five years of age.

Usually a child will suddenly hold his or her breath at the end of a cry. After a few seconds, the child will become blue and then relax and recover. In moderate cases, the child will prolong the breath-holding spell, become blue, and temporarily become limp and unconscious. As soon as the child becomes unconscious, the reflex system that controls breathing will quickly resume the normal breathing pattern. It is this reflex system that the child has overcome during the outburst.

On rare occasions, a breath-holding spell can lead to a **seizure.** In seizures that are due to other causes, it is unusual for a crying episode and blueness to come before the seizure. In febrile seizures (resulting from a fever) and in epilepsy, the blueness follows the seizure.

The best approach to breath-holding spells is the same as to temper tantrums: Ignore them. A recent study indicated that some breath-holding children may be anemic, so over time the spells may be helped by iron supplements. Although these episodes are extremely frightening, damage is quite rare. The problem almost invariably resolves by age five. After that, breath-holding episodes are usually due to contests among peers.

The Preschool Years

In a child's preschool years, his or her most dramatic development is probably in the use of language. Children progress in a few years from the use of two-word phrases to the ability to tell stories and describe fantasies. They begin grasping concepts such as size, numbers, orientation in space, and time.

Play begins to occupy a great deal of preschool children's time. Play accomplishes many things for this age group. Children learn fine motor skills and concepts through play. In the early preschool years, children most often play independently and explore their toys. If placed with other children, they will not interact. As children become older, they begin to play together, although sharing toys does not always come easily. Besides aiding intellectual and social growth, play is a way in which three- and four-year-olds, who seem to have enough energy to run for 36 hours a day, can divert this energy into activities that are less distracting to parents.

Fantasy friends and stories are common at this age. Fantasy is not fibbing; it is a way of learning. Children in the preschool and early school years also lie. They are not necessarily trying to deceive; they often have difficulty drawing a sharp boundary between reality and fantasy.

Preschoolers also experience further emotional development. Parents can provide a tremendous service by beginning to teach children to discuss their feelings. Three- and four-year-olds are sometimes able to tell their parents that they are grumpy or angry or sad. When children can talk about these feelings, it is easier for parents to help them through hard parts of the day. An inability to recognize one's own feelings can lead to problems later in life. We encourage parents to assist their children in developing a sense of their own feelings. This is also an age of sexual exploration, which we will discuss later in this chapter.

Many children attend day care centers or nursery schools at this age. The activities there aid in socialization and help prepare for the activities of formal schooling. Children who do not go to day care or nursery schools still hear a great deal about school from other children or older siblings. Therefore, most children are socially ready for school by the time they enter.

Short Attention Span (Hyperactivity)

There are as many different temperaments as there are children. Some preschoolers have temperaments that many parents consider to be easy. They are social and affectionate, react to new situations with curiosity, and often are considered "even-tempered." Others may be shy, more difficult to warm up, or cautious of new situations. These traits may be viewed as stubbornness. Infants may be innately intense or difficult to comfort.

Some children seem to be unable to focus on any activity for more than a few minutes. Often these children seem to go from one activity to the next with barely enough time to take a breath. Many such children also seem to have boundless energy, are in constant motion, and are viewed as "hyperactive." A child's ability to focus is a gradual developmental process that lengthens with age. However, if a child cannot pay attention for at least 20 to 25 minutes by age five, that very abbreviated attention span can be frustrating for parents. The child also faces a potential for difficulty in kindergarten.

Most parents find it reassuring to learn that their active toddlers, preschoolers, and early-school-age children will gradually develop the ability to sit still and pay attention. However, waiting for this to happen can be frustrating. A short attention span in older children can seriously interfere with both academic and social achievement in school. For these children, we recommend formal evaluation as soon as this problem is reported. (For more information, see Hyperactivity and ADHD, page 296.)

For hyperactivity in younger children, here are some specific techniques that can help.

▲ Don't blame yourself. Children are born with different temperaments, and the very active child is one of the many varieties. In fact, this temperamental style suits many cultures and many adult careers.

▲ Remember that routines are important for all children, but even more so for children with short attention spans.

▲ By all means, follow their lead and allow them ample opportunity to "burn off" their energy. These children often seem to have boundless energy and are literally built for physical activity. However, many of them have difficulty making the transition from one type of activity to another. Therefore, make sure these children avoid strenuous physical activity before going to bed.

▲ Having periods during the day when these children are in a playpen or a quiet area with a limited number of choices can be very helpful. They often have difficulty focusing on one thing at a time, and being allowed to wander from task to task in an unstructured environment can result in overload. Many of these children even ask to be put in a playpen when they sense that their circuits are about to go into overload. Not only is "time-out" in the playpen good for children, but it also gives you some time to do things for yourself. Active children can drain the energy from even the most patient parents.

▲ As with all children, set limits and administer discipline in a firm and consistent manner. Remember that with their increased activity and energy levels, these children seem to be more apt than other children to get into trouble. Confront negative behavior immediately, using a firm tone of voice and avoiding physical punishment. Your child should know that certain behavior is unacceptable. After you convey that message, it is important to reassure your child that you still love him or her but that you will not tolerate any biting, hitting, running, kicking, throwing, and the like.

▲ Use common sense in considering which social situations to enter with your child. Whereas some parents can make it through a quiet dinner in a romantic restaurant with their three-year-old (although we're not sure why they would want to do this), a very active three-year-old will make the same evening miserable. Fast-food restaurants, particularly those that have play areas, are fine for these children. Supermarkets are high-risk zones: The child sees a lot of stimulation, while you want to focus on shopping. We are not suggesting that you and your child remain socially isolated, just that you consider carefully at what time of day your child is best able to deal with highly stimulating situations.

▲ Spend time with your child alone, doing things such as reading or storytelling. It is also important for your child to have time away from older siblings, who tend to excite younger brothers and sisters.

The Early School Years (Ages 6 to 11)

During the school years, children make the transition from being members of a family to being members of both a family and society. Teachers become extremely important figures in the child's life, but playmates remain the most significant people in his or her society.

Friendships

This is a period of organized games, which tend to stress competition and cooperation. Psychology textbooks often stress that this period is one of same gender identity, when 8- to 11-year-olds associate chiefly with members of the same sex. With new societal attitudes toward the dichotomy of gender roles, we expect some of this polarization to diminish. Indeed, the separation between boys and girls varies greatly, depending on the circumstances of the moment. For example, ball games may require the full participation of girls and boys so as to provide the necessary number of players and the necessary equipment. Many youth soccer leagues now offer three divisions: boys, girls, and coed. Even in all-boy or all-girl schools, it is important that children learn both the value and the means of cooperating with members of the opposite sex on meaningful projects.

Because of the importance of friends in this age group, parents must be sensitive to their children's needs if they plan a move. A promise of a bigger house, a room of one's own, or even a swimming pool is negligible when compared with the loss of friends. Fortunately, children make new friends relatively easily, but the parents must be supportive during this transition.

Ethical Codes

Children in the early school years are also developing their own codes of justice. Moral judgment begins at about the age of 6 or 7, when children begin looking at the circumstances surrounding an event to decide whether the event is right or wrong. The moral codes of 7- and 8-year-olds come chiefly from their parents and other members of the adult world. Between the ages of 8 and 12, children begin to talk more with friends and evolve their own codes of justice.

Stealing is frequently a problem in this age group. Some stealing is merely a way for a child to test boundaries and determine proper limits. Most children who steal during these years have a sense of guilt. Occasionally, children may steal as a group or be forced to steal as an initiation rite. Although it is the parents' job to define and maintain the limits that society demands, they should not overreact to the situation. Stealing by a child is a profound disappointment but does not usually herald the beginning of a life of crime. Let your child know firmly, but with love, that such behavior is not acceptable.

In stealing, your child is essentially saying, "Here's what society says, but is society right? How do I feel about this action? The only way I can tell how I feel is to test it." The ability to question society's values is important. The right to question should be encouraged. A mature reaction to the discovery of your child's stealing can be a learning experience for both of you, can establish the limits of acceptable behavior, and can teach the child the relationship between actions and their consequences.

Development in School

Schooling accomplishes many things for our children. At school, children acquire academic skills and learn about the nature of the universe. Besides knowledge, schools foster a child's self-esteem, code of behavior, and ability to function within society. Students discover how to work with other children and begin to appreciate what will be required of them to get along in the larger society. Often, especially in large classes, children do not receive adequate individual attention from teachers. In addition, for a teacher to deal with 30 children, he or she must maintain a tremendous amount of order and uniformity. That environment can be detrimental to your child by preventing him or her from thinking or acting differently. This is clearly undesirable for mature development. Rigidity can stifle creativity. Children require an atmosphere that promotes learning for all, yet at the same time encourages each child's development as a unique individual. Children must learn a combination of competition, cooperation, and creativity. Parents must understand the school program and complement it, so that the child will be well prepared for the wider world.

Children also have different learning abilities and styles. Most schools are geared to teaching the "average" child, and many children—both above and below average—will fall by the wayside. At the first sign of problems, meet with your child's teacher, and if the problem continues insist that your child receive an appropriate learning evaluation and learning plan (see also Chapter 7).

Adolescents (Age 12 and Up)

Father of Two   It's like trying to steer a battleship with the rudder from a dinghy.

Thirteen-Year-Old Girl   When you're twelve you feel like you're trapped inside twelve until you turn thirteen, and then you are trapped inside thirteen.

Seventeen-Year-Old Boy   The best thing about being a teenager is high school, and the worst thing about being a teenager is high school.

Expectations

"The trouble with today's youth is . . . ." How many times have you heard that expression? How many times have you heard the same tired clichés: "They're irresponsible." "They're hung up on sex/drugs/cars." "They never show any respect." Adolescents have suffered from countless generalizations and oversimplifications. By lumping all teenagers together and expecting certain adverse behavior from them, we essentially deny them the freedom to be individuals. When that behavior occurs, we all nod our heads knowingly and feed our own prejudices.

It is interesting to consider how the media portray adolescents. For instance, in the 1950s adolescents were portrayed as angry young rebels. Marlon Brando in *The Wild One* and James Dean in *Rebel Without a Cause* rose to fame in roles portraying youths at odds with the world. When the young people of that era grew up and came to control the media in the 1970s, they portrayed the black-leather-jacket crowd, such as "the Fonz" in *Happy Days,* as polite, well-groomed, respectful superheroes. Whereas parents in the 1960s frowned upon the lyrics and antics of the Rolling Stones, parents now line up to take their children to Stones concerts. The good old days of today are frequently the terrible times of yesterday.

Studies of adolescents have revealed several interesting facts. Most adolescents have attitudes and values that closely reflect those of our society as a whole. Their political orientation is usually that of their parents. The majority of adolescents approve of their parents' attitudes toward discipline, even though they do not enjoy being subjected to discipline. Most adolescents feel that their parents understand them, and most feel that the communication lines with their parents are open.

There is, of course, a wide spectrum here, because many adolescents are at odds with their parents. No individual can be expected to agree with a parent, spouse, or friend all the time. Disagreements produce tension, and because of their unpleasant nature, people often remember them. A thousand productive acts may be forgotten in the wake of one heated argument.

Independence

Adolescence is often a difficult period because of the many complex tasks required of young people and their parents. The adolescent is defining his or her identity while rapidly moving toward legal, economic, and psychological independence. Legal independence is coming at an earlier age than ever before. The old custom of legal majority at age 21 is nearly extinct, and states now recognize the age of 18. Many states say that youths reach the age of majority for making choices about health care at an even younger age; all states allow teens younger than 18 to consent to care for certain medical conditions.

Economic independence requires young people to plan for the future. That ability develops during adolescence. Such planning includes assessing the educational tasks that one must accomplish to reach economic goals. Many adolescents do not have clear-cut goals. Some do not develop these goals until they are in their 20s. Unrealistic or unclear aspirations can lead to lifelong frustrations. Parents can offer support, but telling adolescents what they "should" do is not helpful. Maturation is complex and occurs at different ages for different people. Encourage your child to consider career options seriously. Work-study plans are available in many communities. Vocational counseling is very important for teens.

Psychological independence is, by far, the most important and most difficult part of adolescence. In this period, individuals develop abstract thinking and begin to build a theoretical framework by which they will live. This involves developing a way to deal with the contradictory values of society, as well as ethical and moral values for the adolescent's personal life. During this time, children first begin to recognize the gray zone between black and white with which we all must deal. This is a supremely disturbing discovery. Contradictions about war, pollution, exploitation, and class differences are difficult for anyone to accept, and even worse if you have been raised by parents and teachers to believe in peace, love of fellow human beings, and equality. How do the idealistic teachings of parents and teachers measure up to the reality of the world? This contradiction is extremely difficult for young people to resolve.

Adolescents also come to realize that they must soon move away and separate from their parents. Although many teens talk enthusiastically about leaving home, this is a major source of anxiety. At the same time, adolescents are developing their own personal value systems. Most of these developments have something to do with how they relate to other people. Friendships are extremely intense, and best friends often become inseparable in early adolescence.

In adolescence, people must learn how to develop meaningful interpersonal relationships. Sexuality is only one aspect of these relationships. The sexual drives that adolescents experience cannot be denied. They provide a learning experience, requiring youths to decide on actions that are consistent with their evolving value systems. Younger adolescents sometimes deal with their budding sexuality by engaging in homosexual activities. This can be frightening to adolescents, and even more so to their parents. However, it is a normal developmental phase for many adolescents. Younger adolescents are vulnerable to sexually exploitive homosexual or heterosexual acts. These acts are far more significant than the transient homosexual episodes between peers.

The availability of contraception has become a double-edged sword. It has allowed many adolescents to test their sexuality in a mature and responsible way, but it often leaves some young people without an "excuse" for not engaging in sexual activity. Adolescents need support from parents, and sometimes from professionals, in finding the path that is best for them. Good sex education programs stress the importance of mature choice, as well as the mechanics of contraception. The vast majority of sexually active adolescents have one partner. The level of promiscuity among adolescents actually seems to be lower than that of adults.

Choosing Medical Care

One of the best ways for parents to help adolescents is to encourage them to make their own health care choices. We feel that the best way to ensure good health throughout one's life is to learn responsible decision making. Adolescents often view pediatricians and family doctors as people their parents have chosen. This can discourage them from developing mature medical behavior. In addition, adolescents might be concerned about their privacy and confidentiality. Although very few doctors would violate an adolescent's confidentiality, the fear that a parent-chosen doctor might do so may prevent a teen from seeking necessary medical advice.

The development of free clinics primarily serving youths was testimony to the desire of adolescents to obtain medical care in confidence. Because these clinics sent home no bills, confidentiality was ensured. Most adolescents who have open communication with their parents will discuss their medical concerns within the family, but they should be allowed to decide when to raise these concerns. Youths who are treated as mature individuals capable of making rational choices will develop responsible approaches to medical problems more quickly.

We feel that a doctor who has been seeing an adolescent for several years can provide the best care. Therefore, we encourage parents to let go of the old parent-child-doctor relationship and recognize the importance of confidential communication between doctor and adolescent. Confidentiality between adolescents and their doctors is supported by the American Academy of Pediatrics and numerous state laws.

How can parents best support their children through the intense, often emotional years of adolescence? It's not easy. You gradually grant them more independence, but you are often unsure about how much is appropriate. Your children may be becoming very independent in one area but still show youthful tendencies in another. For their part, youths often become anxious about their own independence. Although they look forward to becoming adults, many of the freedoms of childhood also are appealing. You can help by providing support and by helping your child to acquire the best information possible in matters such as health, education, employment, and sexuality.

What should parents do when problems arise? Many people adopt the attitude that adolescent problems are temporary and will soon disappear. But the percentage of adolescents who are emotionally impaired corresponds rather closely to the number of adults who are impaired. Although many of the minor turmoils of adolescence give way to the different problems of adulthood, the severe ones do not disappear by themselves. Severe emotional impairment in adolescents or adults demands help from doctors, social workers, or counselors. The 6-year-old who cannot function in school, the 16-year-old in trouble with the law, and the 36-year-old who cannot hold a job all need help.

Problem Behaviors

Unfortunately, some problems are worse for adolescents today than they were for their parents. Only half of teenage deaths in the 1950s were due to accidental injuries, homicides, and suicides. Now these three causes represent 80% of the mortality for adolescents. In addition, a disturbingly high rate of depression occurs in adolescents. Researchers have identified three problem behaviors as being responsible for more than half of the serious illnesses and deaths of teenagers.

▲ Substance abuse
▲ Motor (and recreational) vehicle use and misuse
▲ Premature sexual behavior

There are clear-cut associations among these behaviors. The relationship between alcohol and injury, as in driving accidents, is well-known. Substance use is also linked to earlier initiation of sexual activity.

When parents notice a teenager smoking, drinking, or abusing drugs, there is a problem. That's why teenagers rarely do these things in front of their parents. Other signs may indicate a hidden problem with alcohol or drugs. Families that have experienced alcoholism should be especially alert. If you see any of the following signs, get your teenager into a program to discourage problem behaviors.

▲ Decline in school performance
▲ Lack of motivation in school
▲ School absenteeism
▲ School discipline problems
▲ Increased behavior problems
▲ Loss of interest in previous hobbies
▲ Lack of interest in family activities
▲ Changing groups of friends (especially to groups involved in high-risk behaviors)
▲ Friends with criminal histories or behavior
▲ Neglect of appearance, relative to peers

▲ Excessive concern with money
▲ Changes in mood
▲ Depressive symptoms (see page 306)
▲ Running away from home
▲ Driving while intoxicated

Some of these signs, such as changing interests and appearances, are normal for adolescence. It is the *degree* to which adolescents change that might tip you off. Get to know your child's peers, and use your judgment.

It is often difficult, and sometimes impossible, to change a teenager's problem behavior. Your physician may be helpful in steering your adolescent toward an effective community program. Schools are also becoming more involved in this area. Most communities have groups for dealing with substance abuse geared specifically to teenagers. One such group is Alateen, associated with Alcoholics Anonymous (AA). Parents can help by controlling their own behavior—eliminating smoking and excess consumption of alcohol.

Parents must make sure that their teenagers receive appropriate health care, especially when their behavior indicates that they are taking bad risks. Usually, the first step is to arrange a regular health appraisal by the child's physician. Not all doctors are well prepared to confront adolescents about risky behaviors and identify a way to deal with the problem. Most physicians will not treat the problem alone. Instead, they will help you to enroll your adolescent in an appropriate program to help him or her solve the problem.

Discipline

Mother of Two   A parent's most important job is not to make a child happy, but to develop the child's character.

Children require many things from parents. We place tremendous emphasis on good prenatal and child nutrition, safety, immunizations, and other ingredients of healthy child development. However, greater challenges come from the emotional aspects of child rearing. Few parents need lessons in how to love their children, the most important emotional ingredient. But a major dilemma arises in choosing how best to discipline children so that in the end they will be happy, healthy adults with self-discipline. Am I too strict? Is my spouse too lenient? Will I spoil him? Will she learn to limit herself if I impose too many limits? These are all legitimate concerns of parents.

The most important concept is that discipline means giving children knowledge and skills. Discipline is very different from punishment, which is the consequence of an unacceptable behavior. A consistent, positive approach to discipline should minimize the need for punishment. Parents cannot learn appropriate discipline techniques in five minutes, and unfortunately many of today's parents grew up without good parenting models and witnessing considerable corporal punishment. Decades of research has taught us that neither a permissive attitude nor an authoritarian "do it my way because I said so" approach works as well as consistent limit setting with explanations. We encourage your continued learning about these techniques.

Here are some important principles of discipline.

▲ Young infants need a safe environment—entirely the parent's job.
▲ Discipline begins when infants become mobile.
▲ Discipline should be geared to age-appropriate learning.
▲ Catch the child being good. Constantly correcting mistakes is not enough.
▲ Do the right thing yourself. Nobody is as important to your child as you, and children learn by watching parents.
▲ Praise and hug liberally after the discipline discussion. Be sure your child knows you dislike a *behavior,* not him or her.
▲ Children don't need to be hurt to learn. Parents don't need to hurt to teach.

Age-appropriate Discipline
Infants
For infants, safety is of the utmost concern. Infants respond to a sharp "no" or "hot." They will learn your displeasure when your firm voice is accompanied by holding their hands if they scratch or pull.

Older infants and toddlers need the following:

▲ Structured environments that minimize the risk of ruining vases or expensive equipment.
▲ A firm voice in explanation.
▲ Redirection toward acceptable playthings.
▲ To be ignored occasionally. Don't reward attention-seeking behavior (such as tantrums), but do limit problem behaviors (such as biting or hitting).
▲ Praise when they're doing a good job.

Preschoolers
Preschoolers need the following:

▲ Parents with unbelievable patience, fortitude, and stamina.
▲ Clear and consistent rules and expectations repeated and repeated.
▲ Time to get ready: "In five minutes you need to put away your toys and wash for dinner."
▲ Acknowledgment with explanation: "I know you want to stay at Grandma's, but it's time we went home so we can all go to sleep."
▲ Removal now with talk later. A child hitting another needs quiet physical isolation followed by an explanation: "You know we have two important rules. You can't hurt anybody by hitting, and you can't hurt their feelings."
▲ Temporary time-out. Removing a child to a corner for a few minutes can help defuse a situation, give a message, and teach about consequences.
▲ Praise when they're doing a good job.
▲ Praise when they've learned something: "I'm really glad you and your cousin have been playing so nicely this week."

School-Age Children
School-age children need all of the preceding plus the following:

▲ Opportunities to explain.
▲ Opportunities to express themselves.
▲ Opportunities to choose: "I understand you really want to watch the end of this program. However, if we allow this additional 30 minutes of TV tonight, it will mean no more television this weekend." "If you do not make the effort to clean your room today, you will have to live in a dirty room, and I will not make the effort to take you to your friend's party tomorrow."
▲ Opportunities to solve problems: "You seem to have a hard time finishing your homework at night. Why don't you work on a list of suggestions, and then we'll go over them together?"

Adolescents
Adolescents will continue the limit testing they started as infants. Even the best discipline system will be challenged. In addition to the preceding, adolescents need the following:

▲ Discussions on the long-term consequences of today's behaviors.
▲ Limit setting that is agreed on rather than imposed arbitrarily (although parents must ultimately establish the boundaries).

▲ Limits that increase according to their maturity and ability to choose wisely: "You can stay out until 10:30 this year, 11:00 next year, and after that I will evaluate how you use your own judgment to decide."

Punishment

Although we oppose physical punishment of children, we recognize that parents in the heat of the moment may occasionally spank a child. Parents who were punished physically as children need to be aware that they may resort to this damaging behavior and should seriously consider alternatives.

We acknowledge that although all experts agree on a positive approach to discipline, there is still disagreement on physical punishment. However, after years of deliberation the American Academy of Pediatrics stated in 1998 that "corporal punishment is of limited effectiveness and has potentially deleterious side effects." The AAP recommended that "parents be encouraged and assisted in the development of methods other than spanking for managing undesired behavior." Other experts say that you should never have to hurt a child either physically or emotionally to get your point across. Saf Lerman writes, "Parents need to use methods that will make childhood a good experience for their children and parenting a satisfying experience for themselves. When children are being hit and parents are hitting, the process is not beneficial to anyone." Still other experts and authors may tolerate one swat on the bottom with an open hand but decry anything more.

All parenting experts agree that there are better alternatives to physical punishment. Taking away privileges is very effective. It is important to remember such alternatives even at the emotional moment when you discover that your child has misbehaved. Take the situation of a mother who returns home one winter night to learn that her five-year-old twins had summoned the police by dialing 911 while dad was attempting to cook dinner. (Not a true emergency!) After the parents explained why this behavior was unacceptable, one twin agreed not to do it again. The other was less remorseful, arguing that nobody had answered *his* phone call; only his twin sister had gotten through. The mother strongly felt that the children's behavior warranted a punishment, but what? The parents' solution was to take away all the Christmas presents given the previous week, with the understanding that they would have to be earned back. In this way, the parents effectively taught a dramatic lesson about a serious behavior without using physical punishment.

If you find yourself shaking or repeatedly hitting your child, you need help. Perhaps you can enroll in a course that teaches effective discipline techniques. Most communities have helpful child abuse hotlines. Your physician can also be a useful resource.

Sexuality

Like all other aspects of human development, sexual development begins at birth and continues in a logical order throughout life. This process includes the development of gender roles as well as the development of sexuality.

The concept of gender roles is formed early and reinforced continuously throughout life. A child's gender identity may begin in the nursery, when pink or blue cards are used to identify girls or boys. In our society, little boys are handled differently from little girls, even in the first few weeks of life. A close friend of ours, firmly committed to sexual equality in raising children of both sexes, began calling her newborn boy "little tiger," a term she had never used for her daughter. Such subtle and not-so-subtle discrimination of gender roles in the nursery is reinforced by families and schools and continues throughout an individual's life.

Infants

A child's sexuality begins in the first few minutes of life. Achieving pleasure through genital stimulation is only one small part. Showing affection physically by hugging, patting, and fondling the newborn infant is a natural act, affording pleasure to both parent and child. This is probably the first sexual interaction.

Parents often notice that newborn boys have erections. These erections can occur spontaneously or in response to a number of nervous stimuli. There is no reason to believe that infant boys do not feel pleasure during these periods. Certainly by one year of age, both boys and girls are able to reach their genitalia and notice that rubbing will produce a pleasurable sensation. At this age, most parents recognize that their children are merely exploring their bodies and are not concerned about genital manipulation. In the first year of life, infants are more concerned with other stimuli, especially the oral gratification of feeding and sucking.

Toddlers

As infants move into toddlerhood, they continue to derive pleasure from many areas, including interactions with parents, food, toys, and eventually the ability to control bowel movements. However, when a child is three or four years of age, there is often a renewed interest in genital manipulation, and masturbation occurs in both sexes.

Masturbation to orgasm is common in this age group. Parents often have questions about how to deal with masturbation in young children. Certainly, this natural experience is not to be condemned. However, parents may wish to talk to their children about when and where it is appropriate to masturbate. Teaching children how to control their sexual impulses should not be regarded any differently from teaching them not to talk loudly in church.

At this age, it is often common for children to barge into their parents' bedrooms during sexual activity. During these episodes, complex explanations are not needed—just a reassurance that the activity was playful and that any noises did not indicate that anyone was being hurt.

Ages 3 to 6

This is the time when children question how they were born. Explanations appropriate to the level of the child's understanding are important. Again, detailed anatomical dissertations are not what the child wants. Answering a single question at a time is better than embarking on a full discussion.

Children between the ages of three and six have a great deal of curiosity about their genitalia and are frequently anxious to compare theirs to those of their parents and those of children of the opposite sex. Parents should answer questions openly and frankly. You don't need to give a detailed explanation of precise anatomical differences. Little girls concerned about why they do not have a penis should be told that they have a clitoris instead and may be told that they have a vagina in addition. Focus on what the girl *has* instead of why she does not have what a boy has.

When children examine the genitalia of their playmates, especially those of the opposite sex, these activities sometimes lead to conflict among parents. There is no need to apologize for the activity of your child, although you'll probably want to tell other parents that you're sorry they are upset. Especially consider what you say in the presence of the children, for they may begin to think that they have done something terrible. Convey to your own children your feelings about appropriate behavior, as opposed to what Mr. and Mrs. Jones feel is appropriate.

As children reach the age of five or six, they may play "house" or "doctor" with children of the opposite sex. Often they play these games where they may be discovered. Children wonder whether this type of activity is right or wrong, and being found out is one way of testing the situation. Often the children have guilt feelings and need reassurance from their parents that they will not be rejected. An acceptable parental attitude is again to acknowledge the activity without encouraging it in inappropriate social situations and without punishing the child for it.

Ages 7 to 12

Between the ages of 7 and 12, children are occupied chiefly with tasks of learning, developing, and making friendships. These activities take precedence over all others. Genital manipulation persists throughout this stage, but it is less visible and important than at other ages. Although parents may feel that groups such as the Boy Scouts or Girl Scouts and school projects are molding their child's development, children are also learning a great deal about sexual relationships. Schoolchildren have a certain "street knowledge" about the mechanical aspects of sexual intercourse. They all have a repertoire of "dirty" jokes. In rural areas, children often see farm animals and dogs copulating. (We doubt that anyone learns very much from the birds or the bees.)

Children at this age are also astute observers of parental interactions, as well as male-female interactions in general. The most significant impression a child will form about how men and women interact is by observing his or her parents. Parents must provide as good a model in this area as they do in others. It is important for children to witness affection between parents. Naturally, parental battles will occur. When they do, you should explain to your child that he or she is not responsible. Children can adjust to a spectrum of emotions between their parents. They are apt to suffer, however, if they witness only fights or hostile interactions.

When children are between the ages of 10 and 12, most parents attempt a discussion of the "facts of life" with them. Parents should recognize that their children's education in these matters has been going on for many years, rarely with complete accuracy.

Adults often present the "facts of life" differently to girls and boys. Girls tend to be taught about the biology of ovulation and menstruation and the importance of preventing pregnancy. If a girl's mother has been having menstrual difficulties, often the daughter will be apprehensive about her coming periods. Very often children form early impressions about the pain of menstruation. In young children, blood is a sign of pain. Therefore, finding a tampon soaked with blood or seeing their mother change a blood-filled tampon or napkin may suggest to children that mother is being hurt. Explain to them what is going on.

Boys often receive the "facts of life" as a discussion about how to channel their developing drives away from sexual intercourse. In other words, boys are told about masturbation, but girls are not. We do not feel that it is helpful to deny the pleasurable parts of sexual activity. It's important to acknowledge that sexual activity, including masturbation and intercourse, can convey a great amount of pleasure. However, you will probably also want to discuss the personal, emotional, and ethical aspects of sexual activity. Emphasize the long-term benefits that mature interpersonal interaction and sexuality can afford and discuss how much more pleasurable sexual activity can be if accompanied by affection, intimacy, and love.

Adolescents

Recent studies have pointed out that the number of adolescent males having sexual intercourse has changed very little over the past 50 years, although more adolescent women are having intercourse now than 50 years ago. The number of women actively having sexual experiences is approaching that of their male counterparts. This has changed the stresses felt by many women. In the past, they were made to feel guilty if they had a premarital sexual experience. Today many women feel that rather than being pressured into celibacy, they are being pressured into sexual activity. Both men and women at this age need support from parents in dealing with these complex sexual issues.

The emergence of AIDS is beginning to change many adolescents' views on sexuality. The risk of sexual activity has always been present, but the negative consequences have become far more dramatic. Besides AIDS, sexually transmitted diseases (STDs) such as syphilis, gonorrhea, herpes, and chlamydia remain prevalent and, in some cases, are on the rise. Despite these dangers, 47% of high school students report having had intercourse, according to a 2003 survey by the Centers for Disease Control. Disturbingly, more than 7% of students initiated sexual intercourse before age 13, while 62% of high school seniors had experienced sexual intercourse.

Speaking Frankly

Adolescents need information, but they also need to be able to discuss their feelings with adults who will understand the difficult decisions they face and encourage responsible actions—actions that can mean the difference between continued maturation into adulthood and a life prematurely encumbered with a child or terminated by AIDS. Teens need to be able to turn to their parents for guidance throughout this difficult period.

Discussions about sexuality between children and their parents are unusual in our society. We anticipate that few adult readers will have more than cursory knowledge about their mothers' sexual experiences, for instance. Some may feel uncomfortable reading this section, much less using its information to discuss sexuality with an adolescent. Nevertheless, it is important for parents to discuss sex with children.

Virtually all adolescents have sexual interests. The age at which a person's first sexual intercourse occurs depends on many things. Biology is important; some adolescents mature more quickly than others. Personal goals, risk taking, role models, activities of friends, and social pressures are all part of the complex process of sexual decision making. In addition, adolescence involves exploring new feelings and trying on new roles—which can lead to sexual experimentation. Adolescents need to talk with someone about these issues. You can assume they are talking with their friends, and a few are talking with health care providers. But it is best if they can talk about sexuality with their parents as well. Just telling teenagers "no" is not a conversation. It does not give them the understanding to make a responsible choice at the right time.

To have open conversations with your teenagers about sex, you should start several years in advance. By setting up a relationship of trust early, you and your child will feel less awkward when more difficult questions arise.

Parents should encourage adolescents to refrain from sex until they are psychologically mature enough to deal with the responsibilities that accompany it. But encouragement alone is not enough, as our national health records show. The United States is a leader in such biomedical preventive measures as immunizations and zidovudine (AZT) to decrease perinatal HIV transmission, but it's woefully behind most Western societies in preventing adolescent pregnancy, STDs, and the emotional trauma that accompanies both. Our reluctance to discuss sexual behavior in living rooms and schoolrooms has resulted in American teenagers being far less informed than Canadian and many European teenagers and far less reliable in their use of contraception and their practice of "safer sex."

Fortunately, there are signs that our culture is changing. For example, network television episodes in recent years have included many frank discussions about sexuality between parents and children, even a grandmother openly discussing orgasms with her 30-year-old granddaughter. This frank depiction of communication about sexual concerns is an improvement over both silence and the exaggerations of, for instance, some daytime talk shows. If real-life families shared information as responsibly, we would be a much healthier society. Finally, the extensive media coverage of President Bill Clinton's sexual behavior undoubtedly changed our perception of what types of issues can be discussed at the dinner table.

Summary: Parenting Children and Beyond

You are the cornerstone of your child's personality development. You are required to provide constant love and yet set limits. Children need discipline, but it is important to make clear that a specific behavior, and not the child, is being chastised. Parents need to be open to discussing medical choices, sexuality, and other complicated issues with their children.

Parents should teach their children to be aware of their feelings and to respond to them appropriately. They can help children to talk about their feelings, to be able to say, "I am frustrated," "I am sad," "I am depressed." Sadness, depression, joy, and affection are emotions of young children as well as adults.

It is important to state in capital letters that WE ALL MAKE MISTAKES. Making mistakes is part of being human. We are all faced with uncertainty. There is no one approach to all problems, and we must all make decisions in the face of uncertainty. We all do the best we can, we all do things differently, our children all grow up differently, and that's the way things will always be.

Even though your children are officially "adults" and have certain legal rights at age 18, such as voting and confidential health care, your job is far from over when they reach that age. Legally, it is still an additional three years before they are considered mature enough to drink, and realistically it may take them many more years to become financially independent. In fact, parenting never ends. You will always have more experience (which hopefully translates into more wisdom) than your children. You will always have a longitudinal perspective on their traits and behaviors from when they were so young that they can have no memory of events.

As they leave home to start their own lives and families, you will no longer worry about things that now seem so small—that diaper rash, the ear infections, the broken clavicle after a fall from the monkey bars. Because you can no longer direct, you now have to reflect about their decisions and actions. Is their partner right? Is that the correct career decision? You're moving where? Do they even have running water or phone service?

I spoke with several of the parents who contributed quotes to the original edition of this book more than 30 years ago. They were going through pregnancy and raising young children at that time, and they were kind enough to give me their perspectives on parenting adult children now.

Father of Two   *Little people, little problems. Big people, big problems.*

Mother of Three   She was always our best organized and best behaved child; so it's actually OK she waited till she was 21 to have her adolescent rebellion.

Father of Three   It's great. I love visiting all three kids now that they are all in their thirties. But only one of them has health insurance.

Mother of Two   I have come to accept my son-in-law but I know my husband never will.

Father of One   I have come to accept my daughter-in-law but I know my wife never will.

A wonderful perspective on parenting, by the mother of four adult children, is contained in the poem *Lights Turning Green*.

> **Lights Turning Green**
> I wish for you
> clear road ahead,
> and lights turning green.
> Not a destination certain,
> on a map,
> but a road
> where sudden bends
> open vistas to the far horizon.
>
> Crossroads I wish for you too,
> so you can consider new directions,
> take a turnoff just for fun,
> and see where it might lead you.
> A passing lane to get you by
> those who seem to lead the way
> but are really lost,
> and lots of turn outs,
> so you can let traffic speed past,
> not crowd too close behind you;
> and also overlooks, where you can stop,
> see where you've been,
> where you've yet to go,
> and at the same time
> look all around,
> photograph the smallest flowers,

as well as distant
snow-peaked mountains
and shimmering lakes reflecting.
If you need to stop
and turn around,
I hope for ample shoulders,
because proceeding
in the wrong direction
is rarely useful,
though you may only learn
your road is leading
down a dead end
by traveling far enough to see.
Picnic stops too,
so you can rest up,
eat something delicious
and go on at full strength.
And if your lights can't be
always turning green,
I hope you can accept
the need to stop
sometimes
along your way
if only temporarily,
to reassesses,
and also see those opportunities
which don't come at you
straight on,
but from the side, obliquely.
And one last wish:
May your passenger seat
hold someone dear to you,
who is smart enough
to help you navigate,
tune the radio,
pass you a cold drink,
rub your neck,
and tell you,
with a grin,
when you've taken
a wrong turn.

© Lenore Horowitz, 2001

Additional Reading

Your One-Year-Old: The Fun Loving Fussy, Louise Bates Ames and Frances Ilg (New York: Dell, 1983).

Your Two-Year-Old: Terrible or Tender (1980)
Your Three-Year-Old: Friend or Enemy (1980)
Your Four-Year-Old: Wild and Wonderful (1980)
Your Five-Year-Old: Sunny and Serene (1981)
Your Six-Year-Old: Loving and Defiant (1981)
Your Ten- to Fourteen-Year-Old (1989)

The Scientist in the Crib: What Early Learning Tells Us About the Mind, Alison Gopnik, Andrew N. Meltzoff, and Patricia K. Kuhl (New York: Harper Paperbacks, 2000).

Changing Bodies, Changing Lives: A Book for Teens on Sex and Relationships, 3rd expanded ed., Ruth Bell et al. (New York: Crown Publishing Group, 1998).

Infants and Mothers: Differences in Development, rev. ed., T. Berry Brazelton, M.D. (New York: Dell, 1983).

Toddlers and Parents: A Declaration of Independence, rev. ed., T. Berry Brazelton, M.D. (New York: Dell, 1989).

Touchpoints: Birth to Three, T. Berry Brazelton, M.D., and Joshua D. Sparrow (Cambridge, Mass.: Da Capo Press, 2006).

Solve Your Child's Sleep Problems, expanded rev. ed. Richard Ferber (New York: Simon & Schuster, 2006).

The Magic Years, Selma H. Fraiberg (New York: Scribner's Reference, 1996).

The Moral Judgment of the Child, Jean Piaget (New York: Free Press, 1997).

Get Out of My Life, But First Could You Drive Me and Cheryl to the Mall: A Parent's Guide to the New Teenager, Anthony E. Wolf (New York: Farrar, Straus, and Giroux, 2002).

Chapter Six

Today's Family

There is no need to mourn the death of the American family. The family survives, but it is changing as our society is changing. As many functions of the family have evolved, so have our views of the family's purpose. Clearly, for instance, parents no longer produce children in abundance to ensure economic viability, as was required in an agrarian era.

Many of us carry around images of a traditional family with Mom and Dad, two kids, and their dog gathered around the fireplace reading. There is clearly a contrast between this image and the reality of today's family. In fact, although a snapshot of many families might capture the above ideal, a motion picture taken over the past century would reveal changes in almost every family. For example, it may come as a surprise that in a classic study of first-grade children done more than 20 years ago, only 34% lived in households with a mother and a father and no other adults. In contrast, more than 36% lived with only their mothers, 1% with their fathers, 2% with their grandparents, and the remaining 27% with their mothers and other adult relatives. Today a growing number of children (over 540,000) live in foster homes. Adoption, which dates back at least to the time of Moses, is also in transition, as "open" adoptions are becoming more prevalent.

We cannot deny that divorce is a major issue affecting children. But family breakups were not invented in the 1970s. The U.S. government began keeping tabs on divorces in 1867. The rate was 0.3 per 1,000 population then, compared with an all-time high of 5.3 per 1,000 in 1981. There have been periodic surges. For example, immediately after World War II, the rate climbed to over 4 per 1,000 (18 per 1,000 married women), a figure that was not seen again until 1973. The divorce rate has declined steadily and gradually since peaking in the late 1970s and early 1980s.

Today more than 5 million children are living with a divorced parent. This is about 9% of children younger than 18 years old. Many others have parents who are separated. It is estimated that more than a third of today's children will experience the absence of a parent from the home. Divorced parents often share child care responsibility, known as co-parenting. Many parents with children remarry, forming blended families.

Another major change in how children live is the renewed surge of women working outside the home. Although there have always been "working" mothers, the demand for day care today is unprecedented. In our highly mobile society, Grandma may not live close enough to help out every day, and even though Aunt Gigi lives around the corner, she also may be at work. Due to these factors, we are now a nation with millions of toddlers in child care and millions of school age "latchkey children."

In a nation that is still predominantly only a generation or two away from immigrant grandparents, we have grown up with the stresses of leaving relatives and roots behind and with losses through separation and death. The average child born today is expected to move nearly 13 times by age 18. All children and parents experience stressful life events as part of growing up. Coping with these stresses can be both painful and edifying.

In this chapter, we focus on some of the more difficult challenges facing families today.

▲ Adopted children
▲ Child care
▲ Parents divorcing and/or remarrying
▲ Common parental feelings and finding help for them

These challenges are not new. In fact, some of them are as old as families themselves. We try to give advice and point the way to the best solutions for today's families.

Adopted Children

Father of Two   *We decided to adopt an infant after medical problems interfered with our having a second biological child. When our social worker from the state adoption agency cautioned we might react differently to this second child, something she called "differential bonding," I was a bit surprised, because I regarded myself as a competent and caring father who wanted and would love this new child equally. However, several weeks after we brought Michael home, my wife pointed out that our three-and-one-half-year-old was being more affectionate than I was with the baby. The attachment process really was different. I'm glad Theresa confronted me with what was going on, because it seemed to speed up the process, but I'm really grateful to the social worker who anticipated and informed us about this potential problem.*

Mother of Two   *Kristy first learned she was adopted when she was three and one-half. Even though her older sister was also adopted and we thought we had given her just the right amount of information, she became very angry with us. Maybe it was because so many of the other mothers at nursery school were pregnant. Then one of the other children came to school with his newly adopted baby brother. Suddenly, Kristy's attitude changed completely. I think this really helped her understand that this was another way babies come into families.*

Mother of One   *When I first brought Daniel home, I was very anxious that all evidence of his true biological mother be hidden. I even got into a battle with the hospital about the name on his medical record. My attitude has really changed in the last eight years, and now I tell him as much as he wants to know about his parents.*

Father of One   *Now that the baby is here, how do I finally feel about his being a different race? I don't know how I feel. I'm too exhausted from changing diapers.*

Father of Four   *My biologic son is white, my black (adopted) son is white, my other black son is black, and my Asian daughter is also black. She was even elected vice president of the African American group at college.*

Five-Year-Old Adopted Girl   *My mom stole me from my real mom. She said she was just going to borrow me for a short time in the hospital but never brought me back. She lied.*

Six-Year-Old Adopted Boy, Responding to Five-Year-Old Sister's Comment That She Is Taller and Stronger   *Yeah, well I'm older, I'm faster, and I have two moms instead of one.*

By and large, adopted children confront the same medical and social problems as other children. But there are certainly many unique issues about raising adopted children. For instance, they may look remarkably different and be temperamentally different from their parents—even more so than biological children. There are a number of excellent books, newsletters, and support groups that can help people come to terms with the unique psychological features confronting adoptive families. Some of the central issues include telling children they are adopted and helping them understand and sort out their feelings about being adopted.

We are going through a period of increasing enlightenment about adoption. In the past, many well-intentioned adoptive parents concealed information from their adopted children. This resulted in confusion, frustration, and anger. Lies and secrecy have never been a sound model for child rearing. Fortunately, new societal attitudes about adoption are resulting in less pressure on parents to protect their adopted children with secrets.

Open Adoption

In part as a result of the fertility issues confronted by baby boomers who delay childbearing, there has been a growing focus on adoption issues. While surrogate parenting has been receiving extraordinary media coverage, a quiet revolution has been going on. **Private adoption** has been rapidly increasing, accounting for up to half the adoptions in some areas. Private adoptions are open. In other words, biological and adoptive parents are aware of each other, know names, and often meet. In **closed adoptions**, agencies are aware of all parties but usually maintain their confidentiality.

Private adoptions have grown in popularity for several reasons. The wait is considerably shorter for potential adoptive parents. Many mothers who will be relinquishing their infants have a desire to meet or even know who will be caring for their children.

Private adoption is not baby buying. State laws strictly forbid providing monetary compensation to the mother except to cover medical and living expenses incurred during the pregnancy. State agencies also must interview and approve prospective adoptive parents.

A lawyer may be helpful in adopting a child, but having a lawyer is not necessary and can be very expensive. Many parents successfully adopt infants on their own through churches, doctors, friends, and even newspaper ads. **International adoption** is increasing. Children adopted from other countries should be re-immunized, be screened for infectious disease, and have a behavioral assessment (see www.aap. org/sections/adoption).

The new openness about adoption is helping to foster the realization that adopted children will always have two sets of parents: their legal parents (the psychological, or adoptive, family) and their biological parents. Biological parents are part of a child's ancestry, and most of us are curious about our ancestors.

What to Tell Your Child

Although there are no foolproof ways to deal with these issues, we do offer the following practical approaches for telling children about where they actually came from.

▲ Tell the truth.
▲ Don't tell too much.
▲ Tell children things they are capable of understanding.

All children have a natural curiosity about where babies come from and in particular about themselves. However, no three-year-old really wants to hear about sperms, eggs, fertilization, implantation, gestation, labor, delivery, and so forth. Similarly, adopted three-year-olds need not be subjected to the entire saga of the adoption process. Three-year-olds comprehend on a very concrete level. They are looking for simple answers such as "babies come from women's bellies" or "babies come from hospitals."

Children under six cannot integrate or understand any notion such as having two mothers (or fathers). These terms should not even be applied to the biological parents of a young child. If pressed by a young child with a direct question such as "Was I inside your belly?" you can follow the first rule (tell the truth) by explaining, "You came from a woman's belly, and then Daddy and I took you home from the hospital. I'm really glad I brought you home, and I'm your mommy. Would you like to see pictures or clothing from then?" Your preschooler now knows a number of things and still retains a firm sense of who Mom and Dad are.

At around five or six, children can distinguish that they came from "a woman's belly" and they have a mother, whereas most of their friends came from "their mother's belly." This is an age when you can focus on the fact that children can come into families in many different ways. You can use the word *adopted*, but don't make an issue of it. Adjectives such as *special, chosen,* or *unique* and terms such as *our special gift* aren't really necessary. Too many adjectives make children sense differences. Also, biological children at home may resent not having those adjectives applied to them. All children are special.

At this age, children seldom want to know *why* this process occurred. By age eight, however, they certainly want to know the reasons, as they begin making moral judgments at this age. Ultimately, the question of why the other woman gave away her child will arise. At this time, facts, feelings, and the future are important. You can provide some basic information, for example: "She was too young, and it would have been very difficult to be your mother. She wanted you to have a very good mom and dad. With the help of some other people, we all decided that we would be your mom and dad." Supply as much additional information as requested. Also take this time to let your child know that it must have been a difficult but caring act. This is also an important point at which to emphasize that you are Mom and Dad for keeps and are not planning to turn the child over to anyone else.

When children feel frustrated or angry about having to do something they don't want to do, such as cleaning up their rooms, they are apt to say, "You don't love me! I'm leaving here to become someone else's little boy." This might typically be followed by, "I'm going to live with Grandma." For many adopted children, the phrase might become, "I'm going to live with my real parents." It is natural to think of what might have been, but few adopted children persist in these fantasies.

Adolescence is fraught with many issues of establishing a sense of identity. It is inevitable for adoption to play a role in this process. Again, tell as much as you know. Information and pictures are helpful in establishing this additional sense of background. The family should make individual decisions about any meetings between adolescents and their biological parents.

Child Care

The concept of day care is not new. It dates back to 1854, when New York City provided day nursery facilities for unwed mothers required to work as wet nurses. By the end of the 19th century, Maria Montessori began teaching three-, four-, and five-year-olds in such day care centers, beginning a movement in preschool education that is still popular today.

As the times changed, so did the appeal of and interest in day care. The economic and defense necessities of World War II sparked a rebirth of day care, because many young women took the desk and factory positions formerly occupied by men who went off to war. Today women are working due to financial need and by choice. The result is that nearly two-thirds of American households have children under age six regularly cared for by someone other than the core family of parents and siblings. More than 25% of children younger than school age are enrolled in a formally licensed day care center. Although it is common to refer to planned, half-day programs for three- to five-year-olds as "nursery school," and programs for younger children lasting part or all of the day as "day care" (or "infant day care"), we in this book use the term *day care* to discuss all these programs.

Your Child's Needs

Adequate facilities can be found for children of all ages. Infants and toddlers require more attention than older children, and day care facilities for them should have at least one staff person for every four children.

By age three, most children have moved beyond the period of independent or parallel play and are ready to begin playing with other children. Besides enjoying the company of others, three- and four-year-olds usually have a fair language ability as well as some control of their bowels and bladders. This is a good age to start children in day care centers with fewer staff members.

Before deciding on a particular day care center, parents should assess the needs of their child.

▲ Is the child able to communicate his or her needs to others?
▲ Is the child toilet trained?
▲ Does the child have any feeding difficulties?
▲ What are the child's sleeping patterns?

Benefits and Risks

The major concern when contemplating day care is how the experience will affect your child. Within this concern are two separate questions: Will day care adversely affect my child's health? What impact will it have on my child's development, including intellectual, social, and emotional maturation?

There is no doubt that children in day care have greater exposure to a multitude of germs. The more children your child is exposed to, the more likely he or she is to acquire an illness. It is important to pay attention to the proper control of infections by the different facilities you're considering.

Children in day care centers learn at a rapid rate. They also learn to cope with separation from their parents by spending part of the day away from home. To help ease the shock of this separation, parents should introduce their children to the day care center gradually. Spending a few hours a day at the center yourself and gradually decreasing this time often helps. A second child usually has much less trouble if an older brother or sister is already there. Many parents regularly help out and teach at day care centers. This lessens the burden of separation. Children who learn to accept this separation from their parents will generally make a smooth transition to the full-day separation that first grade demands.

A number of studies now indicate that, in general, the separation experience does not interfere with children's attachment to their parents. In the realm of intellectual development, day care seems to enhance the learning of socioeconomically disadvantaged children. Children in day care tend to do better in math and reading early in school and also to become socialized at an earlier age than their peers who stay at home. The nature of socialization has been found to differ across different cultures and, by implication, in different day care centers.

No matter what day care program they attend, all children return home. Thus the most important factor in their development is likely to be you and your efforts to discuss with your child what happened during the day, reinforcing the experiences that are consonant with your values and explaining any objections to experiences that are not.

Choosing a Program

The best program for your child is the one that meets his or her needs. In reviewing day care centers, you should address the following considerations: type, cost, environment, staff experience, and health policies.

Type and Cost

The basic arrangements include care in your own home by a relative, a live-in employee, or a baby-sitter; care in another's home, also known as family home care; or care in a group care center. Facilities range from a neighbor's home to an elaborate institution. Licensing requirements vary from state to state. Always ask whether a facility is licensed and how background checks are performed on staff.

The cost of child care varies considerably. For example, live-in help, depending on accommodations, hours worked, age, experience, and the going rate in your area, can often cost more than $1,500 per month, plus room and board. A home baby-sitter for a single child might be an expensive option, but the cost for two children may not be that much more than for one.

Environment

Location is obviously important. Today's family often includes four or more individuals all needing to arrive at different places between 8:00 and 8:30 A.M. Is a nursery school really worth the added trouble of driving across town?

Consider the facilities and services that the day care center provides.

- ▲ Do the facilities look safe and well cared for?
- ▲ Do the facilities offer children ample opportunities for physical activities and exploration? Are there places where they can play independently?
- ▲ Are climbing apparatuses at a reasonable height and surrounded by sand?
- ▲ Are the equipment and toys appropriate for two-year-olds as well as four-year-olds?
- ▲ Does the center allow for an afternoon nap, which most preschoolers need?
- ▲ Are meals and snacks suitable, nutritious, and reasonably familiar to your child?

Staff Experience

Most important in day care is the staff—their experience, training (Does anyone have a degree in child development? Do staff members have training in CPR? Are they experienced managing problems such as biting or conflicts?), philosophy, diversity, compatibility, and, of course, number. The supervisory staff should be accustomed to children of your child's age. Your child should experience a balance between play with other children and interaction with adults. Most important, staff members should be willing to sit down with you and discuss the individual needs of your child.

Determine whether the staff's attitudes are consonant with yours. Are activities carefully structured for groups or designed to accommodate individual preferences and development? For instance, can your child keep a favorite blanket or other plaything? Ask the staff how they would handle your child if he or she misbehaved. Discussing discipline problems in advance can avoid conflict later on. Some parents find out much too late that staff members' attitudes about child rearing are completely different from their own.

The most useful way to evaluate a day care center is to observe children's behavior there. That will give you a good idea of how it is run. Observe as many activities as possible: group activities, individual instruction, group quiet time, and mealtime (for social interaction, decorum, and nutritional value). Ask about the curriculum and the center's ability to meet the needs of individual students. Finally, talk about the role of parents as participants in the child's care. After choosing a day care program, plan on frequent conversations with the teachers to ensure that your child's needs are being met.

Health Policies

Determine what health policies are in effect at the center, as well as its procedures for handling emergencies. Find out about toilet training procedures. Make sure there are adequate hand-washing facilities for children. In general, children in diapers should have changing areas away from older children.

Facilities should keep the phone number of each child's doctor on file and require a screening exam and up-to-date immunizations. Ask about outbreaks of infections in the previous year. Many infections, such as group A strep, are quite common. Make sure that the center has a system to notify you during such an outbreak. Day care centers should be notified, and in turn notify you, about local outbreaks of the following:

▲ Campylobacter gastroenteritis
▲ Chicken pox
▲ Fifth disease
▲ Giardia infections
▲ Lice
▲ Hemophilus influenzae type B infection

▲ Hepatitis
▲ Measles and German measles (rubella)
▲ Meningococcus
▲ Mumps
▲ Pertussis
▲ Salmonella
▲ Scabies
▲ Shigella
▲ Group A strep infection
▲ Tuberculosis

For more information on this topic, see the "Additional Reading" section at the end of the chapter and www.childcareaware.org.

Divorce and Remarriage

Father in a New Family   *At the end of the argument, Annie really blew up and told me I had to get out of her house. For a few seconds, I felt I had to leave but then realized that this new house was my house, too, and that I had just paid for it. Somehow, with all her kids and her furniture, I sort of believed I was living in her home and not ours.*

Divorced Mother   *It was really hard on [my son] George when he heard his father was going to have a baby with his new wife. At first I thought that George was sad because he was going to have to give up the position he had held for so many years as the baby in the family. But then I realized that he was in utter terror that this child was literally going to take his father away from him.*

10-Year-Old Child   *I like changing from house to house because it's nice being in different backgrounds every now and then.*

11-Year-Old Child   *There are times when going to different houses can be trouble, because at one house you can have most of your things but not the other. Spending a single night at one parent's house is hard, because there really is no reason for it. You go there and only eat dinner, do homework, and go to sleep. When morning comes, you must get up, eat fast, and go to where you are going. But I like spending single nights.*

11-Year-Old Child   *Having two different fathers is not a great deal of stress or nothing to feel sad about unless you like one family more but see [them] less often. But I think of it as just having two normal fathers. Besides, I should be glad that I have two.*

Divorced Father   The kids seem to be doing fine. We talk about things periodically, but the urge to talk is more mine than theirs. They listen tolerantly to my suggestions of their feeling anger and confusion toward me. The other night, [my son] Tom responded to an overture with, "Is this going to be one of those serious talks?" So I'll try to lighten up a bit.

In general, divorce represents a loss to children. The most obvious loss is the amount of time the child will spend with one or both parents, but there is often an accompanying loss in financial status. A mother working part-time may now need to return to work full-time, and new child care arrangements may need to be made.

In addition, it is common for children to believe that they are responsible for the divorce. Younger children often regress and display more infantile behavior, including bed-wetting and night waking, and they may resume or begin tantrums. Older children often have difficulties in school and may withdraw from friends, complain frequently of pain, show signs of depression, or engage in new risk-taking or anti-social behavior.

There is no way to shield your child from the pain and loss that divorce brings. You can help your child cope by answering all his or her questions and anticipating ones the child may be afraid to ask. If true, you should let your child know the following things.

▲ That he or she did not cause the divorce
▲ That each parent will continue to love him or her
▲ How he or she will be able to interact with each parent
▲ Where he or she will live and when
▲ Where he or she will go to school
▲ What will not change (friends, pets, and so on)
▲ What will change, in addition to the loss of the parents functioning as a couple
▲ That he or she should not attempt to patch things up between the parents and that those efforts have been attempted unsuccessfully

Almost all parents have some help in getting through a divorce, usually from friends and sometimes from professionals. Often children's peers are not as capable of lending them support. You are the primary help for your child, but this is one time you shouldn't hesitate to use other resources, such as books or, most important, professional counseling. Your doctor is the best place to start. He or she may refer you to a colleague with greater skills in this area.

As the above quotes indicate, forming new families can be trying. The vast majority of parents who divorce will remarry. Stepparents have had bad press since the days of Cinderella, and adjusting to a new stepparent is far more difficult for adolescents than for younger children. The typical divorce occurs less than seven years after marriage, making younger children most liable to experience the breakup and reconstitution of a family.

When a divorced parent's courtship ends in marriage, a major transition in roles occurs. It is important at this stage to decide clearly on the roles and authority of the stepfather or stepmother versus the biological father or mother. Although a new stepparent often evokes jealousy, children also may perceive that they now have more security or will receive more attention. Because of the tendency of men to marry younger women, a stepmom closer in age to her new husband's children may face authority problems.

Successful transitions do not occur overnight. Give the new family time, but if the stress does not decline, don't hesitate to seek help. Occasionally, the entire family (including the former spouse) may need to gather to negotiate a working system.

Parents' Feelings

There's a saying that goes, "If you're alive, you've got troubles." Having children proves the point. Along with an enormous amount of pleasure comes trouble. This section focuses on helping parents anticipate and recognize trouble and know when to seek professional help.

We can think of parental development in much the same way we do child development. Each milestone achieved by a child implies a response on the part of the parents, which is also developmental. Sometimes the child sets the pace for these transitions. If the child is learning to move around, the parents will respond by "baby-proofing" their home. In other situations, the parents may encourage a child's development, as in shifting him or her from a crib to a bed. Just as there are wide variations in normal child development, there is equally wide variability in the normal response of parents. The parents' job is to be responsive to and supportive of the child's development, while simultaneously monitoring their own development as parents and marital partners.

The Arrival

You are two mature, caring adults, anticipating the arrival of a baby. Your conversation is making a slow shift from politics and daily activities to the advantages of disposable diapers versus a diaper service. You have considered how to reorganize your house to accommodate a child and may have spent vast amounts of money or time on decorating a nursery. You are contemplating when to allow grandparents and friends to come to help out. The big day arrives. Now you two are three. You come home from the hospital, and your fantasies of the first few weeks—being treated like a king and queen, eating healthy meals, napping when baby naps, and having a clean house—are shattered by reality. There's always a crowd of relatives ooing and gooing, and it seems as if you see your baby only in the middle of the night or when he or she is crying. You have had to feed a cast of thousands, and your house is messy and chaotic.

If you are feeling out of control, don't be surprised. The reality of parenthood is almost never what you expect it to be. However, there are some things you can do to help yourself make the difficult transition into parenthood.

▲ Set firm ground rules for visiting friends, relatives, and colleagues; this includes limiting stays and suggesting nearby accommodations.
▲ Don't expect to be able to maintain your household at the same standards you did before the baby.
▲ In the first few weeks, try to use whatever opportunities you have to catch up on your sleep—when the baby is napping or when friends and family can help out with meals or baby-sitting.
▲ Remember that you are still adults who have adult interests and needs. As soon as it is feasible, leave the baby with a friend or relative—even for an hour—and go out together for a walk or drive.

Once the excitement of the first few weeks passes, you will need to make new adjustments. This can be an especially difficult time for a new mother, especially if the father spends most of his time away at work. Confusion, crying, and a sense of isolation are normal. You may be distressed that none of your pre-pregnancy clothes fit or that most of your friends without children are busy with work or other activities. You may find it hard to locate a baby-sitter with whom you feel comfortable or to figure out how to leave your baby—especially if you are nursing—in the care of someone else.

Look for opportunities to lessen your sense of exhaustion and frustration. Try to evaluate your priorities. Although housecleaning, writing thank-you notes, and cooking may seem like obligations you want to fulfill, a nap, an exercise class, a play group with other mothers, or just some free time to take a walk by yourself may be more beneficial. Scheduling time for yourself will enable you to face the demands of baby care with more energy. Although you may want to continue with your life exactly as it was before the baby arrived, try to feel comfortable with making positive changes in your schedule that acknowledge the presence of a new person in the household.

Fathers

For a father, the delight in parenthood may be tempered by feelings of exclusion and jealousy. If you are not the primary caregiver, it is normal to feel that getting to know your baby is taking you longer than it is your wife. Because your wife may be preoccupied with nursing, diapering, and other tasks, you may experience a period of adjustment to her new role as well. Try to work out methods that will make sharing child care satisfying for both of you. Volunteering to help with household chores, as well as offering to spend time alone with the baby, will establish new ties of intimacy within the family. A special task for the father is to support and encourage the marital relationship. A new baby can sap the energy of both parents; a father can be enormously helpful in reminding a mother that she is also still a woman and wife.

Talking about feelings and searching for new solutions together is the first development test for parents. By the time your baby is four months old, you should both have the sense that things are settling down. Ideally, parents should be able to enjoy each other's company alone for an evening without their child.

If feelings of being overwhelmed persist, talk to your pediatrician. For the first few months of your baby's life, you will see this doctor frequently. Part of his or her job is to help you integrate your new baby into your lives. Because pediatricians have observed many parents and have dealt with the common problems this transition creates, they can offer suggestions for how to overcome the hurdles of the first few months. Other resources include support groups, play groups, and many fine books and articles.

Separation

From the first time you leave your child with a sitter to the first time your adolescent goes out alone at night, separation between parent and child is always difficult. It can frequently be traumatic, but generally separation is harder on the parent than on the child and a necessary growth experience.

Some early issues of separation are weaning, leaving your child with a sitter, and letting a child cry himself or herself to sleep. The guideline for all of these experiences is to be patient, loving, and consistent. Try to sort out whether the problems surrounding the issue are yours or your child's. Is your 15-month-old's reluctance to give up nursing for comfort a reflection of your own ambivalence to forgo this intimate and special relationship? If you must call or check up on your child when you go out, are you really fearful about your baby-sitter's competency, or are you worried that your child's independence is a form of rejection?

Bedtime

If bedtime is a major battle scene or your child ends up sleeping in your bed more often than not, you are not providing your child with the opportunity to learn how to comfort himself or herself. Often a stuffed animal or favorite blanket can be an effective object to facilitate a transition from dependence on parents to self-sufficiency. Sometimes it is helpful to buy more than one "lovey" and rotate them. If one is lost or worn-out, you will have a well-used replacement. If, by six or seven months, your child cannot sleep alone in his or her crib—with or without a favorite object or night-light—or if separation situations continue to cause tears and struggles, you may need some professional guidance.

Frustration

All parents become frustrated and angry with their children. These are natural human feelings. Although we all accept anger as a normal part of everyday living, many ways of dealing with anger are unacceptable.

There are many indications that children are often the ones who suffer most, often physically, when family relationships are strained and anger flares. Abuse of children is becoming an increasing societal problem.

We learn how to handle our emotions from our parents. Our temperament clearly has its foundation in the temperament of our parents. It is highly likely that if you remember your parents being impatient with you or having difficulty controlling their tempers, some of this may have worn off on you. For instance, you may have seen a three-year-old throw a puzzle to the floor and shout, "Oh, damn!" That child is probably reacting as his or her parents react to a frustrating situation.

At the end of a long and hectic day, we all deserve to sit down to a peaceful dinner. But more often than not, dinner with a one-year-old child is punctuated by shouts, tossed spoons, and thrown food. On the wrong day at the wrong time, this can be unnerving. It's easy to become exasperated and angry. However, it is important to remember that your one-year-old is behaving exactly as a one-year-old should. If it were a ten-year-old throwing food and utensils, punishment, such as being sent from the table, might be in order. But it is inappropriate to punish a one-year-old who is exhibiting appropriate behavior. What would you do in this situation? Would you start shaking your child violently? If you felt you were going to explode, to whom could you turn, to whom could you talk to prevent an explosion?

Asking for Help

You can deal with any problem of extreme anger and potential abuse most easily once you accept that it is a problem of being human and therefore nothing to be ashamed of. However, it is difficult for most of us to admit that we may need help. Often the first person to turn to is your mate. Neighbors can sometimes help. Although it is often difficult for us to discuss extremely personal problems, a true friendship should give you license to talk openly with a friend about your or the friend's temper problem.

Your doctor is another possible contact. You also may call a parental stress hotline. The fact that so many communities have hotlines reflects a recognition that we all become angry and it is important to keep this anger from harming our children.

The solution to a complex problem is seldom simple. Although most communities have services to help parents and children involved in severe abuse, services geared to *preventing* abuse are in the earliest developmental stages. Most parenting classes focus on preparing expectant couples and individuals, but some deal specifically with the problems of being a parent.

Very often we do not know what to expect when we become parents. Parenting involves more than just adding a family member. It involves readjusting relationships between family members. Some parents find it easier than others to readjust, but no one finds it easy. The time that parents once had to unwind at the end of the day or to talk out problems between themselves may no longer exist once a child is added to the family. And yet this time is important.

We should all be working to make resources available to our neighbors in need of help. If you feel that programs in your community are inadequate, contact your doctor, county department of social services, or members of the local American Academy of Pediatrics chapter (www.aap.org) to inquire about developing such programs.

Psychological Resources

The challenges we have discussed in this chapter—adoption; adjustment to separation, divorce, and remarriage; and parents' potentially overwhelming emotions—can be disruptive enough for your family as a whole or individual members to benefit from counseling. Indeed, psychological and behavioral difficulties can arise in any family, no matter how "traditional" it appears.

One valuable resource is your pediatrician. Many family doctors are now trained to respond to mental health problems, and some take one or two years of additional training in this area. They also see many families and therefore have experience with problems that may seem unusual to you. Most important, your pediatrician can recommend professionals in other fields.

The following three groups of people are licensed to provide mental health services.

1. Social workers are the largest group. A master's degree in social work (M.S.W.) indicates at least two years of postgraduate training. Some states have licensing exams for specialized certifications. Hospital staffs often include social workers. In most communities, a family service agency provides services on a sliding scale of fees. Health insurance companies may not cover social work services.

2. Clinical psychologists have Ph.D.'s. They are often trained to do psychological or educational testing as well as counseling. These tests can provide insights into a person's intelligence, personality, and psychopathology relative to average children or adults. Most insurance companies will pay part of a psychologist's fees; always ask beforehand. Often school systems will pay for educational testing that they recommend.

3. Psychiatrists are M.D.'s who have been specially trained in neurology and psychiatry. A small number—only about 3,000 in the United States—have done the additional two years of training to become board-certified child psychiatrists. For problems that combine psychological and neurological factors (for example, depression and chronic problems in conduct or attention), your child may well benefit from a child psychiatrist's care.

People from all three disciplines can perform psychotherapy (treatment of mental or emotional problems). Indeed, in many states anyone can call himself or herself a psychotherapist. However, among these groups, only psychiatrists can prescribe medications.

A mental health evaluation will probably begin with interviews about you, your relationship with your spouse, and stresses in your marriage. You may be asked about your own upbringing. Questions about sensitive personal areas may feel intrusive. Remember, the more honest and open you are, the more easily the mental health worker can understand your family and share his or her knowledge.

A psychological evaluation of a child is somewhat different from that of an adult. Children often can't express their feelings verbally, so therapists have invented other ways to evaluate their psychological development, even in infancy. In "play therapy," the professional invites the child to play, allowing him or her to communicate many feelings and ideas through this activity. Don't be surprised if your mental health professional has a toy box, puppets, or a sand tray in his or her office.

It is helpful to prepare your child for a visit to a therapist. Children benefit from knowing that Mom and Dad are seeking help as well. Tell your child that you are taking him or her to meet someone who understands and helps children. You may wish to acknowledge being concerned about how the child is feeling: "You've been looking worried to me." Ultimately, it is up to the mental health professional to establish a good relationship with your child. If, after a few sessions, your child is uncomfortable going to visit the therapist, you may wish to ask for a referral to another.

It is harder to measure progress in psychotherapy than in medicine. Some situations can be resolved in a few months, but others may take a year or more. Remember that although therapy requires work and sometimes is stressful, the ultimate goal is to make you and your child feel and function better.

Additional Reading

Surviving the Breakup: How Children and Parents Cope with Divorce, Judith S. Wallerstein and Joan B. Kelly (New York: Basic Books, 1996).

What About the Kids?: Raising Your Children Before, During, and After Divorce, Judith S. Wallerstein and Sandra Blakeslee (New York: Hyperion, 2004).

Chapter Seven

School Days

School is a critical factor in the growth and development of your child. Not only does it teach a child the necessary academic skills for functioning in the adult world, but it also teaches social skills. To help your child get the most out of this experience, you need to understand and complement what your child is doing in school. In this chapter, we briefly discuss some of the common concerns that parents have about the academic and social aspects of school.

School Readiness

Children mature at different rates, so there is no particular age at which it is best for all children to begin school. Some children are ready at age four; others may not be ready until seven or later. Having a child begin school too early may lead to frustration and early failure, hampering the child's future school experiences.

The best learning is an active process, a one-on-one exchange. Parents are in the best position to provide this interaction, although good teachers make sure that every student has some such experiences in the classroom. When an adult is reading to a child and the child asks questions, that is an extraordinary learning experience. The feelings the child acquires when interacting aid his or her emotional and mental development. That experience can't be matched by television, not even by excellent educational programs. Those programs are a supplement to, and not a substitute for, other types of learning. They are a passive technique and not an active exchange.

Many things are important for success in school. For example, a child should be in good general health. (Children with serious diseases will be under medical supervision long before school begins.) Making sure that your child can see and hear adequately is an important prerequisite for his or her starting school. In addition, most states require that children have up-to-date immunizations (see page 173).

Social skills help children do well in school. Sitting in one place all day is not easy, nor is meeting strangers. Children starting school should be able to play well with other children, separate easily from their parents, get dressed alone (except for tying their shoes), have daytime bowel and bladder control, and enjoy games.

Language ability is, of course, very important in school. Children with severe speech defects will require extra help.

Interest in learning is an advantage. It helps if the child likes books, is curious, knows colors, can repeat a few numbers, can hold a crayon, and can draw a square. Many children will demonstrate the ability to grasp complex concepts before they enter school. They may know about the difference between summer and winter and understand concepts such as "over" and "under." They may even be able to tell you the color of grass and the sky without looking at them directly. Children also must be able to follow a series of commands such as "Go to the closet, select a puzzle, and return with it to your seat."

If your child is able to do many of the above tasks, there should be no problem in his or her beginning school. However, if you are concerned that your child may not be able to profit from school for any reason, you should consider a conference with school or medical professionals before enrolling your child.

School Problems

School offers children more than book learning. This is a time for children to begin to experience a world that is different from their home. In school, they have the opportunity to become social beings. Relationships with peers allow children to feel both uniqueness and commonality with other children. They may learn that certain things are required, while others are voluntary.

School offers children a variety of experiences that encourage a sense of self-esteem. They may excel in sports or academics. They may discover a preference for some experiences over others. Because a child's repertoire of skills grows dramatically in school, it is a particularly important area for parents to monitor.

Then comes the first parent-teacher conference. Nothing strikes more terror in the heart of well-intentioned parents than the thought of someone else judging their child. What if all those adorable characteristics, such as climbing on furniture at home, are enough to make the child persona non grata at school? Never fear. There's hardly a more understanding and supportive group than schoolteachers. Regardless of what your child does, they've seen worse. If your child's teacher has concerns, however, it's important for you to consider them seriously. Schoolteachers are good observers of children; often they see things that parents can't or don't want to see.

The identity your child forms in school is an important part of the development of his or her personality and style. Problems in school can be trivial or can indicate potentially greater troubles down the line.

Get to know your child's school, teachers, and classmates. Take the school's concerns seriously. An adversarial stance is not in your child's best interest. If your child acts substantially different at school than at home, find out why. An isolated child with no friends is not a happy child.

How can a parent tell if a child is having problems in school? Obviously, listening to what the school personnel tell you is important. It is equally important to listen to your child. The reams of drawings, tests, and other tidbits he or she brings home are invaluable. Spending a few minutes each day asking your child about school is as vital to your child as your own work is to you. All children voice some complaints: "School is boring" or "Ricky has a club, and he won't let me join!" Talking about these short-term troubles with your child helps him or her work out solutions, and it helps you recognize when a bigger problem emerges. If your child appears excessively anxious about an exam, fearful of relationships with his or her peers, or persistently reluctant to go to school, make an attempt to understand why.

Children with difficulties in school may complain of vague physical symptoms on school days or have difficulty falling asleep at night. It is often very hard for a parent to discern whether a child is really ill or has something else on his or her mind. A good rule is to keep a child home if he or she has a measured temperature (see Fever, page 288). If the child stays home, he or she must stay in bed all day, not play as if it were a weekend. If complaints about a stomachache or headache persist, first check your own behavior: Do *you* tend to experience pain when you are upset? If Mommy or Daddy often has a headache, a child learns that this is a way either to get more attention or to avoid unpleasant tasks.

When problems persist, they may be symptomatic of stress that your child is experiencing. Talk to your child and his or her teachers. If that doesn't resolve the problem, speak to your pediatrician. It may be helpful to have an outside observer evaluate the child.

Learning Challenges

Each child learns at his or her own rate. Many problems can impede a child's learning. Some are so complex that it is impossible to deal with them here. **Dyslexia** is a term that means inability to read, but it is not a single diagnosis. There are literally hundreds of reasons why children may be unable to read. There are just as many reasons why learning in other areas may be impaired. Following is a list of a few factors that may interfere with your child's learning. If you suspect any of the following, consult a professional.

▲ **Vision problems.** Vision testing in children over four years of age is simple. Strabismus, or "lazy eye," can be detected in children as young as two.

▲ **Hearing problems.** Children must not only be able to hear, but they must also be able to identify fine differences in sounds such as *p* and *b*. Suspect hearing and complex language disabilities if the child produces excessive nonsense verbalization after 18 months, is not talking at all by age 2, began talking and then stopped, is not using sentences at all by age 3, or makes no verbal communication of his or her wants.

▲ **Coordination problems.** Much of first grade is devoted to writing and drawing. Children who develop coordination skills slightly later are at somewhat of a disadvantage. This, however, may be merely a maturational lag and is not necessarily something to be concerned about.

▲ **Visual motor ability.** The child's ability to see an object and then copy it involves coordination of eyes and hands. Inability to copy designs may be a sign that visual motor ability is lacking.

▲ **Auditory perception.** Hearing sound accurately is not enough. A child hearing the word *boat* must be able to picture a boat in his or her mind and recall what a boat looks like and what a boat does. Furthermore, the child must be able to describe the images that have been evoked.

▲ **Attention problem.** Some children have difficulty concentrating on the task at hand. They may become easily distracted. Other children may dwell on a task for an unusually long time.

▲ **Maturational lag.** Children mature differently. Not all six-year-olds are capable of learning in the same way. Some will be several months behind others in their learning. This delay does not mean that these children will always be behind. It is similar to the case of the child who does not walk until 18 months of age. Nobody can tell this child from one who walked at 9 months when they are both 5 years old.

▲ **English as a second language.** Children from homes where the primary language is not English are at a disadvantage when beginning an English-language school. These children generally catch up very quickly, but ostracism in the first few months (by classmates or teachers) can seriously hamper a child's confidence and development. Bilingual education programs in areas where many students speak Spanish or another language in the home can be helpful. Being bilingual is extremely advantageous for these children, and the programs are also excellent opportunities for English-speaking students.

▲ **Frequent moves.** Children who change schools may encounter problems. Some of this may be due to differences in curriculum, but much of it is due to the child's need to adjust after losing friends and familiar surroundings.

▲ **Seizures.** Petit mal seizures generally cause short periods in which a child does not respond to the environment. The seizures may last for only two to three seconds, but children may have up to several hundred seizures per hour. During these periods, the child cannot learn. This is a very uncommon cause of learning problems, but one that can be treated effectively, which is why we mention it here.

▲ **Physical differences.** Children with physical defects are often teased by classmates. Although the deformity may not interfere with the child's ability to learn, the feeling of being an outsider certainly does. Physical size may also interfere with learning. A tall seven-year-old who looks like a nine-year-old will be expected to act like a nine-year-old. The discrepancy between adult expectations and the child's ability creates a problem.

▲ **Lack of sleep.** Many children now have television sets in their bedrooms (a practice we deplore), which may result in their staying up quite late at night. Other children who are often tired in the morning may be reading after going to bed. Parents should encourage reading, but not when it interferes with other learning.

▲ **Hyperactivity.** Often one parent will think that a child is overly active, and the other will think not. Hyperactivity can be an extremely subjective complaint. It is often first noticed by a teacher when a child's overactivity or inability to focus interferes with learning. It is important to focus on the quality of the child's activity and not just the quantity. If hyperactivity appears at school and not at home, suspect a learning problem. We all are bored by lectures when we do not understand them. Children having difficulty learning become uninterested in the lesson and consequently find something else to do. There may be other reasons for the behavior, however. Some children have difficulty adjusting to the different standards of behavior at school. Extremely curious children who are learning at a rapid rate may appear to be overactive. Children who speak little English in an English-only classroom can be expected to find something to do other than sit in a seat listening to talk they do not understand. Finally, many medications, including the antihistamines in common cold preparations, can cause hyperactivity responses. (See Hyperactivity and ADHD, page 196, for further discussion.)

Attention Deficit Hyperactivity Disorder (ADHD)

For some children, hyperactivity may be part of a condition known as attention deficit hyperactivity disorder (ADHD). There are several types of ADHD: some children don't listen and are particularly **inattentive**; some are **hyperactive** (in constant motion) and often **impulsive**; some exhibit a combination of these characteristics. There has not yet been identified an abnormal gene, enzyme, or brain program that causes this behavioral condition that can be problematic for children and families. Most children with ADHD will grow into fine adults; we have friends and colleagues who feel their ADHD has helped them achieve success.

Controversy and confusion have for years surrounded children with ADHD. There has been considerable recent effort to establish criteria for accurately diagnosing this condition and to improve the care of children considered to have ADHD. It is hoped that more can be learned so that medications (such as Ritalin) will go only to children who may potentially benefit from them.

For a child with possible ADHD a 10-minute office visit ending with a prescription is not the standard of care. American Academy of Pediatrics guidelines suggest what should be done for six- to twelve-year-olds with school and learning problems; who may have difficult relationships with other children, teachers, and family; and who exhibit other behaviors such as hyperactivity or impulse control (acting without thinking).

▲ Symptoms should be evaluated if they last more than six months and began before the child was seven years old.

▲ Symptoms generally occur in more than one setting (school, home, play situations) and make it difficult for the child to function in these settings.

▲ In addition to yourself, either your child's teacher or physician should observe symptoms.

▲ Your doctor should be interested in performing an assessment of how your child functions at home and how the behaviors may be limiting.

▲ A school assessment should include reports from teachers on established checklists or reports on classroom behaviors and strategies used to help your child. Several are helpful to identify children with ADHD.

▲ Criteria for diagnosing and treating ADHD have been established. See www.aap.org/publiced/BR_ADHD.htm. These criteria should be considered by your doctor before starting any interventions or medications.

▲ Since other conditions are often found to accompany ADHD (learning disability, depression), your doctor should be alert to the possibility of their presence and willing to investigate further.

While recent studies have shown that stimulant medications are very effective in helping with some of the troublesome behaviors of ADHD, we consider them necessary (in many cases) but not sufficient. Helping a child with ADHD is far more complicated than treating a strep throat with penicillin. Developing a plan with the classroom teacher is essential, and a consistent and supportive approach at home will also be needed.

Investigating Learning Problems

A child with learning or school problems needs thorough evaluation. These problems are best handled early. Each child is unique, with particular strengths and weaknesses. It is important to identify strengths and the way a child is best able to learn. Understanding a child's learning style can help parents and teachers to develop a strategy for success in school. Federal law now mandates that states provide learning evaluations and appropriate learning plans for every child with a suspected or confirmed problem. We feel that an adequate evaluation should cover the following areas.

▲ **Medical history,** focusing on the mother's pregnancy, labor, and delivery. Early health and early functioning, such as feeding, activity levels, and behavioral problems, will be discussed.
▲ Assessment of the child's **early development.** This will include questions about the child's coordination, language development, and social development.
▲ **School history,** including questions about day care, preschool, kindergarten, and school failures and successes. If a doctor is performing the evaluation, he or she may request a copy of the teachers' reports, as well as any achievement or psychological testing performed at school. The doctor needs cooperation from the school. He or she may spend considerable time discussing the child's behavior and how certain types of behavior are rewarded or punished.
▲ Extensive **physical, neurological, and developmental examination.** The doctor will check for the impediments listed in the previous section. Depending on the results of the history and physical examination, he or she may suggest additional tests of learning ability, including psychological testing.

Pioneering work by Dr. Mel Levine has resulted in new approaches to neurodevelopmental evaluation. Because children process information and learn in different ways, he asserts that it is a mistake to treat everyone the same when it comes to learning. He has developed programs to help students, teachers, and schools (www.allkindsofminds. org).

Treatment of a school or learning problem requires the cooperation of the doctor, both parents, learning specialists, and the school.

Intelligence Testing

Intelligence testing is about a century old. The techniques were designed to predict school failures, but instruments of prediction, whether crystal balls or written tests, are never completely accurate.

Group testing, the type most often done in schools, is much less accurate than individual testing. Group tests depend greatly on the child's ability to read. A bright child who may be lagging in reading ability will perform poorly on these tests and will be falsely labeled as having a low overall intelligence. An individual tester working with only one child can better determine whether the child's poor performance might be due to a cold, sleepiness, or the child's not applying himself or herself. Individually administered tests usually measure a child's verbal and performance abilities.

Verbal skills tested include vocabulary, general information, understanding, and arithmetic. Performance tests evaluate picture completions, block designs, and mechanical skills. Separate verbal and performance scores, along with a total score, are obtained.

IQ

IQ stands for intelligence quotient. In most IQ tests, a number, such as 105, is the result. This number is derived by dividing the child's mental equivalent age (based on the test) by the child's actual age, then multiplying by 100. If a 5-year-old scored as well as the average 6-year-old, you would divide 6 by 5 (1.2) and multiply by 100 (120) to get the IQ score. A 5-year-old scoring as well as the average 5-year-old would have a score of 100: (5 ÷ 5) x 100 = 1 x 100 = 100.

Tests of younger children are far less predictive than tests of older children. Tests are inappropriate if they do not match the child's experiences. An African American child living in the city has different experiences from the child of a Mexican American migrant farm worker, who in turn has different experiences from a white child living in the suburbs.

Parents should be aware of the frailties of intelligence tests. Your child's IQ will not grant or deny him or her access to schools, jobs, and success throughout life. Although some people would like to use a person's IQ for this purpose, the most responsible use of IQ tests is to help design an educational program suitable for your child. Children who do poorly on group IQ testing often do not do well in the standard group teaching of our school systems either. They may be fully capable of learning but require a different teaching approach. A child who does poorly on a group IQ test should have an individually administered intelligence test. Many low IQs disappear quickly when this is done.

Avoiding School

Tom Sawyer and Huckleberry Finn led exciting lives by avoiding school. Many people today have fantasized about repeating the adventures of these two folk heroes. Almost everyone at one time or another has considered staying home from school or has actually played hooky for a day or two. These thoughts are especially common after returning from vacation or recovering from an illness. Whereas *thinking* about avoiding school may be considered innocent, actually avoiding school is another matter.

Most children who avoid school state that they like school and that they actually want to go. But a morning headache, a stomachache, nausea, or some other symptom keeps them at home. As a parent, you need to evaluate how serious these complaints really are. Most children have a runny nose much of the time. As we explain in the next chapter, runny noses and colds are really not illnesses in children. A minor cold is not a reason for a child to stay home from school.

Even when a child acknowledges wanting to avoid school, that desire is really a symptom. The cause is rarely a terrible teacher, although children often say it is. Sometimes a teaching program that suits most of the children does not meet the needs of your child. More often, the child may be experiencing a learning problem, a problem with friends, a physical problem such as being too small or too tall, or a problem at home. Often parents feel guilty during periods of stress at home and are quick to keep a child home so that they can demonstrate that they still care about him or her.

School avoidance is a complex problem with multiple roots. It must not be treated lightly. Children who miss more than 5% of their school days because of problems not accompanied by a fever or chronic disease are avoiding school. A program to return a child to school will involve the cooperation of the doctor, the teacher, and both parents.

Childhood Athletics

Children have been running, throwing, climbing, and swimming for thousands of years. Such athletic activities bring tremendous benefits to children, teaching them new skills and how to control them. Exercise also is important for conditioning. Adults who follow a regular exercise program are less likely to succumb to cardiovascular disease. Children and adults who are in good physical condition generally feel good about themselves.

Learning how to play a sport is as useful to a child's development as are other learning experiences. There are beneficial socializing aspects to sports. The competition that children impose on themselves is also potentially beneficial. Some of our fondest memories occurred during pickup games of stickball, basketball, or hide-and-seek. We encourage athletics for all children of all abilities. Unfortunately, many aspects of athletics are sorely in need of improvement.

First, most of the sports glorified in our culture—and, consequently, of great importance to children—are sports in which most adults have little opportunity to participate. These include football, baseball, hockey, and others requiring a number of players. By contrast, most people can easily and regularly enjoy sports such as running, skating, and biking on a lifelong basis. We favor athletic programs that emphasize sports with long-range benefits. We want healthy children to become healthy, fit adults.

Second, the sports that receive the most glory are often the most violent, and therefore the most hazardous to a child's health. We prefer sports emphasizing speed, skill, and coordination to those emphasizing violence and mayhem. The growth of soccer in recent years has been a refreshing addition to America's team sports.

Third, competitive sports for adults should be clearly separated from competitive sports for children. The rules that govern professional athletics should not be the model for childhood athletics. Children often have a difficult time dealing with failure. When they think their parents' love depends on their winning a game, that is a psychologically dangerous situation. We applaud the many organized athletic programs for children younger than eight years old that do not keep score.

Fourth, children need to develop in many areas. If competitive sports or any other single skill precludes their full intellectual, social, and emotional development, that sport or skill is to be condemned. A full day of practice for a mature adult is different from a 12-year-old's practice for the same amount of time because of pressure from school, parent, or coach. We do not believe in pressuring any child to practice any sport for long hours daily.

Fifth, school athletic programs spend the most money on the best athletes—the children who need it least. The biggest budgets usually belong to football, basketball, and baseball. Funds for girls' sports have often been smaller than funds for boys' sports, although this is changing. Physical education, as all education, should recognize the principle of equity.

We support organized sports, but we do not feel that the competitive drive to be number one should underlie a child's participation. More than 25 million children are now participating in organized athletic activities. They can all be winners, but they can't all get trophies. You should allow your child to make the decision about the extent of his or her participation, and you should support that decision.

Is Your Child Ready?

When the opportunity for your child to play a new sport comes up, you should ask yourself the following questions.

▲ Does my child have the **coordination** for the sport? The hand-eye coordination necessary for some sports such as tennis and baseball is normally present only in an older child.

▲ Is my child the **proper size** for the sport? There have been several 5-foot 6-inch all-American basketball players, but no 100-pound college football tackles. Children mature at different rates and ages. Children who enter puberty late can be physically injured if matched with opponents of greater weight. Forcing children to compete with younger opponents of the same weight can hurt their egos almost as much.

▲ Is my child playing at the appropriate **skill level**? Most organized sports group children by age. But whereas older players may be excluded from younger teams, younger players are often permitted on older teams. Even an athletic child will encounter difficulties playing against older, stronger children.

▲ Is my child in the proper **condition**? Size is not everything. A child wishing to join a team in mid-season may have the size and coordination but not the stamina to play successfully.

▲ Does my child have any **medical conditions** that might be limiting? Many schools have rules that prohibit children with certain problems (listed below) from playing contact sports (football, basketball, wrestling, ice hockey, lacrosse, boxing, soccer, and rugby). Often these children can participate in noncontact sports.

The following conditions often disqualify children from contact sports, although a doctor or the courts may permit a child with some of these problems to participate.

▲ Brain concussion
▲ Head injury with residual skull defects
▲ Absence of an eye
▲ Detached retina
▲ Glaucoma
▲ Lung infection (tuberculosis or pneumonia)
▲ Certain heart rhythm disturbances
▲ Severe heart defects
▲ Severe or recent heart inflammation
▲ Certain types of undescended testes
▲ Missing kidney
▲ Bone infection
▲ Hemorrhagic blood disease

Temporary conditions that often disqualify students from formal sports competition include the following:

▲ Active infections
▲ Perforated eardrum
▲ Hepatitis or enlarged liver or spleen
▲ Healing fracture
▲ Injured growth plate of bone
▲ Pregnancy

Conditions that may disqualify certain students from some sports and for which individual decisions are most appropriate include the following:

▲ Physical immaturity
▲ Diabetes
▲ Severe visual handicap
▲ Hearing loss
▲ Asthma
▲ High blood pressure
▲ Absent testicle
▲ Seizure disorder (epilepsy)

Children with HIV infection can participate in all sports but are discouraged from wrestling because of the likelihood of bleeding and potential transmission of the virus.

Sports Safety

Children should continually be taught sports safety as a basic skill. This is the best insurance against serious injury. They should also learn to warm up and stretch appropriately for a sport. They must heed pain as a warning sign of injury and allow proper healing time. Finally, they must consider the implications of a minor illness on their participation. An earache may ground a swimmer, or a swollen knee may put a runner on the bench. An archer, however, could participate with these problems but not with a fingernail or eye infection.

Supervising adults should be prepared to deal with common emergencies. During interscholastic competition, where the risk of injury is relatively high, professional help should be nearby. Following are some often forgotten problems.

▲ **Contact lenses.** The safety record of soft contact lenses is excellent, and they are recommended by many doctors for older competitive athletes. The use of hard contact lenses is permissible in some circumstances. Sport goggles with safety lenses and straps are often a less costly alternative.

▲ **Heat exhaustion and heatstroke.** Athletes need water during workouts. Loss of water and salt from the body through prolonged sweating can cause heat exhaustion. Under severe conditions, heatstroke can occur, resulting in a rapidly elevated body temperature. Heatstroke can be fatal.

▲ **Weight loss.** Losing weight to place in a certain weight category, as in wrestling, should be restricted to loss of fat. We discourage weight reduction of more than 2½ pounds (1 kg) per week. Trying to lose weight through dehydration is dangerous and can compromise a child's strength. A substandard diet to maintain a certain weight deprives a growing child of the food necessary to grow normally.

Children should be encouraged to have fun. That's what sports are for. If children, their parents, or their coaches take sports too seriously, the sports may not be healthy, and they won't be fun.

Additional Reading

A Mind at a Time, Mel Levine, M.D. (New York: Simon & Schuster, 2002).

Revealing Minds: Assessing to Understand and Support Struggling Learners, Craig Pohlman and Mel Levine (San Francisco: Jossey Bass, 2007).

Chapter Eight

Working with Your Doctor

In the normal course of growing up, your child will need various kinds of medical attention—from physical examinations and laboratory tests to psychotherapy and surgical operations. In this chapter, we discuss some of the encounters that your child will have with medical professionals and provide guidelines to help you choose a doctor or other health care worker to meet your family's needs.

Finding Someone to Care

A Mother   The doctor is such a mixed blessing. You have this kid whom you know so intimately . . . you know him as nobody else does. And then there is this guy who has all this medical knowledge who knows things about your kid that you don't know, and there can be a subtle something in this relationship between the mother and the physician that can undermine altogether her confidence in herself and her mother role. . . . Pick the doctor with care, and don't accept an autocrat.

Medical Practitioners

A variety of professionals provide medical services to children and their parents.

▲ **Pediatricians** are doctors who have spent at least three years after medical school in formal training for the management of childhood and adolescent problems. The pediatrician is no longer a "baby doctor"; many treat a large number of adolescents.

▲ **Family practitioners** (general practitioners) are doctors who spend part of their formal medical training in the management of children's problems and who are trained to treat the whole family. Those who have become family practitioners recently have had training in the psychological as well as medical aspects of family interactions.

▲ **Internists** (specialists in internal medicine), though not trained in the care of children, are familiar with many diseases that occur not only in adults but also in children, and sometimes they see children referred by general practitioners.

▲ **Emergency room physicians.** Physicians trained in emergency medicine generally have 6 months of formal pediatric training. Large
centers may have pediatricians with additional emergency medicine training.

In addition to physicians, several groups of practitioners are capable of dealing competently with the common problems of childhood.
Nurse-practitioners have an R.N. degree and have attended a program
(usually from six months to a year and a half in length) that gives them
further training in the management of common medical problems.
Some nurse-practitioners spend their entire time with children. Others,
called family nurse-practitioners, spend part of their time with children. **Physician's assistants** have graduated from a one- or two-year
training course, enabling them to work alongside doctors in the management of common problems.

The most important factor in selecting a medical care provider is
your confidence in the individual. Confidence develops with time and
experience; don't rely entirely on first impressions. Asking friends for
their opinions of local providers can be a good way to get started.

Marks of Good Care

Look for the following attributes; they are hallmarks of good medical
and pediatric care.

▲ Does the practitioner **listen** to you? He or she must perceive the
same problems that you do.
▲ Does the practitioner encourage **questions**? Are your questions
taken seriously?
▲ Do you receive satisfactory **answers** to your questions? The quick
reply "She'll grow out of it" may not always be enough.
▲ Does the practitioner take an appropriate **medical history**? Be wary
of practitioners who listen for only a few seconds before deciding
on a course of action. Decisions based on a partial story are often
wrong. Injuries and simple problems may not require many questions, but a complicated illness does.
▲ Does the practitioner do a careful **physical examination** before ordering laboratory tests? Some practitioners will hear that a child
has fallen off a bicycle and order a whole series of X rays before
performing an examination. With some severe injuries, sending
the child for X rays may be dangerous. Also, every X ray involves
radiation exposure. A good medical history and physical examination will suggest a diagnosis to most competent practitioners. Laboratory tests should be used only when necessary to confirm the

diagnosis. Not only will test-oriented practitioners waste your time and money, but dangerous reactions may result from many tests.

▲ Does the practitioner take throat cultures for sore throats and order other appropriate **lab tests** before prescribing antibiotics and other medications?

▲ Does the practitioner try to solve the **underlying problem**, or does he or she merely make sure there is no biological illness? Being told that your child does not have meningitis, sinusitis, or a seizure disorder may ease your anxiety. But if your child is having headaches three times a week and is missing school because of it, the practitioner's job is not yet done. Your doctor's job is to help your child return to an optimal level of functioning, not merely to monitor the return to normalcy of laboratory tests.

▲ Is your practitioner concerned about the child's **development** and safety? About preventing illness rather than just treating it?

▲ Is there a **backup person** available when the practitioner is out of town?

Second Opinions

Second opinions are sometimes warranted, but remember that you can always find a number of different opinions about any given problem. Much has yet to be learned about illness, and there are many different ways of interpreting what we already know. Two explanations for the same phenomenon may sound totally different to you. We strongly recommend a second opinion if you aim to ensure the correctness of a serious decision. If, however, you are merely trying to find agreement with your own opinion about how to manage a problem, you are playing a dangerous game. You may well find a practitioner who will agree with your interpretation, but the real issue is which solution is best for your child.

Physicians also rely on other physicians, particularly specialists, for assistance with complex problems. Health plans vary in the types of specialists available to see your child. Work with your doctor to make sure you get the best referral.

Internet Information and Misinformation

Decades before the information explosion of the internet, we set out to provide parents with knowledge to assist you in understanding your children and making sound medical decisions. Thirty years after writing the first edition of *Taking Care of Your Child*, our goal is the same: to provide the highest quality information available. Unlike many current sources of information for parents, we have no advertising or corporate sponsors. This gives us the freedom to offer recommendations based on current science and the latest medical research. Some issues in child health care are black and white, but more are in the gray zone. In this edition, as in the past seven editions, we identify those recommendations that are universally accepted and, when in the gray zone, we delineate the controversy and where we stand. We encourage you to get as much information as you need to make a decision. There are hundreds of good health books and thousands of health websites (see below). Your doctor or nurse practitioner can also help you sort things out and make medical decisions. After all, that is their job description. Your relationship with these medical professionals is more important than your relationship with your computer.

With a keystroke and a mouse click you can now get information on your computer from tens and often hundreds or thousands of sites for a variety of diseases. At this writing there are countless health sites and a Google search of asthma resulted in more than 32 million references. No health care professional can keep up with all medical advances, and information acquired by patients on the Internet has, in our experience, often changed medical management. But getting good information can be daunting.

Information You Can Trust

The best information on the Internet is often provided by your tax dollars. A number of government sites are accurate, useful, and up-to-date. Below are some of our favorites and the type of information they provide.

▲ www.cdc.gov   Information on infectious diseases from the Centers for Disease Control.
▲ http://yosemite.epa.gov/ochp/ochpweb.nsf/homepage   Information about environmental risks to children.
▲ www.cdc.gov/nip   The latest on immunizations. Talks about safety as well as risks.
▲ www.cdc.gov/travel   Health recommendations for travelers.
▲ www.nih.gov   Information on many diseases from the National Institutes of Health.
▲ www.nhlbi.nih.gov/guidelines/asthma/index.htm   The latest available guidelines for children with asthma.
▲ www.ahrq.gov   The federal agency working on health care quality. Often sponsors research and issues new guidelines on childhood problems such as attention deficit hyperactivity disorder (ADHD).
▲ www.medlineplus.gov   Information from the National Library of Medicine.

Many universities also provide health information websites. A website is as good as the people developing the information. Some sites have strict criteria for including evidence-based information; some material on these sites is written by leading experts in their field. Other sites rely on experienced (or not so experienced) clinicians to develop material. In general, university sites are solid without much commercial interest.

Professional organizations, such as the American Academy of Pediatrics (AAP), often have excellent websites (www.aap.org). The AAP information is generally provided by committees made up of a number of experts and their recommendations are revised and updated when appropriate. (Author RHP served on two of these committees and chaired one.) Not all sites ending in .org are of the same quality. Many are produced by groups with a mission to provide objective information about a childhood problem. Some excellent sites were developed by parents dealing with their own child's illness. Unfortunately, some sites are platforms to advance one side of a complicated issue. We advise caution and recommend you know something about the organization when considering its advice.

The biggest challenge with the Internet is navigating through the dot coms. Regulation is limited because no United States government agency can regulate sites operated from outside the United States. Consequently, there is a tremendous business in providing prescription medications directly to consumers. This is a practice with potentially lethal consequences. Even worse, fantastic remedies and cures can be offered without the type of assurances of safety and efficacy afforded by the Food and Drug Administration. The quackery of nineteenth century medicine shows is being reawakened by the Internet.

Most dot com sites have commercial sponsors or accept advertising. This may interfere with the site's ability to provide information that is truly unbiased. In fact, one of the oldest and largest health websites was accused of deception by a leading medical journal for describing a list of hospitals as "the most innovative and advanced health care institutions in the country" when it was discovered that each institution had paid $40,000 to be on the list. While efforts are underway to assure voluntary compliance with high standards of content, truthful advertising, and consumer privacy, there is as yet no true regulation. Caution and common sense are needed to separate the substantial number of high quality sites from those that are no more than health infomercials.

Children and the Internet

The Internet is not only a source of health information for parents but also a new way for children to learn. From online encyclopedias and lectures to the latest scientific breakthrough, the Internet has it all for today's students. Just as there is some danger associated with a young child walking four or five blocks to the public library, the Internet has its own risks. And just as we tell our children to be wary of strangers they meet, we need to tell them to be wary of strangers on the Internet. Most people behave reasonably and decently online, but some are rude, mean, or even criminal. The online industry has tried to be responsive and most Internet browsers allow parents to block unknown or potentially offensive sites. However e-mail, instant messenger programs, and other chat rooms have certain risks. The following helpful material was excerpted from information developed by the White House and the Department of Education several years ago.

Teach your children that they should:

▲ **Never** give out personal information (including their name, home address, phone number, age, race, family income, school name or location, or friends' names) or use a credit card online without your permission.
▲ **Never** share their password, even with friends.
▲ **Never** arrange a face-to-face meeting with someone they meet online unless you approve of the meeting and go with them to a public place.
▲ **Never** respond to messages that make them feel confused or uncomfortable. They should ignore the sender, end the communication, and tell you or another trusted adult right away.
▲ **Never** use bad language or send mean messages online.

Also, make sure your children know that people they meet online are not always who they say they are and that online information is not necessarily private.

Child Health-Supervision Visits

Child health-supervision visits are also called well-baby or well-child visits. They represent opportunities for you to affirm that all aspects of your child's health are going well. You and your doctor will exchange biological, developmental, psychological, and social information during these visits. Developing a rapport with your doctor early on is of paramount importance.

The first well-baby visit generally occurs within the first two weeks after birth. By that time, parents have come to know some of the unique characteristics of their babies and often have many questions. At least three more visits in the first year and two in the second will be required. For older children, an annual visit is routine. Immunizations will be given during these visits. You can schedule additional visits periodically when and if you have concerns.

During the first series of well-baby visits, the doctor will put considerable emphasis on detecting physical and biological abnormalities through frequent examinations and screening tests (such as for thyroid disease), as well as on preventing diseases with immunizations. Your doctor also will be interested in how you and your infant are adapting to each other.

As your child grows, the doctor will continue to show an interest in physical problems. He or she will check older children for vision and hearing problems and adolescents for sexual development. However, it is likely that the doctor will devote more time to prevention (injuries, obesity, smoking), parenting issues (such as discipline), and your own concerns about behavior, day care, schooling, sex education, and the like. The time spent on these issues is just as important as the time devoted to looking for physical abnormalities during the first few visits.

The preventive child health visit, a cornerstone of pediatrics that has helped infants and children for a century, is coming under increasing scrutiny. The successes of preventive care have been remarkable. Immunizing infants has virtually eliminated diseases that terrorized families 20 years ago; counseling parents to have babies sleep on their backs has cut the rate of Sudden Infant Death Syndrome in half; and recommending that infants and children sit in the backseat of cars has dramatically reduced automobile accident deaths in all age groups. However, physicians complain that they are expected to deliver an ever increasing list of safety and other preventive messages in shorter and shorter time slots, while parents express frustration that appointments never seem long enough to adequately address their concerns. Numerous studies point out that when parents express concerns about child development, there is often considerable delay in adequately addressing the problem.

There is growing consensus that the nature of preventive child health visits should change, perhaps to focus on age appropriate themes such as infant nutrition, toddler discipline, school readiness, and adolescent risk taking. Each child is different, and no single strategy for preventive care will fit all. For now, you should consider each visit an opportunity for you to share your concerns about *any* aspect of your child's development or health. This includes any of the major problems of today's children such as obesity, learning disorders, and depression and risk-taking behaviors in adolescents. If you are worried about these or similar issues, consider making a separate appointment to address the concern rather than waiting until the next annual visit.

Many issues are far more complicated to diagnose and treat than an ear infection. Considerably more time may be needed to understand and to manage your child's problem. If you feel you did not have enough time to address your concern, ask for another visit in the near future or for a referral to another professional with expanded expertise in your area of concern.

Measurements and Checks

Besides a check on development, the most important parts of a well-baby examination are the simple measurements of the infant's height, weight, and head circumference. These measurements are useful in detecting nutritional problems and metabolic or glandular growth disturbances.

Following are some of the areas your child's doctor will measure and examine.

Head

Head measurements are important because they can indicate several correctable problems in the development of the skull and brain during the first few months of life. One of these is **craniosynostosis**, an early fusion of the bones of the skull, preventing further growth. Another is obstruction of the fluid system bathing the brain, known as **hydrocephalus**.

Hips

Examining the hips is especially important in infants. Hips may be dislocated, partially dislocated, or unstable, and this examination should be repeated after a month or so. Congenitally dislocated hips are very easily treated in the first few months merely by using extra-thick diapers. Tell your doctor if your child was breech or anyone in the family had hip dysplasia. Failure to detect this condition until later may result in surgery or casting.

Feet and Legs

The feet should be examined carefully in newborn infants and during the first few months of life. Foot abnormalities such as **metatarsus adductus**, when detected early, can be corrected with a few weeks of casting. Metatarsus adductus causes an exaggerated curving of the outside of the child's foot. Children often have a certain degree of toeing in, which is normal until age two. Toeing in also may result from the twisting of one of the bones in the lower leg or the rotation of the thigh bone at the hip joint.

Genitals

Genital examinations are important. Boys should be checked for unde-scended testicles and foreskin problems. Girls should be checked for problems with the external genitals. We feel that regular external examination of girls will make the first internal (pelvic) exam some-what less frightening.

Spine

By the time your child reaches school age, your doctor will be check-ing for curvature of the spine (**scoliosis**) by having the child perform a toe-touching maneuver.

Eyes

Periodic examination of your child's eyes is necessary. Infants are capa-ble of seeing at birth, and their eyes can follow you around the room. Infants begin focusing clearly at about six weeks of age, and at this time the wandering of their eyes diminishes. **Strabismus**, also known as a wandering eye or weak eye, is not normal after six months. You can check for strabismus by having the child focus on any bright object and alternately covering and uncovering one of the child's eyes. When the eye is uncovered, it should not move. Any movement is a sign of a weak eye muscle and should be checked by the doctor. Untreated strabismus can result in blindness in the weak eye. Three- and four-year-olds should be tested during doctor visits.

Ears

Hearing disturbances can interfere with a child's development. New-borns are startled by sounds and later turn to locate the sounds. Many newborn nurseries now perform hearing screening, but parents are usu-ally the first ones to suspect a hearing problem. They may notice that an infant will not turn in response to their voices or has difficulty learning to talk. A child won't learn to talk if he or she can't hear. Precise hear-ing can be most readily tested after 12 months of age. If you are con-cerned about your child's hearing, be sure to have an evaluation done.

Teeth

Adequate dental care requires regular visits to a dentist, as well as rou-tine flossing and brushing. A good doctor, however, also will check the development of your child's teeth.

Blood Pressure

Blood pressure measurements should be done at least once every two years.

Heart

The casual statement by a doctor that a child has a **heart murmur** is enough to strike terror in the heart of many parents. Some perspective is needed. A murmur is just the sound of blood rushing through the heart. In fact, a heart murmur can be heard in almost any child when he or she has a fever, is excited, or has just exercised. This does not mean your child has heart disease. Such murmurs occur in the part of the heart cycle known as the systole and are frequently called "innocent," "benign," or "functional" murmurs. They will usually disappear as the child gets older. Don't worry about them. If, however, your doctor hears a murmur in a certain (diastolic) part of the cardiac cycle or a particularly loud murmur, or if the child is growing poorly, is blue (cyanotic), or is short of breath, further evaluation is required. Your doctor will explain this situation to you.

There are many other aspects of well-child examinations. The doctor may pick up on almost any problem during such an examination, but most important problems are noted at home first.

Your Doctor, Your Child's Doctor

Nine-Year-Old Girl   Before the doctor gave me stitches, she came at me with a huge syringe with a giant needle. I was afraid she was going to inject it into me, but all she did was wash out my cut. She should have told me what she was going to do so I wouldn't have gotten so scared.

Seven-Year-Old Boy   After the shots, I got a cat face drawn where the holes were. It was like a medal and award of endurance.

Twelve-Year-Old Girl   Why do they have to talk about "shots"? It just makes things seem even scarier.

Eight-Year-Old Boy to Physician Having a Lengthy Conversation with His Mother   Hey, talk to me. I'm the patient.

"Children should be seen and not heard" is a familiar expression that few would accept as a policy for dealing with children. Unfortunately, too many children are treated in precisely this fashion in the doctor's office. Doctors may seem too busy to talk with children. Yet most doctors caring for children, especially pediatricians, chose their professional specialty because they genuinely like children.

Often doctors may not be able to initiate a dialogue because of a child's anxiety. The fear of shots, for example, is universal among children. We feel strongly that if children are to develop competence about dealing with their health, illnesses, and the medical profession, they should have experience communicating during an office visit. Once children are school-age (and assuming, of course, they are not too ill), they should begin expressing their own concerns to the doctor, as well as participating in discussions of any plans that directly involve them.

You can help. Answer as best you can any questions your child has before a visit to the doctor. Encourage the child to speak up and ask questions. You may need to introduce an opportunity for the child to ask the doctor a burning question. Children often do not respond to a doctor's questions for a couple of simple reasons.

▲ The panic of the moment has made them forget their age, their sibling's name, or whatever information the doctor is requesting.
▲ They do not understand the question.

You can be helpful as an intermediary. Don't jump in with answers, but calm the child and translate terms. Help the child achieve his or her own communication skills.

During the visit, your child may participate in the examination process, as well as in decisions about follow-up care. Discuss, for example, who will be responsible for remembering medicine or who will decide about when the child can return to school. Ultimately, you must decide when your child should begin to have time to speak in confidence with the doctor and opportunities to telephone him or her directly. We recommend gradually transferring responsibility, so that by the middle-school years your child is spending some private time with the doctor, and by adolescence he or she is spending most of the time alone with the doctor.

The First Pelvic Examination

The first pelvic examination in girls arouses much concern because of its social and sexual connotations. When should the first exam be performed? How often are such examinations necessary? Briefly, here are some things to consider in making this decision.

Pelvic examinations are performed in adult women to detect problems, such as cancer, before symptoms appear. These problems are so rare in childhood and adolescence that routine pelvic examinations are seldom necessary. Individual circumstances should determine the need for the first exam.

Currently, professional organizations and government task forces recommend all sexually active adolescents be tested for sexually transmitted diseases (STDs). However, new tests are available for detecting

STDs by checking the urine. With cervical cancer being found in only 1 in 500,000 teenagers, pelvic exams are required less frequently.

If a child requires a pelvic examination prior to adolescence, the procedure should be done by the family doctor or pediatrician with the mother present. Having the family doctor perform the exam eliminates the stress of introducing the child to a strange doctor and office. Only occasionally will a gynecologist be necessary.

During adolescence, the decision about which doctor to use is more difficult. Some adolescents view the pediatrician as a "baby doctor" and feel that they should see a gynecologist, internist, or family doctor. Many pediatricians spend a great deal of time practicing adolescent gynecology, but the choice should be left up to the young woman.

Whoever the doctor is, confidentiality is extremely important. The mother should not be present during the examination or during discussions between the doctor and the adolescent unless the adolescent asks her to stay. Do not demand that either the doctor or your daughter tell you exactly what happened. These are adult conversations and must be treated as such.

You can be most helpful by explaining the procedure to your daughter before you get to the doctor's office. Discuss the reasons for the examination and the purpose of each step. Make it clear that there may be some discomfort but no cutting or severe pain. If your daughter doesn't understand the procedures, she may imagine it as something harmful and fear damage to her sexual organs. Not only do these fears make the examination more difficult, but they may also result in psychological harm.

The doctor usually performs the pelvic examination with a nurse in attendance. Amenities are important. The metal "stirrups" on which the heels rest can be wrapped, and the speculum can be warmed. A sheet will usually be placed as a drape over the knees so that the patient feels less exposed.

The full examination consists of inspection of the outside genitals, palpation (feeling) of the internal organs, inspection of the inside of the vagina, and the taking of test samples as indicated, not always in that order. The young woman should not douche for 24 hours before the exam because douching may make diagnosis of some conditions impossible.

Inspection of the outside genitals includes the genital lips, clitoris, and anal opening. Rashes, sores, small growths, or other problems may be identified.

Palpation of internal organs includes the vagina, the mouth of the womb (cervix), the womb (uterus) itself, and the ovaries. Usually, this is performed with two gloved fingers inserted into the vagina.

Internal inspection requires a light and a speculum. The speculum is metal or plastic and gently spreads the walls of the vagina so that the doctor can see inside. The speculum is not a clamp and should not pinch or hurt. It will be lubricated with water or a substance resembling petroleum jelly to make insertion easier. Specula come in several sizes; smaller ones will be used in young girls or virgins. The procedure should always be performed gently, with all actions explained in advance. The patient can assist by relaxing as much as possible. Taking slow, deep breaths or thinking of an enjoyable leisure activity may help.

The manner in which a gynecological examination is performed will help a young woman judge the quality of care she is receiving. An examiner who is abrupt and rough or who doesn't explain what is happening is insensitive to a fault. Pelvic examinations are medically essential in many situations, but an examiner who is not sensitive to the complex considerations of psychology and human dignity that are involved cannot be giving good medical care.

Laboratory Screening Tests for Children

Eye tests and hearing tests are the most important screening examinations for children. Some of the more common laboratory examinations are discussed here. Except for tuberculosis screening, we do not feel that these tests need to be done routinely for all children; they are needed only for particular children.

Tuberculosis

Tuberculosis is still common in some parts of the country and is on the rise, particularly in low-income, inner-city areas. While it is no longer considered necessary to screen all children *regularly* for the disease, most schools require PPD tests for entrance. Infants and children should be tested if they are known to have been exposed to tuberculosis or to people at high risk for tuberculosis (such as people with AIDS).

Anemia

One way to screen a child for the most common form of anemia, iron-deficiency anemia, is to ask what the child is eating. Children fed a nutritionally balanced diet are almost never iron deficient.

Children who have experienced a number of infections may become iron deficient. In the presence of a diet with adequate iron, this condition will spontaneously resolve after infection. We see iron-deficiency anemia most commonly in children about one year old whose diets consist mainly of milk. Milk is low in iron. By one year of age, the child should be eating lots of different things. Detection of most other types of anemia at an early age is usually suggested by a family history of spherocytosis, sickle-cell disease, and other illnesses. Some doctors routinely screen all infants for anemia, but many only selectively screen their patients.

The test results for anemia may be expressed in two ways. **Hemoglobin** is a measure of the amount of protein that carries oxygen in red blood cells. **Hematocrit** is the percentage of one's blood that is composed of red blood cells. An abnormally low value for either indicates anemia.

Sickle-Cell Disease

Sickle-cell anemia is a severe genetic blood disease occurring almost entirely in blacks. For a child to have **sickle-cell** (anemia) **disease**, a sickle gene must have come from each parent; two genes are required. Someone with a single sickle-cell gene is a "carrier" and is referred to as having "sickle trait." The two-gene disease causes anemia, infections, and other problems. The one-gene trait seldom causes problems; some individuals have had problems at high altitudes.

It is now routine to screen for sickle-cell disease in the newborn period. We believe that sickle-cell screening should be available to adults who are planning a pregnancy and would like to know whether they are carriers of a single sickle-cell gene. Fetal screening also is available. All parents who know that they carry the sickle-cell trait should have their infants screened, because this may result in early detection and treatment of children with sickle-cell disease.

Urine

Controversy surrounded the question of routine urine examinations to detect bacterial infections that are not causing symptoms, especially in girls. Most studies suggest that treatment of these asymptomatic problems is of no benefit. In general, treatment of "diseases" that are not causing trouble often does more harm than good. Use of the urine for other screening (for example, protein or sugar) is also unwarranted and urine screening is no longer recommended by the AAP. For children who have had urinary tract infections in the past, a periodic analysis of the urine may be in order.

Diabetes

Juvenile diabetes mellitus is a different disease from adult-onset diabetes mellitus and cannot be detected by screening. The first episode will bring the child to the doctor with increased urinary frequency, excessive thirst, nausea and vomiting, shortness of breath, or coma. Prior to this time, screening tests will produce negative results.

Cholesterol

Blood cholesterol and heart disease are linked, but an elevated cholesterol level is only one of many factors that contribute to heart problems. Children should not be routinely screened for cholesterol. Childhood cholesterol levels correlate poorly with adult levels. Many children have been tyrannized by a value that is a poor predictor of an event at least 40 years away.

If one parent has had a heart attack before age 45, however, the family should have a cholesterol screen and a comprehensive approach to treating the condition. This will include discussions about exercise, cholesterol, diet, stress, and anxiety. We believe that some attention to these factors, including a diet moderately low in saturated fats, is indicated for everyone, regardless of the cholesterol level. (For further discussion, see pages 199–201.)

Lead

Lead poisoning in children has been slowly decreasing in the United States. The decline in the use of lead-based gasoline and the limitation of lead in paint sold after 1978 have been helpful. However, many children still have blood levels of lead high enough to interfere with their intellectual growth and functioning. As a result of studies suggesting that problems may arise with lower levels of lead than had been previously thought, in late 1991 the Centers for Disease Control and Prevention (CDC) recommended that all children should be screened.

Unfortunately, this screening involved considerable expense, discomfort, anxiety about borderline levels, and follow-up for many children with marginal elevation. Consequently, many physicians did not routinely screen all children, and the CDC reversed its position. We support the current CDC recommendation for screening high-risk groups and for encouraging communities and states to make recommendations based on local conditions. We also believe that physicians should be familiar with local surveillance data and intelligently advise you about your child.

The CDC priority groups for screening include children ages 6 months to 6 years who meet any of the following criteria:

▲ Live in housing built before 1960
▲ Live in housing with remodeling going on
▲ Have siblings or friends with lead poisoning
▲ Are exposed to lead because of household members' jobs or hobbies (such as metalworkers, plumbers, auto repair workers, and potters)

▲ Have environmental exposure by living near lead smelters, battery plants, or industries releasing lead
▲ Children enrolled in Medicaid

Screening for the Cause of Frequent Illness

All children contract a large number of colds (upper respiratory infections) in the process of growing up. We do not like to consider these episodes as sickness or illness. Many parents are surprised that we would call a three-day episode of a temperature of 100°F (37.7°C), a runny nose, and a slight cough anything but an illness. The point we are trying to make is that respiratory infections are a normal part of growing up and actually provide benefits to the child. We regard common respiratory infections in children as a type of immunization. Like other immunizations, viral infections may have side effects, such as fever, runny nose, and cough. Children usually fare better with a given viral respiratory illness than adults do.

In careful studies conducted at several university medical centers, infants and young children have been found to develop between six and nine viral infections per year. The older the child, the fewer the infections, but even first-graders average about six viral episodes per year. We are not usually disturbed by a child who has nine viral infections a year unless they interfere with the child's daily routine or are slowing growth or maturation. Two bouts of pneumonia or two bouts of skin abscesses are more significant medically than nine colds. Certain types of pneumonia or other unusual findings may occur in children with AIDS, but frequent colds should not cause anxiety. In a child who is having frequent illnesses, the question is not so much how frequent, but how serious. (For a further explanation, see the decision chart and discussion under Frequent Illnesses, page 316.)

Don't be afraid to send your child to school with the sniffles if he or she feels like going. For most illnesses, the period when the child is most contagious is the period *before* he or she gets sick. It is regrettable that children are often sent home from school at the first sign of a cold, as the cold can serve to immunize the other children against that virus. Here's a good general rule.

▲ Fever above 101°F (38.3°C)—home in bed
▲ No fever—school

Hospitalization

Each year, 1 in 30 children will leave the familiar surroundings of his or her home, the companionship of friends, and the support and care of parents to enter a frightening social system and institution—the hospital. In this foreign environment, the child is not only expected to recover from an illness but to demonstrate good citizenship as well. These expectations are, to say the least, a tall order for a sick six-year-old.

Psychological Effects

Parents worry about the psychological consequences of a hospitalization, as well as their child's prompt and full recovery from the problem necessitating the stay. Fortunately, most hospitalizations are brief. Long-term psychological problems have been found primarily in children who have experienced numerous prolonged hospital stays at an early age.

During a hospitalization, it is common for children to experience considerable anxiety about separation from parents, mutilation, and especially death. Being "put to sleep" (anesthetized) can easily be construed as permanent. Some behaviors are common, such as increased crying and activity level. Occasionally, a child will become depressed or have other psychological disturbances in the hospital.

Immediately after discharge, it is quite common to see a child regress to immature behaviors such as thumb sucking, bed-wetting, baby talk, clinging, crying, increased dependency, and a decreased attention span. Sleep problems occur frequently, and some children become aggressive. Anxiety may be manifested in a refusal to leave home or an excessive fear of doctors or nurses.

By contrast, some children may have positive psychological responses to a hospitalization. This is particularly true of 8- to 11-year-olds, who often gain self-esteem by making it through a procedure and show accelerated learning.

It is clear that the way a child experiences a hospital stay and what a child learns from this experience can be influenced by both medical professionals and parents. Your child may participate in a variety of hospital-sponsored preparation procedures, including puppet therapy, coloring books, or films designed to help children cope with stressful procedures. Most important, however, are the comfort, reassurance, and information you give your child.

Common Concerns

If you have any concerns about your child's hospital stay, make sure your doctor and the hospital staff address them. If you are overly anxious, your child will pick up on this and become anxious, too. Here are some tips for addressing the concerns of children in various age groups.

▲ **Ages 0 to 3.** Allow the child to handle (where possible) new and strange equipment. Bring favorite cuddlies or dolls. Assure the child that you will return.

▲ **Ages 4 to 7.** Bring a favorite toy. Encourage the rehearsal of responses to the procedure. Help the child distinguish attainable goals. For instance, blood tests cannot be avoided but can be made easier if children help by holding still or by choosing which arm they prefer. Assure the child that he or she will not be mutilated or permanently separated from home. Reassure him or her that the hospitalization is not a result of evil thoughts or a form of punishment. Explore any misconceptions. Some common ones include the following: all diseases are contagious, procedures that hurt (or don't hurt) aren't therapeutic, and blood is a fixed quantity that can be permanently depleted.

▲ **Ages 8 to 12.** Explore concerns about how the hospitalization will affect the child's status with his or her peers. At this age, children may not grasp the value of preventive measures and may be confused about an upcoming surgery if they feel fine physically.

▲ **Ages 13 to 18.** Explore the adolescent's concerns about his or her body image and independence. Adolescents have a tendency to deny or minimize the severity of illness. They also may desire more information than the doctor has provided about the cause or origin of the illness and the future consequences of it. In addition, many have real concerns about the financial impact of a hospitalization on the family.

Remember that almost all children are interested in the immediate events that will affect them. Finding out when they must leave for X rays can be quite important to their peace of mind. Here again, you can be an important intermediary between your child and the doctor and can increase the likelihood that your child will learn from this experience.

Surgery

Discuss any recommendations for surgery with your family doctor. You should understand why the operation is being done and the possible implications and complications. Many procedures that required a hospitalization several years ago (for example, hernia repair) can now be performed as day surgery, in which a child is admitted to the hospital in the morning and discharged the same day. In this section, we discuss some of the more common operations performed on children.

After circumcisions, tonsillectomies and adenoidectomies are together the most frequently performed operations on children in the United States today. Because they are operations on separate organs and because they are done for different reasons, we discuss them separately.

Tonsillectomy

The tonsils are located on both sides of the back of the throat and can be seen quite easily when your child's mouth is open. Tonsils consist of lymphoid tissue, which is useful in fighting infections. Because children between the ages of four and seven years develop so many colds (upper respiratory infections), the tonsils are largest in this age group. Large tonsils are natural; they are enlarged because they are busy fighting infections. Occasionally, the tonsils themselves may become infected, but only when there is an infection of the entire throat.

Removing a child's tonsils does not reduce the child's chances of developing a sore throat. Nor does it reduce the child's chances of developing a cold. Nor does it reduce the child's chances of developing an ear infection. Why, then, are so many tonsillectomies done in this country? This is indeed a difficult question to answer, especially because children die unnecessarily each year as a result of tonsillectomies.

There are, of course, some good reasons for a tonsillectomy. If the tonsils are so large that they interfere with the child's breathing, they should be removed. Snoring or sleep difficulties should prompt a sleep study. This condition is exceedingly rare, however. When such airway blockage occurs, the problem is detected by evaluation of the heart and lungs. Merely looking at the tonsils will not reveal an obstruction of breathing. Although we have never seen it occur, it is conceivable that very large tonsils may interfere with eating or swallowing. This may also require their removal. In addition, if a serious abscess forms in one of the tonsils, it is likely that this abscess will recur. A recurrence may be prevented by a tonsillectomy.

Adenoidectomy

Tonsillectomies have been traditionally accompanied by adenoidectomies. Surgeons often decided that since a patient was going to be placed under anesthesia anyway, the adenoids might as well be removed. The adenoids, however, are located in a different region and have their own functions. Adenoids can create problems, but removing the adenoids when only a tonsillectomy is indicated will increase the chances of a bad result from the operation. In addition, removing the adenoids can lead to ear problems in certain children.

The adenoids cannot be seen by looking at the throat. They are in the back of the nose above the palate and near the opening of the eustachian tube, which drains middle-ear secretions into the nasal passages. Adenoids contain lymphoid tissue, and they enlarge as they fight infection in the upper respiratory tract. If they become too large, they can block the opening of the eustachian tube and increase the likelihood of an ear infection.

Adenoidectomies used to be considered for children who had frequent ear infections. Today ear tubes generally accomplish the same function, providing adequate air circulation in the middle ear. If the ear infections are caused by allergies, children generally do not profit from an adenoidectomy. Children who may benefit are generally those who have had a severe impact from ear infections, such as hearing loss. Some children will actually have more ear infections after an adenoidectomy. It is sometimes possible to identify these children before the operation.

Severe obstruction of breathing or interference with sleep may also be reasons to consider removing the adenoids. A sleep study is generally recommended before proceeding with surgery.

Ear Tubes

Ear tubes (ventilation tubes) are small plastic tubes that are inserted through the child's eardrums. They are placed in children who have frequent earaches to provide adequate airflow in the middle ear. Aeration aids the healing process and prevents the middle ear from becoming sealed off (an ear infection generally does not develop unless the middle ear is blocked).

The placement of ear tubes is a very simple procedure that is usually done as day surgery after the summer swimming season is over. Indications for ear tubes include the following:

▲ Documented hearing loss with speech delay
▲ Recurrent ear infections that have not responded to medical therapy, including prophylactic antibiotics
▲ Presence in the middle ear of a material that is too thick to drain under normal conditions

Considerable controversy surrounds the indications for this procedure. Discuss the benefits, potential harms, costs, and alternatives thoroughly with your physician. The purpose is to reduce infection and to ensure adequate hearing.

Repair of Umbilical Hernia

An umbilical hernia results from the failure of stomach muscles to grow together in the area surrounding the belly button. Umbilical hernias are very common in black children but do not pose any risk to their health. Generally, these hernias disappear within the first few years of life. Those that don't disappear slowly heal by the time the child is of school age. Because these hernias are of no risk to the patient and because they usually heal themselves, we do not advocate surgical repair, except in rare cases where cosmetic improvement is psychologically important. In general, time is a better and safer healer than a scalpel.

Undescended Testicles

It is common to find that one or both of a boy's testicles are not in the scrotal sac. The testicles are often in the inguinal canal, located just above the scrotal sac. One of the most common reasons for the testicles to find their way up and out of the scrotal sac is the presence of an examiner's cold hands. Occasionally, the testicles may withdraw all the way into the abdominal cavity. (Some Japanese wrestlers can accomplish this feat voluntarily.)

Testicles that are permanently located within the abdominal cavity should be brought down surgically. Doctors differ on the best time for doing this, but the procedure should be done by one year of age.

It is of the utmost importance to determine whether the testicles can or cannot descend into the scrotal sac normally. The best way to decide this is to have your child sit with his legs crossed (the Buddha or lotus position) and check for the presence of the testicles within the scrotal sac. We do not recommend hormonal treatment for bringing testicles into the scrotal sac. It usually doesn't help and may have side effects.

Hydrocele and Inguinal Hernia

Hydroceles and inguinal hernias both cause swelling of the scrotal sac. It is difficult to tell the two apart, and a doctor's visit is necessary.

A **hydrocele** is a fluid sac within the scrotal sac and is often present in newborn boys. The fluid does not create any problem for the child and will be reabsorbed in time. Some doctors prefer to remove the fluid from the scrotal sac with a needle. Nature will work just as well, though not as quickly.

An **inguinal hernia** will also cause swelling of the scrotal sac. Hernias generally first appear after the newborn period and often following a vigorous bout of crying. Severe problems such as intestine blockage can result from inguinal hernias, because a hernia is a small portion of the child's bowel that has found its way through the inguinal canal and into the scrotal sac below. Unlike inguinal hernias in adults, which doctors are able to feel on examination, hernias in children can be evaluated only when the scrotal sac is swollen. The child should see the doctor when the sac is swollen.

Appendectomy

Appendicitis is discussed under Abdominal Pain, page 465.

Circumcision

Circumcision is discussed on pages 33–34.

Transfusions

Transfusions are seldom required, except for such conditions as severe jaundice or anemia in newborns, destructive (hemolytic) anemia in infants and children, and after the loss of blood due to trauma or surgery. Although blood used in transfusions is evaluated to make sure it is compatible with your child's blood and free of severe viral infections, there has been some concern over the risk of acquiring AIDS through blood transfusions. Since the spring of 1985, all blood has been screened for antibodies to HIV, which causes AIDS. Newer and more precise tests are currently used. Due to the nature of the test, it is still a rare but real possibility that a unit of transfused blood will contain undetected HIV. Transfusion with blood from a family donor whose medical history you know can be reassuring but has not been shown to reduce this low risk even further.

Preventive Care

We believe that the best approach to dealing with serious problems is to prevent them. Only 3% of the money we spend on health care is for prevention. We think that greater national emphasis on disease prevention and health promotion, as well as on changes in personal behavior, will have enormous health benefits.

This chapter and the next discuss major problem areas in which prevention is essential. We realize that most of our readers will rely heavily on Part IV of this book to help them respond promptly and appropriately to new medical problems and to save time and money. But the information in these two chapters is no less valuable to your child's overall good health.

Chapter 9 addresses three areas in which parents can help their children avoid medical difficulties later in life.

▲ Immunizations
▲ Allergies
▲ Dental care

Immunizations

Infectious diseases were historically the most significant wasters of human life, but now they have been controlled by many methods, including improved nutrition, sanitation, and housing and, more recently, the development of immunizations and antibiotics. Immunizations are undoubtedly the most significant contribution of science to the control of disease. Smallpox has been eliminated from the face of the earth by the worldwide campaign of the World Health Organization; the last case in the world occurred in 1977 and the disease was declared eradicated in 1980. Polio, which crippled 20,000 Americans a year in the early 1950s, no longer affects children in the United States, thanks to immunization campaigns.

We are in a critical period in this nation's history with regard to immunizations. Many people have become complacent about immunizations because of the rarity of the diseases they prevent. In addition, there have always been problems in the use of immunizations. However, the risks of the vaccines are usually minimal when compared with the risks of the diseases they prevent. Because the bacteria and viruses responsible for causing infectious illnesses may be spread by contact with people, animals, or airborne droplets, avoidance is often impossible. Fortunately, protection by immunizations is simple and effective. We feel that immunizations are vital to children's health.

Principle

The principle of immunization is to develop your body's defense system to a point where it is capable of foiling any attack by a particular agent. To accomplish this, a small dose of the modified infectious agent is given. For some immunizations, the virus has been modified in a laboratory so that it causes a very mild infection. Other immunizations use a dead virus that is chemically the same as the living virus but cannot cause infection. Still others use part of a virus or bacteria. The body's defense system builds up an immunity to this modified agent, which in effect creates an immunity to the infecting agent.

The practice of immunization dates back several thousand years to attempts by a Chinese monk to prevent smallpox. Immunization methods were developed long before the nature of the infecting agents was known. Edward Jenner, who is credited with the modern development of immunization in the late 18th century, borrowed the idea from English farmers who had been using cowpox to protect themselves from smallpox for centuries. Jenner performed a study validating what the farmers had been doing.

Many vaccines are for a specific illness, but some, such as the DTP (diphtheria, tetanus, pertussis) injection, are combination vaccines that protect against two or more diseases. There are no particular medical advantages or disadvantages to combination vaccines, but they do reduce the number of shots your child must receive.

Vaccine Safety

Modern virological techniques allow the manufacture of vaccines that are effective against many illnesses. But all immunizations carry with them the possibility of side effects from the immunization itself. No immunization is 100% effective or 100% safe. While the media have reported claims of a potential link between the MMR vaccine and vaccines containing mercury (thimerasol) and autism, *extensive* scientific reviews have *not* found any association.

Vaccines containing a live virus are not recommended for children taking high levels of steroid medications, receiving chemotherapy, or with immune-system disorders.

It is important that you maintain your own records of your child's immunizations. Do not rely on the doctor, health department, or clinic where the immunizations are given.

Questions

If you have questions, such as those listed below, about a particular immunization, your doctor or health department should be willing to explain in detail the current risks, benefits, and recommendations for that immunization. You can also consult the Centers for Disease Control web page at www.cdc.gov/nip.

- ▲ How effective is this immunization?
- ▲ What are the possible side effects?
- ▲ Who is likely to experience a side effect?
- ▲ Will people in contact with the immunized person also become immunized?
- ▲ How long does the immunity last?
- ▲ Is the immunization safe for pregnant mothers?
- ▲ Is it safe to immunize children whose mothers are pregnant?

Diphtheria

Nature of the Illness. Fewer than a hundred cases of diphtheria are reported each year in the United States. Diphtheria affects the throat, nose, and skin and is contagious. Complications of diphtheria include paralysis (in approximately 20% of patients) and heart damage (in approximately 50%). Diphtheria can be treated by a combination of penicillin and serum injections. However, despite treatment, approximately 10% of persons who contract diphtheria will die from it. Only immunization can successfully prevent diphtheria.

Nature of the Immunization. Diphtheria immunization has been available since 1920. A portion of the toxin (the chemical product of the bacterium that causes damage) is altered with formalin to render it harmless. This modified toxin, known as a toxoid, stimulates the body's defense system to produce an antitoxin. Immunity persists for many years after several inoculations. Although the person may come in contact with bacteria and even become infected, the toxin will be neutralized by the antitoxin within the person's body, and the infection will cause no harm.

Reactions to diphtheria toxoid are extremely uncommon. Generally, they are limited to a slight swelling at the injection site. This reaction can be decreased in older children and adults by giving them lower concentrations of the toxoid, known as "adult-type" diphtheria toxoid.

Diphtheria toxoid should be begun, in combination with tetanus and pertussis (whooping cough), at the age of two months. The combination vaccine is commonly referred to by its initials, DTaP (aP stands for acellular pertussis). The primary schedule consists of three immunizations given several months apart in the first year of life.

Pediatrix vaccine is a combination of DTaP, polio, and hepatitis B. A booster shot should be given one year after completing the initial series. An additional booster shot should be given when the child enters school at 11–12 years and every 10 years thereafter.

Tetanus (Lockjaw)

Nature of the Illness. Tetanus is a dangerous illness. The tetanus bacterium and its spores are found everywhere. They are present in dust, soil, pastures, and human and animal wastes. Symptoms consist of severe muscle spasms, often of the neck and jaw muscles, causing lockjaw. The symptoms are caused by a toxin produced by the tetanus bacterium. Tetanus bacteria grow only in the absence of air, so wounds that are created by punctures or sharp objects, possibly introducing bacteria underneath the skin, are most likely to cause tetanus. After tetanus develops, it may be treated with antibiotics and tetanus immune globulin, but mortality may be as high as 40%. Tetanus can and should be prevented by immunization.

Nature of the Immunization. The tetanus immunization is a toxin produced by the tetanus bacterium and modified in the laboratory so that it has very little of its toxic potential. Local reactions are rare and usually cause only mild discomfort for a short time.

Of all the vaccines available, tetanus comes closest to 100% effectiveness after the initial series of shots. Tetanus shots are needed only every 10 years after the initial series unless a particularly dirty wound is suffered. (See Does My Child Need a Tetanus Shot?, page 262.) The vaccine is part of the DTaP combination, which also immunizes against diphtheria and pertussis.

Pertussis (Whooping Cough)

Nature of the Illness. Pertussis is a bacterial infection that still occurs in thousands of children each year. It is the only vaccine-preventable disease that is increasing. It has a high mortality rate among young infants. Pertussis causes extremely long and severe bouts of coughing. The prolonged coughing so robs the child of air that he or she breathes in violently, causing a whooping sound. Pertussis is contagious. Treating with antibiotics can stop the spread.

Nature of the Immunization. Pertussis vaccine has been administered since the late 1940s. For years, the only available pertussis vaccine (DTP) consisted of killed pertussis bacteria. Many minor reactions were common with this vaccine. About half of all children developed a fever. A similar number experienced pain or fretfulness.

Concerns about the safety of this pertussis vaccine led to the development of our current vaccine, called the "acellular" pertussis vaccine (DTaP), which is not made from whole pertussis bacteria cells. This vaccine works well and produces only half the local and nervous system reactions as the whole-cell vaccine. There is also about a 50% reduction in the number of children who develop a fever. A new preparation of Tdap (Boostrix) is now given routinely to 11–12 year olds.

Polio

Nature of the Illness. Polio is a contagious viral illness and a devastating disease that was familiar to almost everyone a few decades ago. Besides the paralytic form, which crippled tens of thousands and caused more than 1,000 deaths annually as recently as the 1950s, polio also causes meningitis and respiratory infections. No antibiotics are effective against polio. The only way to prevent polio is through immunization.

Nature of the Immunization. In 1955, Dr. Jonas Salk introduced the inactivated poliovirus vaccine (IPV). This injected vaccine caused a dramatic decline in the frequency of polio in this country. In 1961, the Sabin vaccine was introduced, in which live poliovirus was prepared in such a way as to markedly weaken it. This live poliovirus vaccine was known as the oral poliovirus vaccine (OPV) because it could be taken by mouth.

The only problem with the OPV was its rare side effects. One or 2 people in 10 million will develop paralytic polio either because of receiving the oral vaccine or by coming in contact with a person who recently received it. Consequently, in the year 2000 the American Academy of Pediatrics (AAP) and the Centers for Disease Control (CDC) recommended exclusive use of IPV in the United States. The IPV is not known to cause paralytic polio; the OPV is no longer available.

Measles

Nature of the Illness. Measles, one of the "usual" childhood diseases, is now quite rare. Before the 1966 introduction of an improved measles vaccination, there were 400 deaths annually due to measles. Far more often than causing death, measles caused devastating complications, such as brain infections, pneumonia, convulsions, and blindness.

Despite the extraordinary success of measles immunization programs, several hundred cases are still reported annually, and there are periodic outbreaks. A resurgence of measles occurred in 1990, with nearly 30,000 cases and 130 deaths reported. The disease spread because there are still many unvaccinated people and because the vaccine given at 15 months is only 95% effective. Consequently, it is recommended that children receive a second dose, and most college entrants will be required to have documentation of two doses.

Even uncomplicated cases of measles can be serious. (See Measles, page 422.) Fortunately, most infants are protected against measles during the first few months of life because of antibodies they received from their mothers' blood (if the mothers have had measles). This immunity wears off by the fourth month of life.

Nature of the Immunization. The most widely used vaccine today is the Schwarz strain, which causes a rash in an estimated 5% of children and a fever in an estimated 15%. There has been concern over the possibility of allergic reactions in children allergic to eggs or the antibiotic neomycin. Consult with your doctor about allergy testing before the immunization if your child has had these reactions. Symptoms generally consist of fever, mild irritability, or rash and may not appear for 5 to 10 days. Overall reactions to the measles vaccine have been minimal.

The vaccine is most effective when given after the first year of life. Current recommendations are to immunize children initially at age 12 to 15 months, with a second dose at 4 to 6 years. Measles vaccine is combined with mumps and rubella in the MMR vaccine.

Rubella (German Measles)

Nature of the Illness. Rubella is a mild illness, usually with a mild fever and a mild rash. Many people do not even know they have the illness. The danger from rubella lies in the risk to a developing fetus during early pregnancy.

In 1964, during the last rubella epidemic in this country, more than 20,000 children were born with deformities caused by the rubella virus. The deformities included heart defects, blindness, and deafness. Many fetuses escape these devastating effects, but the large number who have suffered greatly make efforts to eliminate this disease worthwhile.

Nature of the Immunization. The purpose of a rubella immunization program is to prevent pregnant women from becoming infected. Before rubella immunization became possible in 1969, more than 80% of women had already been infected and therefore were not at risk of producing an infant deformed by rubella. Women who have had rubella infections can become reinfected with rubella a second, third, or even fourth time. It is doubtful, however, that these reinfections pose any threat to the fetus.

Rubella vaccination has resulted in a 99% reduction of rubella among children and newborns. Rubella is combined with measles and mumps vaccines in the MMR vaccine, given at 12 to 15 months. A second dose is given at 4 to 6 years.

Mumps

Nature of the Illness. Mumps is a contagious viral illness. It infects and causes swelling of the salivary glands. Swelling can be on one or both sides and is often painful. Meningoencephalitis (inflammation of the brain and its coverings) occurs but is far less frequent and less serious than with measles. The greatest concern with mumps is the possibility of inflammation of the testes in males and of the ovaries in females. Inflammation of the ovaries is far less frequent than inflammation of the testes. Inflammation of the testes is usually one-sided. Although it is commonly believed that the inflammation can result in sterility, this is very seldom the case.

Nature of the Immunization. The mumps vaccine is a live weakened virus. Exposure to the mumps virus usually gives two types of protection: one carried by the blood serum antibodies, and the other carried by the white blood cells. Mumps immunization provides protection through the blood serum antibodies for at least 12 years and possibly much longer.

Infants should be immunized at 12 to 15 months for mumps, measles, and rubella with the MMR vaccine. Children are immunized again at 4 to 6 years.

Hemophilus Influenzae Type B

Nature of the Illness. *Hemophilus influenzae* type B (HIB) is a bacterium capable of causing serious illnesses such as meningitis, epiglottitis, and arthritis in young children. Most of these serious infections occur in the first four years of life. A considerable number of deaths and permanently damaged children have resulted from HIB. A major breakthrough in the control of this leading cause of meningitis in young children occurred in 1985 with the release of a vaccine. As a result, serious infections from HIB have plummeted. Once the leading cause of meningitis in young children, it is now rarely responsible for such serious infections.

Nature of the Immunization. The vaccine is made from a purified chemical that is part of the bacterium's capsule. The presence of this chemical tricks the immune system into mounting a response that is reasonably effective in preventing future infections with HIB. To enhance effectiveness, the newest version of the vaccine is linked (conjugated) to other proteins. These conjugate vaccines are effective for preventing disease in young infants. The HIB vaccine is often combined with the hepatitis B vaccine in one immunization.

Pneumococcal Disease

Nature of the Illness. The pneumococcus bacterium is responsible for some common infections, such as ear infections, as well as some more severe diseases, such as pneumonia and meningitis. There are many strains of pneumococcus, making immunization difficult. For years a polysaccharide vaccine was used for some children, including those with sickle-cell disease or immune deficiency, who were particularly susceptible to serious pneumococcal infections; however, it was not very successful in children younger than two years. All children were at risk of meningitis from pneumococcal disease and several thousand cases occurred each year. Fortunately, a new pneumococcal (conjugate) vaccine licensed in 2000 greatly reduced cases of serious disease, and all children should receive it starting at two months. Some children older than two years may need the vaccine for some chronic illnesses.

Nature of the Immunization. The vaccine for young children is a protein conjugate vaccine (PCV). It protects against meningitis and other serious infections and has few side effects. Older children with certain conditions may need the pneumococcal polysaccharide vaccine (PPSV).

Hepatitis B

Nature of the Illness. There are many types of hepatitis. All are infections of the liver and result in jaundice (yellowing of the whites of the eyes and the skin), nausea, and weakness. Most children recover, but some develop chronic liver problems. Each year the hepatitis B virus causes infection in more than 200,000 people in the United States, and 4,000 to 5,000 people die as a result of chronic problems from hepatitis B. This virus is acquired principally through contact with infected blood or from intimate contact of moist body surfaces, as during sexual intercourse. Infants can be exposed to hepatitis B as they are born. Therefore mothers are tested during pregnancy. Infants and children may also get it from close contact with family members.

Nature of the Immunization. In November 1991, the Advisory Committee on Immunization Practices of the Centers for Disease Control and Prevention recommended vaccination of all infants in the United States. One dose is given in the first 2 months after birth, a second dose 1 to 3 months later, and a final dose at least 2 months after the first but not before age 6 months. (Special policies apply to infants of mothers found to have certain markers for hepatitis B in their blood during routine prenatal screening.)

For children who were not immunized as newborns, vaccinations can start at any age. As the principal way to acquire the infection is through sexual intercourse, we strongly support immunization prior to the time when some adolescents become sexually active.

Vaccines for children are now available for hepatitis A (a liver infection not quite as serious as hepatitis B). Hepatitis A vaccine is now recommended for all children between 12 and 23 months. Two doses are required, at least six months apart. Your physician or health department can advise if additional shots are needed in your area.

Chicken Pox

Nature of the Illness. Chicken pox, generally a mild viral illness of childhood, produces a rash and slight fever. In rare instances, it can be complicated by more serious problems such as arthritis, meningitis, pneumonia, Reye syndrome, or bacterial infection. Chicken pox is considered serious because some of these bacterial infections, especially streptococcal infections, have caused deaths in children, with more than 40 deaths annually.

Nature of the Immunization. A live-virus vaccine was recommended for routine use in 1996. Concern had been expressed that immunity might decrease after many years, making adults more susceptible to the illness. Although this was a legitimate concern, there is as yet no evidence that it will happen. Current recommendations call for all children to be immunized with two doses after 12 months of age. Because this vaccine contains a live virus, it is not recommended for children who take high levels of steroid medications for asthma or other conditions or children with other immunodeficiencies.

Influenza

Nature of the Illness. Influenza is a respiratory tract infection caused by the influenza virus, which produces severe muscular symptoms as well. Many illnesses may mimic influenza, and the term *influenza* (or "the flu") is applied liberally to those involving coughs, colds, and muscle aches.

Nature of the Immunization. Influenza virus vaccines are live weakened virus vaccines. Each year's vaccine represents the most likely strains to cause infection during the coming "flu season"; hence the vaccine is given every year. Influenza virus vaccines are currently recommended for all children after 6 months of age, pregnant women, and close contacts of young children and the elderly (family members, hospital staff, nursing care staff). They also are recommended for children with chronic illnesses, particularly respiratory illnesses such as asthma, and cardiac disease. The influenza vaccine is available in two forms—a shot and nasal spray. The nasal spray can be given to healthy children over age 5. If your child is under age 7 and has never received the influenza vaccine, he or she will get two doses one month apart.

Smallpox

Smallpox, a disease that has killed millions of people over the centuries, has been eliminated through immunization. Smallpox vaccinations are no longer given. (See also "Parenting in an Age of Bioterrorism," page 23.)

Meningococcal Disease

Nature of the Illness. Meningococcus is a bacterium that causes meningitis as well as a widespread blood infection. The latter often ends in shock death. Fortunately, the disease is rare, but outbreaks do occur.

Nature of the Immunization. The vaccine consists of purified parts of the bacterium's cell wall. It is now recommended for children older than 11 years and is often required for college admission.

Rotavirus

Nature of the Illness. Rotavirus is a very common cause of gastroenteritis and infects the majority of children in the United States before age five years. In addition to diarrhea most children will have vomiting and half will develop fever. It is more severe than other causes of viral diarrhea, and an estimated 1 in 70 infected children will require hospitalization.

Nature of the Immunization. The immunization is a "reassortant" virus that was created by combining portions of nucleic acid from 5 different parent rotavirus strains. Unlike a previous immunization for rotavirus (RotaShield), the current vaccine (RotaTeq and Rotarix) has not been complicated by an increased rate of intestinal blockage (intussusception) in infants. It is administered orally at 2, 4, and 6 months.

Human Papilloma Virus

Nature of the Illness. Human papilloma virus (HPV) infection is very common and the majority of women in the United States will have been infected by age 50. There are many strains of HPV and most will not cause serious illness. However some strains are responsible for cervical cancer while others cause genital warts. Like most sexually transmitted infections, prevention is possible through safer sex practices. In addition, routine Pap smears will allow early detection of pre-cancerous lesions that should allow for stopping the advancement of cervical cancer. Despite the widespread availability of routine pap smears, adherence to medical recommendations is variable and there are over 9,000 cases of invasive cervical cancer in the United States each year, with more than 3500 deaths.

Nature of the Immunization. In 2006 the FDA approved the licensure of a vaccine (Gardasil) effective against four strains of HPV, and the national Advisory Committee on Immunization Practices (ACIP) recommended three doses for girls over age 9 years. Two of the strains are estimated to be responsible for 70% of worldwide cervical cancer cases, and two of the strains are responsible for the vast majority of genital warts. The vaccine was documented to be effective in preventing pre-cancerous lesions and presumably cervical cancer. The vaccine is prepared similarly to hepatitis B vaccine and consists only of virus protein particles and not a whole virus.

As this is a relatively new vaccine questions continue to be asked about the occurrence of rare adverse effects. (In 1998 the FDA approved RotaShield vaccine against rotavirus as safe and effective but after widespread use it was shown to cause intestinal blockage—intussusception—and was withdrawn in 1999). In addition it is clear the vaccine is not effective for 30% of the cases responsible for cervical cancer, its duration of protection is unknown as the study used to obtain approval was 15 months long, it is unknown whether there will be a shift in the epidemiology of the virus or changes in sexual behavior of recipients. For all of these reasons, as well as the availability of other preventive measures for avoiding cervical cancer, many parents and teenagers have elected not to be immunized against HPV.

Immunization Schedule

Figure 9.1 lists the current immunization schedule of the CDC, AAP, and AAFP. In addition, children who are not immunized according to schedule can catch up at any time. This is especially important after age 2 for hepatitis B, tetanus-diphtheria, MMR, chicken pox, and pneumococcal disease. (Also see www.cdc.gov/vaccines.)

Figure 9.1: Immunization Schedule

Vaccine	Age (months)									Age (years)		
	Birth	1	2	4	6	12	15	18	24	4–6	11–12	13–18
Hepatitis B	Hep B	Hep B			Hep B							
Diphtheria, tetanus, and pertussis			DTaP	DTaP	DTaP		DTaP			DTaP	Tdap	
Hemophilus influenzae type B			HIB	HIB	HIB	HIB						
Poliovirus			Polio	Polio	Polio					Polio		
Pneumococcus			PCV	PCV	PCV	PCV			PPSV			
Rotavirus			RV	RV	RV							
Measles-mumps-rubella						MMR				MMR		
Chicken pox (varicella)						Chicken pox				Ch. pox		
Meningococcus										Meningo-coccus		Meningo-coccus
Hepatitis A						Hep A		Hep A				
Influenza					Influenza (yearly)							

Range of acceptable ages for vaccination

Vaccines may not be needed; check with your doctor

Adapted from the Centers for Disease Control, United States Public Health Service

Allergies

Allergies, with some exceptions, do not pose the serious health threat presented by the viral and bacterial illnesses discussed in the previous section. Still, the chronic nature of allergies can make them a lifelong health concern for sufferers. And asthma, which is often an allergic response, is a major—and potentially deadly—health concern. Although there is no vaccine to eliminate allergies, prevention and relief of symptoms are possible.

Allergy was first described at the turn of the century by a pediatrician named Clemens von Pirquet. The term *allergy* means "changed activity" and describes changes that occur after a person comes in contact with a foreign substance. Pirquet noticed two types of change.

▲ One change is beneficial: the development of protection against a foreign substance after having been exposed to it. This response provides the scientific basis for most immunizations. The protection our body gains from our first exposure to a substance prevents us from developing an infectious disease when we're exposed to the substance a second time.

▲ The other type of response is known as a hypersensitivity response. It is generally not beneficial and is the response for which the term *allergy* is generally used.

A hypersensitivity response is possible even on the first exposure to a substance, and all persons are capable of allergic responses. For example, anyone given a transfusion with the wrong type of blood will have an allergic reaction.

However, the term *allergy* is overused. When your eyes smart in a smoggy city, they are not allergic to the air but are experiencing a direct chemical irritation from the pollutants. Similarly, skin coming in contact with some plants or chemicals may be directly damaged; this is not an allergic response. Doctors often blame a milk or food allergy for vomiting, diarrhea, colic, crying, irritability, fretfulness, or sneezing in infants. Although allergies can cause these symptoms, so can countless other things.

Over the next few pages, we discuss common allergies (such as those to foods, insects, drugs, pets, pollens, and dust), common allergic problems (such as asthma, hay fever, hives, and other skin problems), and medical treatments available.

Food Allergy

Almost any food can produce an allergic response. Only breast milk appears to be incapable of causing an allergy. Even in this case, certain foods in a mother's diet may be detected in the breast milk and can cause an allergy in an infant.

There are many causes of digestive upset in children, however, and food allergy is blamed for much that it does not cause. For example, some children are born without an important digestive enzyme known as lactase, which is necessary to digest the sugars present in milk. Other children lose the ability to make lactase after the age of three or four. The absence of lactase can produce diarrhea, abdominal pain, bloating, and vomiting after a child drinks milk. This is only one example of a digestive problem that can be confused with food allergy. There are many others.

Symptoms of Food Allergy

Food allergy may produce swelling of the mouth and lips, hives, skin rashes, vomiting, diarrhea, bloody stools (feces), asthma, runny nose, and shock (extremely rare). Of course, many other allergens besides food can cause these problems, making it difficult to prove that a particular food is the culprit. The best approach for detecting food allergy is for the parent to think like Sherlock Holmes. If your child's lips swell only after eating strawberries, you have your suspect.

If several foods are suspected, eliminate them all from the diet, then add them back one at a time and watch your child for a reaction. If eliminating the suspect foods will prevent your child from having a balanced diet, consult your doctor about a plan of action.

Foods Responsible for Allergy

As infant formula is based on cow's milk, it has been blamed for (but infrequently linked to) almost every symptom in infants, including allergy.

Cow's milk does cause allergic responses in some infants, with diarrhea and even bloody stools. This situation is a clear indication for the removal of cow's milk if the severe diarrhea is documented by a doctor through tests analyzing the stools (feces). These tests are simple and should be repeated after the child has been taken off cow's milk. Sometimes a repeat challenge with milk is suggested to see if symptoms recur.

Controversy exists over the relationship between early exposure to cow's milk and the later development of asthma. Some doctors maintain that avoidance of cow's milk will delay or eliminate the development of asthma. Cow's milk may have some effects on children likely to develop allergies but probably should not be of particular concern for children with no family histories of allergy. As discussed on page 53, hydrolyzed formulas may benefit infants from families with allergic disorders.

Other foods that have been associated with allergic reactions in children include wheat, eggs, citrus fruits, beef and veal, fish, and nuts. Severe reactions are very rare in children; parents need not be anxious about giving their children new foods. A family with a strong history of allergy can introduce new foods to an infant once every few days so that if an allergy develops, the cause is obvious.

Soybean Substitutes for Milk

The amount of soybean formula produced in this country exceeds the amount necessary to provide for children with cow's milk allergy or an intolerance to cow's milk because of the lack of lactase. There are two possible reasons to buy soybean preparations. First, parents may buy these products because they like them. They are nutritious and an excellent source of iron, and children tolerate them well. However, they tend to be more expensive than cow's milk. The other reason for the high consumption of soybean formula may be that parents have been instructed to substitute it for cow's milk formula at the slightest suspicion of an allergy.

Many stories of children getting better on a soybean preparation result from the child's spontaneous recovery from whatever was producing the troublesome symptom—rarely cow's milk allergy. If you wish, you can switch back to a cow's milk formula to see if symptoms recur. If they do, a soybean formula is probably warranted. (Also see "Bottle Feeding," pages 52–53.)

Asthma

No Smoking!

Asthma is a potentially severe disorder that is often triggered by an allergic response as well as by other "triggers," including viruses, mold, and changes in temperature. Asthma is characterized by the following changes in the lungs.

▲ Swelling of the air passages
▲ Spasm of the muscles in the walls of the smaller air passages in the lungs
▲ Excess production of mucus

The swelling and muscle spasms cause asthma's most prominent symptom, wheezing. (See Wheezing, page 354.) All wheezing in children is potentially serious and should be evaluated by a medical professional, at least for the first few occurrences. The swelling and mucus production of asthma further narrow the air passages. This can aggravate the difficulty of getting air out of the lungs and also cause a troublesome cough.

Asthma tends to occur in families where other members have asthma, hay fever, or eczema.

An asthma attack can be triggered by irritants, such as cigarette smoke, an infection, a change in weather, an emotionally upsetting event, exercise, or exposure to an allergen. Common allergens include house dust, dust mites, pollens, molds, foods, shed animal materials ("animal danders"), and even insects such as cockroaches. It is sometimes easy to identify airborne allergens to which a person is susceptible. Some children will wheeze only around cats, others only during a particular pollen season. (Pollens usually cause seasonal hay fever, or *allergic rhinitis*, rather than asthma.) Most often there is no clear reason for a particular asthmatic attack. If asthma is severe, it is desirable to identify the offending allergens if possible.

Infections (see Wheezing, page 354) and foreign bodies in the air passages can mimic asthma.

Treating asthma involves a partnership consisting of you, your doctor, and your child. You should see your physician at least once a year to review your child's asthma management plan, or more often depending on the severity of the child's case. Everyone should understand his or her part in managing this chronic condition. Children should be given jobs appropriate to their age. Younger children should report symptoms promptly. Older children may be responsible for taking medicines.

The increase in asthma in the United States has led to widespread media coverage. This increase has also led to a proliferation of education programs, many of which are excellent. Talk with your physician about education resources. Be wary of the several hundred thousand items now on the Internet—their quality varies.

The treatment of asthma depends on the severity of the problem. Some children have only one or two episodes of asthma and are never troubled again. Other children have daily attacks, which severely compromise their growth, development, and ability to function well in school and at home.

Some doctors maintain that children never truly outgrow asthma, but the evidence suggests otherwise. More than half of the children diagnosed as having asthma will never have an asthmatic attack as adults. Another 10% will have only occasional attacks during their adult lives.

Therapy provides relief of symptoms, often dramatically so, but it also must work to remove the cause, be it allergic, infectious, or emotional. Our approach to asthma involves three components: allergen avoidance, physical control, and medication.

Allergen Avoidance

Occasionally, an offending allergen, or "trigger," is easy to identify. More often no offender is found, and a general approach to reducing allergen exposure is advisable. A relatively clean and dust-free house is all but essential for the allergic person. An asthmatic child's room should be particularly allergen-free, because sleeping requires 8 to 10 hours in the room. **Plastic covers on the mattress and pillow case are essential.** We do not recommend changing the entire household furnishings to reduce allergen exposure, except in severe cases. Even then, removal of items should progress on a rational basis after suspected allergens have been identified.

Rugs, furniture, drapes, bedspreads, and other items that are particular dust catchers should be vacuumed regularly. We are very concerned about old carpets in children's rooms. If you have finished flooring beneath wall-to-wall carpeting, we suggest that you get rid of the rug.

Clothing attracts dust, pollen, and other troublesome particles. Keeping nonseasonal clothing outside your child's room or in plastic storage containers may be helpful.

Children and pets may do fine together, although it is best not to allow pets to sleep in an allergic child's room.

Toy animals should be kept clean. Washable ones are best. A home without stuffed animals seems to some like a morning without sunshine and orange juice, but avoid products that may be stuffed with animal hair.

Change heating and air conditioner filters regularly.

Irritants. Other important causes of asthma include tobacco smoke and air pollution. Children with asthma should live in a smoke-free environment. There should be absolutely no smoking at home, and your child should avoid all public places where smoking is permitted.

Other Factors. Aspirin can trigger asthma. We no longer recommend aspirin for children.

Viral infections are responsible for many asthma attacks. We recommend an annual flu shot for children with chronic asthma.

Because infections can trigger asthma, a physical examination is important during the first attack or any frequently recurring attacks. Antibiotics should not be given unless a bacterial infection is found.

Physical Control

Exercise can trigger asthma in some individuals, especially in sports that call for sudden bursts of energy. Warming up slowly before playing and staying in good physical condition can minimize the wheezing caused by exercise.

Asthmatics can participate in athletics. Athletes with asthma have been Olympic gold medal winners in sports ranging from swimming to the heptathlon. Swimming appears to be far and away the best exercise and best sport for the asthmatic child. Exercise programs with long and steady energy requirements, such as swimming, seem to work best for asthmatics. In addition, swimmers come into contact with far fewer allergens than do participants in most other sports. There are also excellent medications that children can take immediately prior to exercise to control wheezing.

Medication

Prevention (Controller) Medication. For children who wheeze only occasionally (once a week or less) and seldom wake at night (once a week or less), no daily preventive medicine is required. Children troubled by symptoms two or more times a week should take regular preventive medications.

Several drugs are currently used daily to prevent asthma attacks. In general, these drugs control the swelling (inflammation) of the air passages. Most are inhaled directly into the lungs. Corticosteroids (different from steroids used illegally by some athletes), the most commonly used preventive medicines, are inhaled into the lungs and do not have the same risks as steroids taken by mouth. Inhaled corticosteroids include beclamethasone (Beclovent, QVar, Vanceril), budesonide (Pulmicort), triamcinolone (Azmacort), fluticosone (Flovent), and flunisolide (AeroBid). Some physicians prefer to start with cromolyn or nedocromil because they are so safe, though they are less effective and require more frequent administration. A new group of medicines known as leukotriene modifiers are considered an alternative to the above drugs. Zafirlukast (Accolate) is now available for children over 12 and montelukast (Singulaire) for children over 6. For more severe asthmatics, the dosages of the above drugs are increased or several drugs are given together. Sometimes prevention medications are combined with quick-relief drugs.

Quick-relief Medication. Drugs that open the air passages are known as bronchodilators. Some of these quick-relief medications (methylxanthines such as theophylline) have been used for more than 75 years. But the current approach calls for using a type of drug known as a beta agonist. Among these highly effective inhalants are metaproterenol (Alupent), albuterol (Proventil, Ventolin), and levalbuterol (Xopenex).

Older children can be trained to use handheld metered-dose inhalers. These should be used with a spacer device. Younger children may need to use plastic inhaling chambers or nebulization machines.

Quick-relief *oral* drugs are of two types: beta agonist drugs, such as metaproterenol (Alupent) and albuterol (Proventil, Ventolin), and theophylline. These drugs are accompanied by more side effects than inhalants, are seldom used, and are no longer recommended.

Combination products (controller and quick-relief) also are available. These include fluticasonel salmeterol (Advair) and budesonide/formoterol (Symbicort).

Antihistamines are not useful in asthma, and their drying effect may cause plugging of the airway.

Always obtain a written Asthma Action Plan from your doctor so you know how to adjust medicines. Also see www.nhlbi.nih.gov/health/prof/lung/asthma.

Supportive Therapy. Severe asthma is stressful for parents and other family members, as well as for the affected child. Assistance is often required to manage the emotional consequences of asthma for the whole family. Do not hesitate to seek this assistance. Social workers and other counselors can be invaluable resources.

Allergic Rhinitis

Allergic rhinitis is the most common allergic problem. A stuffy, runny nose; watery, itchy eyes; headache; and sneezing are all common symptoms. The cause in infants is often dust or food, and in adults dust or pollen. Most individuals are troubled only in pollen season. Ragweed, the cause of hay fever, is particularly troublesome. The problem seems to run in families.

Treatment is directed toward both symptomatic relief and avoidance of the offending allergen. The first line of symptomatic relief is the use of tissues or handkerchiefs, but often this is not enough. Drugs that can reduce symptoms may be prescribed or purchased over the counter, but may have side effects.

Antihistamines block the action of histamine, a substance released during allergic reactions. They have a drying effect and reduce nasal stuffiness. They also may be useful in reducing itching, helping motion sickness, and decreasing vomiting. The antihistamines used most often in allergic rhinitis are either "first generation," such as diphenhydramine (Benadryl) and chlorpheniramine maleate (Chlor-Trimeton); or "second generation," such as loratadine (Claritin), fexofenadine (Allegra), or cetirizine (Zyrtec). The second generation drugs cause less drowsiness and have become less expensive since being available over the counter. Individuals respond differently to different drugs, and a trial of the different types of antihistamines may be necessary to determine the most effective type for your child.

The most common side effect of antihistamines is drowsiness, which may interfere with a child's schoolwork. Antihistamines should not be used as sleeping pills, because the drowsiness they produce decreases the amount of deep sleep necessary for normal rest.

For severe cases, nasal sprays containing steroids, cromolyn, or antihistamines may be recommended.

Eczema

Atopic dermatitis, commonly known as eczema, is an allergic skin condition characterized by dry, itching skin. Itching often leads to scratching. The scratching then produces weeping, infected skin, which dries and crusts. This weeping and crusting condition is what doctors refer to as eczema. Sufficient scratching will produce a thickened, rough skin, which is characteristic of long-standing atopic dermatitis.

Atopic dermatitis runs in families with asthma and allergic rhinitis. Like asthma, a variety of conditions can aggravate it. These conditions include infection, emotional stress, food allergy, and sweating.

Infants seldom exhibit any signs of this problem at birth. The first signs may be red, chapped cheeks. Often infants rub these itchy areas.

As the child grows older, atopic dermatitis can change location. It may be found on the backs of the legs and fronts of the arms. Adults often have problems with their hands. This is especially true of people whose hands are in frequent contact with water, which tends to have a drying effect on the skin and thus aggravates the cycle.

Therapy is based on the avoidance of allergens and good skin care. Following are some specific tips.

▲ Avoid wool, which tends to aggravate itching.

▲ Avoid excessively warm clothing, which will cause sweat retention and aggravate itching.

▲ Keep the child's fingernails clipped short.

▲ In moderate to severe cases, avoid bathing the child with soap and water, because these tend to dry the skin. Instead, use nonlipid cleansers. Some cleansers with cetyl alcohol, such as Cetaphil lotion, prevent drying of the skin.

▲ When inflammation is prominent (the skin is red and oozing), apply a wet dressing of Burow's solution or give a total-body oatmeal (Aveeno) bath.

▲ Avoid all oil or grease preparations. They occlude the skin and increase sweat retention and itching.

▲ Apply lubricating lotions to dry skin. You can make your own by combining Crisco and glycerin, or you can purchase Keri, Cetaphil, Aveeno, Lubriderm, or Aquaphor (lotions), Keri or Nivea (creams), or Eucerin (creamy paste).

▲ Avoiding cow's milk is often suggested. Make sure this works for your child before permanently changing to a more expensive substitute. When putting your child on any milk-avoidance diet, make no other changes in food or other care for a full two weeks unless absolutely necessary.

Itching is often worse at bedtime. Antihistamines reduce itching but should be used only if necessary.

Steroid creams also are useful against itching. Steroids should be used only as long as needed. Weaker preparations are used on the face.

Other prescription creams such as pimecrolemus (Elidel) and tacrolimus (Protopic) have been linked to skin cancer and we do not recommend them.

Antibiotics are often necessary to clear up badly infected skin. There is no benefit from either skin testing or hyposensitization.

Emotional factors may need attention and may be the key to successful therapy.

For more information on treating eczema, see Eczema, page 388.

Allergy Testing and Shots

The purpose of allergy testing is to help the doctor decide what is causing the allergy. Skin testing and RAST tests are both sensitive ways to check for allergies. An allergy test is not a treatment, and it is not always accurate. Once the results of an allergy test are positive, the doctor must choose between two treatment approaches: avoidance and hyposensitization (desensitization).

Avoidance is sometimes, though not usually, possible. Seldom is a child allergic to cats and nothing else, and usually such an isolated allergy is noted by alert parents and children without testing. Avoiding dust, pollen, trees, and flowers is next to impossible, so hyposensitization is sometimes reasonable if the problem is severe.

Hyposensitization involves injecting a tiny amount of the offending allergen into the child. Gradually larger and larger amounts are injected until the child is able to tolerate exposure to the allergen with only mild symptoms.

Hyposensitization works in many cases, but several problems may arise. Local reactions at the site of the injection are common but can be minimized by injecting the allergen through a different needle from the one used to withdraw the material from the bottle.

Hyposensitization requires weekly injections for months or years. It may be considered for children with moderate or severe asthma or severe hay fever, but it is probably unwarranted for children with mild asthma or mild allergic rhinitis.

Dental Care

Helping your child establish good dental hygiene practices at a young age is a highly valuable prevention measure. Dental neglect will lead to a lifetime of painful, expensive, and often embarrassing problems—all of them preventable. Just a few good dental habits will reward your child with better health and a better quality of life.

Children's teeth begin forming during the fetal stage. The mother's diet provides the essential nutrients for tooth development. Calcium and phosphorus are the basic building blocks of teeth and are found abundantly in milk and dairy products. Vitamins C and D are also important, as are small amounts of the element fluoride. Drugs, especially tetracycline, should be avoided during pregnancy partly because they may stain or weaken teeth.

Teething

In teething, children instinctively seek hard surfaces against which to rub their gums. Most children begin teething actions several months before the eruption of the first tooth. The first tooth usually appears on the lower jaw and is one of the front teeth, known as incisors. These incisors appear in most children by 8 months of age, but teething may begin as early as 4 months or as late as 15 months. Usually, the two lower central incisors come first, followed by the four upper incisors. Many children will have these six teeth in place shortly after their first birthdays. The next teeth, appearing between 18 and 24 months, are the first four molars and the remaining two bottom incisors. Before the child's second birthday, the pointed teeth, also known as the canine teeth, usually appear between the incisors and the molars. After the child is 2 years of age, the remainder of the first set of teeth, the last four molars, appear.

Many parents wonder about massaging children's gums before their teeth erupt. There is some evidence that the bacteria that cause tooth decay will stick to gums less often if the gums are gently massaged.

The eruption of teeth and the practice of teething has led to much folk wisdom. Some is accurate, but there are common misconceptions. For example, teething does not usually cause a high fever. Children experience many mild viral infections within the first three years of life, and some of these infections will occur simultaneously with the eruption of teeth and during periods of increased teething activity. Teething hurts, but it is not the cause of high fevers, extreme irritability, or a marked change in your child's daily activities.

Teething is important and necessary and can be done on almost any hard rubber object. Certain pacifiers, such as the Nuk pacifier, can be used in teething infants and may have the advantage of ensuring proper tongue thrust for proper jaw development. Parents should be careful to avoid cleaning a dropped pacifier by sucking it clean; transferring your mouth bacteria to your infant can cause tooth decay.

Children should never be allowed to teethe on a bottle full of milk. Milk is for the feeding of young infants and not for pacification or teething. Major problems may be caused by allowing an infant to fall asleep with a bottle of milk in his or her mouth. The milk will remain in constant contact with the teeth, providing an ideal setup for tooth decay. Studies also have shown that children who lie flat in bed with a bottle in their mouths drain some milk into their eustachian tubes and consequently may experience a higher incidence of ear infections.

Tooth Decay

Although dental problems are less dramatic than some other health problems, they remain a serious concern, because they are the most frequent health problems in children. Virtually every child in this country will need dental work at some point. More than 25 million adults in the United States have no teeth at all. Dental cavities (caries) and, more important, gum disease can be prevented.

Genetics is one important factor in the development of cavities. People who have never had a cavity should in part thank their parents. More important than what we acquire from our parents, however, is what we do to ourselves. If our teeth never came in contact with food, our teeth would never develop cavities. Given that all of us do eat, it is important to know the components of food that cause tooth decay: sugar and starch. Normal mouth bacteria require sugar and starch to survive. An excess amount of these bacteria can lead to rapid decay, as they produce an acid that is capable of eating through the hard enamel that covers our teeth.

Once the bacteria have eaten through the enamel, they set up housekeeping inside the soft portion of the tooth. They are extremely resourceful and can live quite well in the absence of air. But they still need sugar and starch to survive. Their food supply now has to come to them. Only sugar and starch in extremely minute, dissolved form can enter a small hole in the surface of the enamel. That is why highly refined sugar is such a problem in fostering tooth decay. We now eat more than 15 times as much refined sugar as people did a century ago. A lost "baby" tooth placed in a glass of sugary soda will dissolve almost overnight! A certain amount of the acid that mouth bacteria produce is neutralized by our saliva. This is why our teeth do not rot quite as quickly from drinking soda as they do when allowed to sit in it overnight.

A sound program of cleaning teeth to remove trapped food particles is critical. This includes brushing, flossing, and using a water jet. Finally, a diet that is high in roughage provides us with a natural toothbrush. It is the custom in many European countries to serve the salad at the end of the meal. This makes good sense, because salad serves as a natural toothbrush and clears away the sugars.

Brushing Your Child's Teeth

Brushing should begin whenever your child seems receptive. Most children will enjoy brushing their teeth with their parents during the imitative years (from age one on). A two-year-old will not be very proficient at brushing his or her teeth and will need help from Mom or Dad. By age three and one-half, however, children will have acquired the fine skills necessary for doing a good job by themselves. Parents can help by encouraging brushing as a family activity and regarding tooth care as a pleasurable experience, not a chore.

Choice of Toothpaste

Several toothpastes have been recommended by the American Dental Association (ADA) for their effectiveness in preventing cavities. The potential for preventing cavities lies in the fluoride content of these toothpastes. The fluoride content of our foods and water supplies is slowly increasing, and the importance of using the right toothpaste is slowly diminishing. We still recommend a toothpaste that is ADA approved. Here are some other tips.

▲ So-called glamour toothpastes may contain caustic materials that gradually wear out the tooth enamel.
▲ To reinforce brushing as a pleasurable experience, your child should enjoy the taste of the toothpaste being used.
▲ Watch young children brush, and don't let them swallow or eat toothpaste. Children younger than five are reluctant to spit, so go easy on the toothpaste. If swallowed, this can be a source of excessive fluoride.
▲ Regular nonfluoride brushing is better than sporadic fluoride brushing, but regular fluoride brushing is best.
▲ Soft toothbrushes are preferable.
▲ Although brushing vertically is currently not recommended, it is the thoroughness of the brushing that is most important.

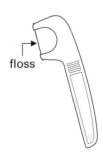

floss

Dental Flossing

Dental floss is an excellent tool for removing particles from between the teeth and encouraging healthy gums. Flossing is now being recommended for children with their first teeth. Floss suspended in special holders can allow parents to floss children's teeth. However, once children have developed their permanent teeth, they should be encouraged to use dental floss. Again, the best way to encourage children to floss is to floss yourself. Dental floss without wax is slightly preferable because particles of wax can become dislodged and remain between the teeth.

Water Jets

Water jets are an effective method of removing particles from between the teeth. Children who don't like dental floss often enjoy using a water jet. Dental floss does a better job of cleaning if it is used correctly, however. Some children are frightened by the noise of the water jet. Allow them time to adjust.

Fluoride

Fluoride is a compound of the natural element fluorine. Fluorine is extremely effective in preventing tooth decay in children. Some people have promoted it as a miracle drug, and others have attacked it because of its potential to cause tooth damage in extremely high doses. Fluoride compounds will decrease, but not eliminate, tooth decay.

Fluoride is found naturally in many water supplies and in many vegetables as well. In addition, most cities and towns in the United States fluoridate their water supplies. Because of these fluoridated water supplies, many packaged and canned foods have measurable amounts of fluoride. Even if your community does not have a fluoridated water supply, you are undoubtedly receiving a fair amount of fluoride in the packaged foods you buy.

Areas Without Fluoridation

In areas where the water supply is not fluoridated, infants should receive prescription fluoride drops starting after 6 months of age. Children between the ages of 3 and 10 years should receive about 1 mg (usually one tablet) of fluoride each day. Fluoride is recommended through age 10 or so, until the permanent teeth are in. Too much fluoride can discolor the teeth, so do not exceed the recommended doses. These doses are slowly being decreased because of the increasing amount of fluoride in packaged foods. Fluoride is a prescription item, and your doctor should be aware of the latest developments in its use.

The First Trip to the Dentist

The time of your child's first visit to the dentist depends on the nature of the child's teeth. Some pediatric dentists recommend 6 months after the first tooth. Examine your child's teeth yourself periodically. It is not difficult to see small holes in the teeth. Usually, teeth will not begin developing cavities before age three. If you think you see holes in your three-year-old's teeth, by all means make a dental appointment. Although baby teeth are lost and replaced by permanent teeth beginning at about age six, severe damage to baby teeth can cause both dental pain and potential loss of adult teeth. Losing baby teeth prematurely may result in permanent teeth coming in crooked. If your child's teeth appear all right, a dental visit may be postponed until age three or so, when the child will be less frightened by the examination. We recommend a yearly visit to the dentist thereafter.

Permanent Teeth

Permanent teeth begin forming in the first few months of life, but they do not erupt until the fifth or sixth year. Permanent teeth arrive in approximately the same order as baby teeth. The number of teeth will increase from 20 primary (baby) teeth to 32 permanent teeth. The eruption of permanent teeth generally does not end until an individual is in his or her 20s and the third molars (wisdom teeth) appear. There is no reason to have wisdom teeth routinely removed. If wisdom teeth become impacted or grow into other teeth, dental care may be necessary, but many people have all 32 teeth.

Additional Reading

One Minute Asthma: What You Need to Know, 8th ed., Thomas F. Plaut (Amherst, Mass.: Pedipress, 2008).

American Academy of Pediatrics Guide to Your Child's Allergies and Asthma. Michael J. Welch, M.D., editor (New York: Villard Books, 2000).

Chapter Ten

Healthy Habits at Home and Away

Good health is a way of life. This chapter presents, as simply and clearly as possible, the groundwork for a healthy life. Some of this information you already know, and much of it you have heard before. The emphasis here, as in the previous chapter, is on prevention. Three areas are discussed.

▲ Injuries
▲ Avoiding adult diseases
▲ Missing children

Injuries and many adult diseases can be effectively prevented. When one considers that injuries are the number one killer of children and teenagers and that AIDS is increasing rapidly among adolescents (the number of cases more than doubled between 1998–2008), the importance of prevention is obvious. As parents, we cannot protect our children from every danger. But by creating the safest possible environment at home; by teaching our children how to limit risky behaviors and observe safety techniques; and by helping them to make good decisions about diet, exercise, and self-protection, we can go a long way toward ensuring that they thrive.

Injuries

Injuries are the number one threat to your child's health. More children are seriously injured or die as a result of accidents than of cancer, infectious diseases, and birth defects combined. In adolescents, injuries and deliberate violence (homicide and suicide) account for more than 70% of deaths.

Household

Young children spend most of their time at home. This provides them with the greatest opportunity for getting into mischief. Playpens may be somewhat restrictive, but they can be an island of safety when you must spend time on the phone or at the front door.

Remember that as children grow, the opportunities for accidents increase. You must keep one step ahead of your child at all times. Before you know it, crawlers become climbers, and they will be able to get up to that previously unreachable cabinet.

Older children should be taught safety responsibility. They should know how and when to dial 911 for emergency assistance. For burns, they should know to plunge the burn into cold water immediately. If on fire, they should not run (which fans and increases the flames), but **stop, drop, and roll** on the floor. Teach them a plan for exiting the house during a fire.

Here is a checklist to help you evaluate the safety of your home. Review this important list every year.

Throughout the House

▲ Keep electric cords in good repair. Put away extension cords when they are no longer needed.

▲ Cover electric sockets not in use with plastic safety shields.

▲ Build a guardrail around space heaters, Franklin stoves, and other hot items. Keep fireplaces adequately screened, and keep any combustible liquids used in fireplaces out of reach.

▲ Beware of poisonous plants, such as poinsettia leaves, daffodil bulbs, and castor beans.

▲ Keep long cords from venetian blinds, mobiles, and so on well out of a small child's reach.

▲ Lock windows above the ground floor, or protect them with gates.

▲ Block stairways with nonfolding gates as soon as a child becomes mobile.

▲ Block tables with sharp corners, and clear them of objects that could fall and hurt a small child.

▲ Do not put your child in a baby walker, because his or her enhanced mobility can lead to numerous dangers. Each year more than 27,000 emergency room visits are due to baby walkers.

▲ Always strap babies into infant carriers and place the carriers on solid, level surfaces. Never leave a child unattended in a carrier.

▲ Check all fire escapes, balconies, and terraces for danger of falling.

▲ Install a smoke detector in the house and keep its batteries charged. If possible, install a smoke detector on each floor and carbon monoxide (CO) detectors near sleeping quarters.

Kitchen and Dining Room

▲ Lock the following materials out of reach: oven cleaners, drain cleaners, ant and rat poisons, insect sprays, furniture polish, bleach, lye, and other poisons.

▲ Turn pot handles away from the edge of the stove.

▲ Remove electric cords on appliances such as coffeemakers from the sockets immediately after use.

▲ Keep electric irons away from children.

▲ Place a fire extinguisher near the stove, out of a child's reach.
▲ Keep small children away from dangling tablecloths when a hot meal is on the table.

Bathroom

▲ Dispose of razor blades safely.
▲ Set the hot water heater to around 120°F (49°C).
▲ Lock all medicines out of reach, including aspirin, iron tablets, and sedatives.
▲ Flush prescription drugs left over from previous illnesses down the toilet.
▲ Lock all bathroom cleaners, especially drain cleaners, out of reach.
▲ Keep the toilet lid down so that infants cannot fall into the water.
▲ Never leave a child unsupervised in the bathtub.

Nursery

▲ Never leave an infant unattended on a changing table.
▲ Do not leave an infant who is too young to turn over on his or her stomach.
▲ Do not put anything on a cord, such as a pacifier, around a baby's neck.
▲ Do not string toys across a crib, because the cord is a strangling hazard.
▲ Periodically check and tighten all connections on a crib. Cribs should have no more than 2½ inches (6 cm) between slats and between mattress and frame, so a baby's head cannot become wedged in those spaces. Remove tall knobs from corner posts, because they can catch the clothing of an infant climbing out of the crib and cause strangulation.
▲ Take rattles, squeeze toys, and other small objects out of the crib when the baby is sleeping.
▲ Do not use infant cushions, which have been banned by the Consumer Product Safety Commission. An infant could suffocate while lying facedown on one of them.
▲ Install spring-loaded lid-support devices on toy chests so that the top cannot fall on a child's head.
▲ Do not leave infants in mesh-sided playpens or cribs with the sides down. The baby may roll into the narrow space between the mattress and the mesh, become caught, and suffocate.

Parents' Bedroom

▲ Keep cosmetics and perfumes out of reach.
▲ Keep mothballs and shoe polish out of reach.

▲ Dispose of all plastic bags (especially dry-cleaning and trash bags) so that children have no chance of suffocating inside them.

▲ Never leave an infant unattended on a flat bed.

Child's Room

▲ Check toys for sharp edges.

▲ Check toys for small parts that can be easily removed and swallowed, including marbles.

▲ Discard all broken toys and pieces of balloons.

▲ Check all connections on a bunk bed. There should be no spaces measuring more than 3½ inches (9 cm) between mattress and frame.

▲ Lock model glue away from toddlers.

Workroom

▲ Keep small children away from large buckets, including diaper pails.

▲ Store guns and bullets separately, and lock them away. Handguns are a frequent cause of accidental death in children. Their potential benefits are far outweighed by their real risks. Consider getting rid of any handgun kept in or around the house.

▲ Lock electric tools and tools with sharp edges out of reach.

▲ Lock paints, solvents, automobile fluids (especially antifreeze, which tastes sweet), pesticides, fertilizers, and snail bait out of reach. Never store them in soda bottles or other tempting food containers.

Yard and Garage

▲ Never leave a child unattended in a stroller.

▲ Invest in a helmet for your child. Helmets reduce serious injuries in bicycling, skateboarding, skiing, surfing, and horseback riding.

▲ Keep children away from rotary lawn mowers, and make sure those mowers have protective shields.

▲ Remove the doors from old refrigerators or freezers in which children could play, and dispose of the appliances properly.

▲ Build fences around swimming pools, and watch children playing in them.

Although children spend most of their time in the home, there can be an increased risk of accidents away from home. The surroundings are unfamiliar, and homes without children or with older children often have hazards not present in homes with young children. This is one reason why it is important for babysitters and grandparents to call the national poison control number at **1-800-222-1222**.

Although it is important to make your child's environment as safe as possible, it is also important for the child to gain experience with his or her environment and to learn to make personal safety decisions. This requires a testing of the environment and some painful experiences. The adult world is not totally safe, and there are perils in both underprotection and overprotection. Common sense is your best guide.

Automobiles

Automobile accidents are the number one killer of children. There is absolutely nothing more important for your child's health than protection in the automobile. Drive prudently and use seat belts or safety restraints. (Air bags *supplement* seat belts; they do not replace them.) The average infant or child car seat costs considerably less than the average doctor's office visit. A car seat can be used for many children, then passed on to a friend or relative. It is the best health bargain of all time and required by law in every state.

Car Seats

In selecting an infant or child car seat, be sure to purchase a model with a label certifying that it has been "dynamically crash tested." Understand how it must be installed. Many seats require anchoring that will involve placing a bolt through the floor of the car. If a seat requires a tether strap and anchor bolt, it will not protect your child without them. Also, seat belts that lock only on impact are inadequate for holding seats in place when the car goes around a sharp turn or over a minor bump. Special clips are available for these seat belts to allow them to accommodate infant seats. Seat prices vary considerably. Many communities have rental programs, but we consider a child seat a vital purchase, because your child will need one for four to five years. See www.aap.org/family/carseatguide.htm.

There are three basic seat types.

1. Infant car seats face backward. Because air bags can be dangerous to small people, install an infant car seat in the backseat. Even in cars without air bags, the backseat is generally safer for children. Infant car seats should be rear facing until 12 months and 20 pounds (9 kg). For current information on car safety seat models see www.aap.org/healthtopics/carseatsafety.cfm.

2. Some infant car seats convert to seats for small children, and we recommend them. Initially, they are installed in the reclining position facing backward. As the child grows, they are repositioned to face forward. These seats are good from birth to age 5 years or

about 40 pounds (18 kg). There are a number of models to choose from. A padded chest protector is another benefit of most of these seats.

3. Seats that require anchoring are ineffective unless you install them properly. Some parents have found highly recommended seats so complicated to use that they were forced to buy a different seat.

It is important to purchase your infant seat before you bring your baby home from the hospital. Make the first ride a safe ride. Also, bring along towels or blankets to prop your tiny child up in the seat. Remember, even the best seat will not protect your child if it is not used.

Other Measures

Harnesses, seat belts, shoulder straps, and booster seats can be used for older children. Booster seats must be used with a lap *and* shoulder belt, never a lap belt alone. Children over 40 pounds (18 kg) can use seat belts. Children under 4½ feet (137 cm) tall should not use shoulder straps, since they can cause neck injuries. Place the strap behind the child. Some new car models have shoulder belt adapters for younger children. The best way to teach a child to use a seat belt is to use one yourself. The child will quickly learn that when you enter a car, you automatically put on your seat belt.

Airbags have killed young children. Children younger than 13 years should always sit in the back seat.

We must add an extra word of caution about leaving small children unattended in cars. With a car's windows rolled up on a warm day, it can take only minutes for a child to suffocate or die of heat exhaustion. Also, leaving a child alone is an invitation to abduction. Finally, parents who would never leave pills or solvents within reach of children at home often leave shopping bags full of these same dangerous products with children in cars. Children display remarkable ingenuity in removing "childproof" caps. NEVER LEAVE A SMALL CHILD ALONE IN A CAR!

Finally, parents should be community advocates for full implementation and enforcement of traffic laws designed to protect children, including speed limits, minimum drinking age, and license suspension for drunk driving.

Bicycles

For a child, a bicycle is a friend, companion, horse, and source of transportation and exercise. It is important that a child learn the basic principles of bicycle safety, which will provide lifelong benefits for general and automotive safety as well.

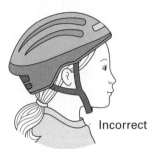 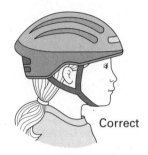

Incorrect   Correct

Proper position for bicycle helmets. The helmet should be worn level, so that it covers the forehead (right). A helmet that is pushed back on the head (left) provides little or no protection in a crash. Children—and adults—should always wear a helmet.

Many excellent books about bicycle safety are available for children. However, books should be used to supplement, not substitute for, parents' teaching. You will want to teach your children the following rules.

▲ Always wear a bicycle helmet.
▲ Know how fast the bicycle can be ridden safely. How fast is too fast going down a hill? How quickly can the bicycle stop when the brakes are applied? Remember, bicycles traveling at faster speeds require a much greater distance to stop.
▲ Understand and obey traffic signs and signals.
▲ Make sure the bicycle is ready to ride. Children should be taught to check the handlebars, the tires, and the brakes before beginning a ride.
▲ Ride on streets where it is safe to do so. If children must ride on the sidewalk, are they careful of other people? Are they careful about riding near automobiles where doors may suddenly open? Are they careful when riding around small children and animals?

Children should not be allowed to ride their bicycles in the street until they are about 10 years of age and can demonstrate good control of their bikes and knowledge of the rules of the road. The exact age depends on the child's maturity and skill and on local traffic patterns. Riding in the street around sundown is especially hazardous. Depending on the traffic flow in your neighborhood, street riding may need to be deferred to an older age, or it may never be safe.

As parents, you are familiar with the hazards of your neighborhood. Teaching a child how to balance a bicycle is not enough. You also must teach the child to maneuver the bicycle safely. And you must teach a child to stop at stop signs by doing so yourself.

The bicycle design and equipment revolution of recent years has made superb equipment available at reasonable prices. You should have no trouble finding the perfect bike for your child. We recommend a good local bike shop. They can help you with fit and riding tips.

Skates, Skateboards, and Scooters

Children zooming past you may have wheeled propulsion other than bicycles. Skateboards, in-line skates, and scooters provide potential for both fun and fractures. Each year there are about 550,000 injuries from in-line skating, skateboarding, and roller skating severe enough to require emergency room (ER) visits. More than one-third of the visits are for wrist injuries, with about one-fourth of injuries being wrist fractures. Facial lacerations occur in 1 in 10 in-line skating injuries. Fortunately only about 1 in 200 skaters or boarders is injured badly enough to visit the ER.

Protection helps! People without wrist guards were 10 times more likely to fracture their wrists. Elbow guards also reduce injuries. Head injuries account for only 5% of injuries, and we'd like to see this figure stay low. Have your child wear an approved helmet or bicycle helmet. In addition, bear in mind that skateboarding requires the development skills of a child at least 10 years old.

Water Safety

Children and water are a natural combination. The beach, swimming pool, bathtub, and lake offer more opportunities for fun than all the toys ever invented. However, water tragedies are all too common.

Young children must be watched carefully near water. It is easy for parents to fall asleep while lying on the beach or at poolside, and even short lapses in supervision can have fatal consequences for children. Drownings also occur frequently in bathtubs. Use your common sense in deciding when your child is old enough to be left alone in the tub.

"Waterproofing"

More and more swimming classes are being offered for children as young as six months of age. Although these "waterproofing" classes do not actually teach infants how to swim, they do teach them to kick sufficiently to get to the surface. This will help if a child falls into the far end of the pool with the parent watching. The infant can reach the surface and kick long enough for the parent to reach the child. However, organized programs for children under age 4 years are not recommended by the American Academy of Pediatrics. Excess water swallowing in this age group has led to seizures. Also, both you and your child may develop a false and fatal sense of security. You must remain alert and observant.

Swimming Lessons

It is important for all children to learn how to swim. The local YMCA, Red Cross, and many other organizations provide these services either free or at a minimal cost. If you are a competent swimmer, you will enjoy the time spent teaching your child how to swim. Water safety is as important as bicycle or automotive safety. Children should be taught never to swim by themselves and never to go too far from the shore without at least one experienced adult swimmer. Children should never swim in irrigation canals or other fast-moving water. Finally, children should never dive headfirst except in designated pool areas.

First Aid for Drowning

We prefer to talk about prevention, but it is also important to know what to do if you are the first one on the scene of a drowning. The techniques for resuscitation of a drowned child cannot be learned by reading a few pages in a book. The Red Cross offers an eight-hour multimedia safety course that we recommend highly to all individuals interested in being able to deal with emergency situations themselves.

Dogs

Children and their parents are too often unaware of what constitutes good pet safety. It is natural for small children to be afraid of dogs. Even medium-size dogs tower over toddlers and weigh as much as a seven- or eight-year-old. It is the parent's responsibility to teach a child how to act around dogs, even if the family does not own one, because all children come in frequent contact with dogs.

Every year thousands of children are bitten, sometimes severely, by dogs. Very few of these dog bites are by vicious dogs or dogs with rabies. Most often a bite comes from the friendly old dog next door, almost invariably because the child has unknowingly threatened the dog in some fashion. Even the friendliest dogs bite children.

Here are some hints to help prevent dog bites.

▲ Explain to children that they should not squeal in loud, squeaky voices around dogs. Dogs have sensitive ears, and such sounds will often terrify a dog, which will then react to protect itself.

▲ Teach children not to make sudden moves around dogs. A dog may interpret these movements as an attack, and the dog may react to defend itself. At other times, a dog may respond to a quick move in a playful fashion, which may include nipping. When playing with each other, dogs sometimes nip at each other in fun. (Parents and children do not consider dog nipping as much fun. This is a cultural difference between dogs and humans.)

▲ Children should not wave sticks or throw stones around dogs. Again, a dog may sense an attack or try to retrieve the stick out of the child's hands.

▲ Children should be cautious about running behind lying or sitting dogs. If a child steps on a dog's tail, the dog may react to protect itself.

▲ Children should be taught how to approach a dog. A child should approach a dog slowly, allow the dog to sniff a hand for a few seconds while talking calmly, and then proceed to pet the dog gently.

▲ Avoid dangerous breeds. While most pit bulls are wonderful pets, if they become agitated there is greater potential for damage than from many other breeds.

Finally, let's protect puppies, too. Small children often love puppies, and because a child is bigger than a puppy, most parents consider this a safe relationship. However, children of two, three, and even four years of age often delight in swinging a puppy by the tail and throwing it. This type of puppy abuse may produce a very nervous or even vicious older dog. Remember also that because dogs grow more quickly than children, the abused puppy may become a vicious adult dog in only a few months, and the child will suffer.

In general, we feel that age five should be considered the minimum age for a child to get his or her own puppy. The child should be old enough to demonstrate responsibility in keeping up with the routines of feeding, grooming, and cleaning up after a pet before acquiring a dog. Parents remember the joys of their own childhood pets and tend to rush into getting pets for their own children. This can lead to troublesome situations.

Growing Up Healthy/Avoiding Adult Diseases

The origins of the most serious medical problems of adults can usually be traced to behaviors and attitudes developed in the early years. Heart attack, stroke, high blood pressure, obesity, diabetes, cancer, emphysema, drug side effects, alcoholism, suicide, and homicide are the major national killers of adults, all with links to childhood.

There are effective ways of reducing the likelihood of encountering every one of these problems. It is your responsibility to transmit to your children the habits and attitudes that will serve them over a lifetime.

Smoking

No Smoking!

With each new edition of *Taking Care of Your Child*, the tobacco toll rises. We previously wrote that tobacco was responsible for 20% of cancer deaths; now it is known to cause 20% of *all* deaths. When pregnant women smoke, they are more likely to have miscarriages, stillbirths, and undernourished newborns. Their infants are more likely to succumb to sudden infant death syndrome (SIDS). Toddlers and children of smoking parents are more likely to develop asthma, respiratory infections, ear infections, and hearing problems.

Teenagers are particularly vulnerable to the ravages of smoking. If they have one smoking parent, they are more than twice as likely to start smoking as teenagers with nonsmoking parents. Ninety percent of all adults start smoking as teenagers. This is not surprising, given that adolescence is a time of experimentation and peer pressure—not to mention the pressure generated by the $2.5 billion spent annually by the tobacco industry on advertising, much of which targets youths.

In addition to all of the above problems caused by smoking, there is another disturbing problem: fires caused by cigarette lighters. Each year children under 5 years of age manage to start more than 5,000 fires at home, leading to about 150 deaths and numerous serious injuries.

There are many things you can do.

▲ The examples and attitudes of parents are critically important here. If you don't smoke, chances are your children won't either. If you do smoke, don't do it in front of your children. Children respect their parents' judgment and often imitate them. You can improve their chances of not smoking by not smoking around them.

▲ Don't tolerate behaviors in others that will jeopardize your children. You can be respectful of smoking relatives who visit by asking them to smoke elsewhere for the sake of your children. Send all your ashtrays to the local recycling center.

▲ When choosing a baby-sitter, make sure he or she understands and adheres to your no smoking policy.

▲ Always eat in no smoking areas of restaurants. If the smoke is still troublesome, take your child and your business elsewhere.

The decline of adult smoking in America is a reassuring and healthy sign. Nearly twice as many adults smoked in 1964 as smoke today. Despite this trend, almost half of American households still have at least one smoking adult, and smoking is actually increasing among young persons! Recent news indicates that daily use of cigarettes in 12- to 17-year-olds increased by 50% during 1988–1996, but declined from

1999–2003. In 1999 70% of all 12–17 year olds had tried smoking, while 59% tried smoking in 2003. We now have over 4 million teen smokers. Unfortunately the latest (2008) report indicates that smoking is no longer declining in teens and each day 3000 underage teens begin to smoke.

Obesity

Perhaps the most significant epidemic threatening American children is obesity. This year's projections indicate that children born in 2008 will be the first group ever with **life expectancies shorter than their parents**. Since the first edition of this book the rate of obesity in 2- to 5-year-olds has more than doubled from 5 to 12%. Things are even worse for older children, who have a rate of 17%, and adolescents whose rate has more than tripled from 5 to 16%. In addition, a third of all children are considered overweight or obese. A recent study has shown that the arteries of obese children are now equivalent to the arteries of a 45-year-old adult. For decades we have known that obesity and dietary fat intake are associated with the early onset of arteriosclerosis. Excess total body weight increases the load on the heart, and dietary fats appear to cause arteriosclerotic plaques to form more quickly. For every pound greater than 10 that an adult is over his or her ideal weight, life will be, on average, one month shorter. In addition to reducing arteriosclerosis, maintaining a normal body weight enables many individuals to avoid diabetes.

Unfortunately, we are seeing a dramatic increase in diabetes in children due to their weight. It is critical to reverse this trend. However the challenge will be formidable as the increase in adult obesity has mirrored what is happening to children. Simply put, the dietary habits of families are hurting children. For you to help your child avoid the multiple hazards of obesity your entire family will need to develop a healthy approach to balancing nutrition and exercise. Recognizing this crisis, some health plans have now developed programs that may be helpful in your family's approach to nutrition.

Nutrition

In Chapter 3 we give tips on good nutrition (see page 58), and in Part IV, we describe how children may become obese adults. (See Overweight/Obesity, page 302.) More important are the attitudes we develop in childhood toward food. Here is some specific advice.

▲ Watch portion sizes! Super-sizing is a major cause of obesity.
▲ A well-balanced meal is still the best policy. Children don't buy groceries. If they are eating too much junk food, you are responsible.

MyPyramid Plan

Eat these amounts from each food group daily. This plan is a **1800** calorie food pattern. It is based on average needs for someone like you. (A **10** year old **female**, of average height, of average weight, physically active **30 to 60 minutes** a day.) Your food needs also depend on your rate of growth and other factors. See a health care provider who can track your height and weight over time to identify your specific needs.

▶ Grains	6 ounces	tips
▶ Vegetables	2.5 cups	tips
▶ Fruits	1.5 cups	tips
▶ Milk	3 cups	tips
▶ Meat & Beans	5 ounces	tips

Click the food groups above to learn more.

MyPyramid.gov
STEPS TO A HEALTHIER YOU

Food pyramid. The art is a facsimile of the screen a parent would see after requesting information for a 10-year-old girl who is moderately active.

▲ We advise moderation in eating eggs, ice cream, and butter. We also recommend low-fat rather than whole milk for schoolchildren. (Infants and toddlers should have whole milk, however.)

▲ Parents should eat sensibly. If you have a weight problem your child also is at risk. Consult your physician and a local weight control program.

▲ Rules do not have to be rigid. Arteriosclerosis develops over a lifetime, and good habits are not altered much by temporary indiscretions; children should eat cake at birthdays but not every day.

Exercise

Controlling heart attacks requires more than dietary control. Adequate exercise also protects us from heart attacks. Exercise must be regular—at least four or five times a week—and lifelong.

We are a nation of television watchers, video game players, and desk sitters, and these behaviors are bad for us. Billboard ads stating "It's a nice day; why are you outside?" and television networks beckoning "All we want is eight hours a day" are not amusing. Some of our most serious adult diseases, such as arteriosclerosis and hypertension, are sometimes called "diseases of civilization." Everything from hemorrhoids to stomach ulcers to middle-aged spread can be related to our lack of serious physical exercise.

Good physical exercise is a workout for the heart and blood vessels, not just the muscles. To work the heart, the exercise must be steady, be moderately strenuous, and last at least 30 minutes. Bicycling, swimming, and running meet these requirements.

Exercise, when regular and sustained, makes the heart more efficient. This reduces the resting pulse rate, a sign of greater efficiency, and also reduces blood pressure. At any exercise level, a healthy heart will not have to work as hard as an unhealthy heart.

The best way to encourage your children to exercise is by example. Exercise regularly yourself, and exercise with them. Your whole family will benefit.

Stress

Stress contributes to the high incidence of heart disease. Stress cannot be avoided. Even young children experience stress, either in their own lives or through their parents. But people can deal with stress effectively. By encouraging communication, parents put themselves in a position to recognize and respond to their children's stress. And by helping their children cope, parents teach children that they need not confront all their problems alone.

AIDS

It is natural to be concerned about the risks of HIV (human immunodeficiency virus) infection and AIDS (acquired immune deficiency syndrome) to our children. However, children face far greater health risks than these. The risks of injury while riding in an automobile or on a bicycle are substantially greater than the risk of HIV infection. Similarly, the risk of acquiring a serious infectious illness such as meningitis while attending day care or school is substantially greater than the risk of HIV infection. Fortunately, just as infant safety seats, seat belts, bicycle helmets, and immunizations can reduce your child's risks from many potential problems, there are some things you can do to minimize your child's risk of HIV infection.

First, do not panic. In 2007, only 28 cases of AIDS were diagnosed in children under age 13 in the United States, a remarkable drop from the 894 cases in 1992 due to treatment of HIV-infected pregnant women.

Although some women have acquired HIV infection through behaviors known to place them at risk, such as injecting drugs, many unknowingly have acquired HIV from partners. It is estimated that about 50% of the women of childbearing age with HIV infection have no knowledge of any behaviors placing them at risk. Because of the availability of effective medical treatments, it is now recommended that all pregnant women be screened for HIV infection.

A number of children acquired AIDS through transfusions of blood that carried the HIV virus. Most of these children acquired their infection prior to April 1985, when blood screening for HIV began. It is currently estimated that the risk of blood containing HIV that has not been detected by today's testing procedures is 1 in 500,000, a real but nevertheless very small risk.

To date, there has been no known transmission through casual contact (for example, being coughed on by a person infected with HIV). Because HIV is transmitted through blood, it is theoretically possible that toddlers biting hard enough to draw blood might acquire AIDS. For older children participating in sports, there is also a theoretical possibility of being exposed to infected blood and the AIDS virus in close body contact (possibly in wrestling). Although these situations are theoretically possible, there have been no cases reported to date. Again, we emphasize that the risk of a child's encountering serious infectious diseases and injuries in day care and school is far greater than the risk of his or her getting AIDS.

It is with this information in mind that we endorse the recommendations of numerous national policy-making groups that children with HIV infection be allowed to attend day care and schools. The risk to other children in these schools is thus far zero. Even if news of a transmission is reported, it is important for parents to remember that the risk of AIDS remains substantially less than the risk of a whole host of other health problems associated with schools.

There are steps you can take to minimize your child's risk of HIV infection. Because HIV is a sexually transmitted disease (STD), we anticipate the continuing spread in adolescents engaging in sexual activity. This trend is alarming. Most individuals diagnosed with AIDS in the 20- to 24-year-old age group acquired HIV infection in their teenage years. Now, more than ever, it is imperative for parents to develop an openness about discussing sexual behavior with their children. As we have discussed in our section on sexuality (see pages 99–104), these discussions can begin in early childhood. Both your tone of voice and what you say about sexual development and behavior are very important. Children have a natural curiosity about anatomy, physiology, and reproduction. You should answer their questions matter-of-factly at an early age. If you do, when they approach the years of sexual activity, it will be easier for you to discuss with them both your values about sexual behavior and frank information about the variety of options for preventing STDs. You should also inform your children of their legal right to obtain confidential services relating to sexually transmitted diseases.

Virtually all our children will become sexually active at a certain stage of their adolescent or young adult life. Responsible behavior is what we advocate. Fostering good decision making about all aspects of life is essential to ensure good decision making about sexual behavior. At a certain stage of life, saying no is responsible. At a later stage of life, safer sexual behavior (that is, protected intercourse with condoms and foam) will eventually save many lives. (See Chapter K, "Adolescent Sexuality.")

Homicide

For people in their late teens and early 20s, only accidents cause more deaths than suicide and murder. Murder is constantly dramatized as a purposeful crime, but it usually is not. Most frequently, it is spontaneous and results from temporary rage or miscalculation, often aggravated by alcohol or other drugs. Fully 75% of all murder victims are known to their attackers, and a high percentage of best friends and family members are involved.

The murderer often has not learned to assume responsibility for his or her actions, has grown up in a family where violent rage is common and sanctioned, and possesses a weapon capable of causing rapid death. When a teenager murders, there is often a handgun in the home. In many cases, the adolescent has had legal problems before committing the violent act. There is a pattern to senseless destructive behavior, and its origins often lie early in life.

Suicide

Suicide is becoming a more common problem in our society. It is no longer unusual to find seven- and eight-year-olds attempting and committing suicide. Among adolescents, it is the third most common cause of death.

Most people think of committing suicide at some time. It is sometimes, but seldom, a sign of mental illness. Because suicide is against the law and violates religious and moral codes, it is often a problem that families keep hidden. A suicide gesture or attempt, no matter how minor, is extremely serious and is a signal for a family to obtain professional help.

There are many reasons why a person attempts suicide. Often a major life change or stress is at the root of the problem. Suicide may be one of a variety of coping strategies the person explores. It is in this exploration stage that children can be helped the most by your support.

Adolescents who attempt suicide are often isolated. They are loners, withdrawn. They have few friends and, frequently, only one close friend. Many have serious problems in school. A significant number are failing or experiencing discipline problems. Many live alone.

Following a seemingly minor altercation with a boyfriend, girl-friend, or parent, this adolescent will attempt suicide. At other times, an attempt may follow an extremely angry exchange with a parent. The motivation behind such an act is complex. It may be an attention-seeking device, a manipulative act, an attempt to hurt a parent, or a reaction to a loss, anger, or guilt. It is always a cry for help. If an adolescent is crying for help, it not mean that the parents have failed; it means that help from a doctor, social worker, or other skilled counselor is needed at that moment.

Any child or adolescent who talks of suicide should be taken seriously. If a child says, "You'll be sorry when I'm gone," pay attention. Most suicide attempts are unsuccessful, but 10% of people who attempt suicide once later kill themselves. Children and adolescents involved in frequent serious accidents also should receive professional counseling.

Substance Abuse

Nicotine and alcohol are the traditional American drugs, but there are others. Everyone likes to think that the other person's drug is terrible, while his or her own habit is not. We see self-righteous zealots who are "drunk" their whole adult life on tranquilizers. We see alcoholics who find a son's marijuana use offensive. And we see young women who despise a parent's alcohol consumption but use "speed" to get up and "reds" (barbiturates) to get down. Medically, all drug habits are psychologically equivalent.

It is clear that children emulate their parents, so developing appropriate attitudes and behaviors about alcohol and other drugs must begin at home. Parents should begin open discussions about street drugs as soon as they leave their children alone on the street. Peer pressure can be enormous for school-age children and adolescents, and parents must promote appropriate decision making by discussion and example. Parents also should ensure that a school program exists that reinforces this message.

Illegal Drugs

When parents worry about "drugs," they are usually concerned about illegal "street" drugs such as cocaine, amphetamines, marijuana, and heroin, as well as steroids used to enhance athletic performance. All of these substances are either banned or restricted to supervised medical use. Taking such drugs is dangerous for three reasons.

▲ The drugs are by and large highly addictive. People who take these drugs feel compelled, physically or psychologically, to keep on taking them whatever the consequences (loss of money, loss of job, loss of friends, health problems, and so on).

▲ It is possible to suffer severe, permanent harm from overdosing on these substances.

▲ Because these drugs are illegal, obtaining them is associated with violent crime.

Parents should warn children about these drugs and show them a good example by never using them. If a child does start taking illegal drugs, parents should help him or her into treatment. Breaking an addiction is never easy, but it can be done. Additional information is available at www.aap.org/healthtopics/subabuse.cfm.

Remember that for children, alcohol and tobacco are illegal drugs. It is illegal to sell these substances to children under a certain age, usually 21 for alcohol and a younger age for cigarettes. Nevertheless, teenagers can obtain these substances rather easily, and such surreptitious, risk-taking behavior often leads users to "harder" substances.

Alcohol

Alcohol is a useful sedative and serves some social purposes. As a drug, it is even relatively safe when used as directed. If we were to prescribe it as a prescription drug, the label would read, "Caution: May cause drowsiness and altered judgment. Do not attempt productive work or driving after taking this drug. Do not exceed recommended dosage of 1½ ounces (43 g) daily. May be habit-forming. Long-term or excessive use has been associated with ulcers, gastrointestinal hemorrhage, cirrhosis of the liver, inflammation of the pancreas, and atrophy (wasting) of the brain." Again, parents set the example, and again, we counsel moderation.

More and more adolescents are now turning to alcoholic beverages. Chronic alcoholism is now becoming common in adolescents. A chronic alcoholic needs help at any age.

Medication Abuse

There is another side to the national drug problem that is of major medical importance. One out of six hospitalizations is for a drug side effect, and one out of seven hospitalized patients will have a drug reaction while in the hospital. We think that history will record our drug dependence as one of our society's worst features and will remark on the curious concept that there is a pill for everything. You will note from the discussions in Part IV that, except for bacterial infections, there is a satisfactory pill for almost *nothing*. The average American goes to the doctor and to the medicine chest far too often. We spend fortunes on overpromoted patent medicines and on prescription drugs of low value. We get taken. And unless we are careful, our children will get taken, too.

Consider two boys, each of whom scrapes his arm. The parents of one clean the injury and apply a bandage. The parents of the other take him to the emergency room of the hospital, where an intern, trying to be helpful, prescribes an antibiotic, thinking the scrape might be infected. After five days, both scrapes are healed, but the family that used the emergency room has lost more than time and money. Now they credit the antibiotic with the cure—for an infection that never was! The emergency room will now be necessary for every scrape. The other boy has learned that a scrape will heal if cleaned and left alone. He will develop a certain measure of confidence in the body's natural healing properties. Children learn drug dependence from their parents. You should never encourage your child to use any drug, no matter how harmless, unless he or she really needs it.

Missing Children

Worry about a child's being abducted is a valid anxiety for parents. Over the past two decades, our society has become increasingly aware of this serious and terrifying problem. Unfortunately, the intense news coverage of child abductions in recent years has helped to create an atmosphere of fear and paranoia, while not doing enough to educate parents about the true nature of this complex problem.

It is important to realize that the vast majority of child abductions occur within the family, often in cases involving divorce and child custody. Only a very few children are abducted by nonrelatives. The U.S. Justice Department puts that figure at about 4,600 each year. Of these, 200 to 300 will end up in every parent's nightmare scenario: held for a prolonged period or murdered. Although even this relatively small number is disturbing, you should keep in mind that your child faces a far greater risk of being injured by an automobile while walking to school than of being abducted by a non–family member.

Preventing Abduction

It is impossible for any parent to make his or her child abduction-proof, but there are some things you can do that may slightly reduce your chances of having to confront this tragedy. Educate your child in an age-appropriate manner about the possibility of this situation and set firm guidelines (rules) for the child regarding interaction with persons when you are not present: with whom, when, and where it is acceptable.

General Guidelines

The National Center for Missing and Exploited Children (NCMEC) says that the traditional "Stay away from strangers" advice is difficult for children to grasp: "It is more beneficial to . . . teach them to respond to a potentially dangerous situation, rather than teaching them to look out for a particular type of person." NCMEC also recommends that "kids need to be empowered with positive messages and safety skills that will build their self-esteem and self-confidence while helping to keep them safer."

We still believe it is important to caution children and to teach them to use a "No, Go, Tell" approach for dealing with adults and others, familiar or unfamiliar to them. Anytime a child is touched, asked a question, or asked to keep a secret and the child feels something bad or wrong has happened, he or she should say **no**, then **go** and **tell** a grown-up the child trusts about the incident. Teach your child that he or she has certain rights—not to be touched, not to be asked to keep secrets—even with an adult. Give your child permission to be assertive by using "No, Go, Tell" to exercise those rights.

Although it may be difficult to keep track of an active toddler or young child, it is particularly important not to let him or her out of your sight in a department store or shopping mall. Allowing a child to get lost in the crowd may invite real danger. If, after a few minutes, you cannot locate your child, notify store authorities immediately. Prompt action may save your child's life.

Warn of adults who claim they are police but are not in uniform or patrol cars. Even uniformed police seldom talk with children unless they are creating a nuisance or taking risks.

Warn your children that adults with friendly puppies or dogs are not safer than other strangers.

Never allow your child to wear a sweatshirt or T-shirt or carry any item with his or her name imprinted on it. This is a common way for abductors to achieve familiarity.

Older children (those over eight) can use the buddy system to walk to and from school, church, and other neighborhood locations. Make sure your child travels with a group of children having at least one other same-age child. If your child is under eight, insist that an older sibling or adult accompany the child to his or her destination.

Always have a backup location to which your child can go if you are detained and cannot be home to meet him or her.

Report any suspicious people you notice on your neighborhood school grounds or playgrounds to the police. It is far more reasonable to report such persons to the police than to assume they are harmless or that your imagination is running away with you.

Cars, Car Pools, and Other Dangers

Tell your child never to approach a car when a driver has requested directions.

If your child must use public transportation, teach him or her to wait for the bus at bus stops used frequently by other people or at bus stops that are in front of stores or schools or near the home of a person whom you trust. In this way, if someone does bother your child, he or she can run into the store, school, or home for refuge.

Tell your child never to stand on the curb right next to the street. A possible abductor in a car or van could drive up and pull the child into the vehicle without much trouble.

When setting up car pools with the parents of your children's friends, make sure you meet them and feel comfortable with them. If you are uncomfortable with a particular person, you should not use this car pool, and you should check out your feelings with other parents.

If your child is picked up from school or an activity by a car pool, caution the child never to go with anyone who is not a regular driver. Individuals have been known to learn parents' names and can easily con young children into a ride. If your work situation is such that you must ask friends or neighbors to pick up your child, make sure that you establish some system with your child, such as a code word that must be provided by this neighbor before the child will travel with him or her. Generally, children who are older than seven years of age are capable of this sophisticated screening process. For younger children, it is best to inform them never to get in a car with anyone who is not a family member or neighbor whom you have approved.

Never leave a child of any age alone in a car. This is double jeopardy. Heat exhaustion and abduction are real risks.

Telephone Help

Many children now carry cell phones. You should be certain your number and those of other important contacts are available.

Children without cell phones should memorize, as soon as they are able, your home and business phone numbers and the phone number of a trusted friend. Instruct your children always to call you or another trusted person if they need to stop anywhere on their journey home.

Response to Possible Abduction

The success of law enforcement agencies in recovering young children abducted by strangers is related to how quickly they are informed about a child's absence. As awareness of the child abduction problem has increased, police departments in general have become more sensitive and more expert in their handling of these emergencies. Some have even developed special bureaus with officers assigned solely to missing children situations.

Avoid products and services from companies that prey on your fear of losing your child. Items such as home fingerprinting kits and anti-abduction alarms that children wear or carry are of little or no value, offering a false sense of security at best.

Your best response to a missing child emergency is to contact local authorities right away. According to NCMEC, 99% of missing children are found and returned to their families by local police departments.

If your child is late returning home or meeting you somewhere, it is important that you notify the police promptly (after checking other logical places your child could be). Expect the police to question you about your child's behavior prior to the incident, and be honest in your answers. It is often assumed that a child who is missing, especially an older child, is a runaway. Be adamant if you know that the possibility of your child's running away is essentially zero. You, not the police, are the best judge of your child's patterns and behavior and whether or not this incident is a deviation from the norm for your child.

In addition to notifying your local law enforcement authorities, you may want to contact NCMEC (1-800-843-5678; www.missingkids.com). This organization, created with the aid of the U.S. Justice Department, maintains a data bank of missing children and provides other services to assist public and private efforts to locate missing children.

Chapter Eleven

The Home Pharmacy

As a society, we have relied far too long and far too often on drugs to solve our problems. Drugs have, of course, saved many lives. Medications for bacterial infections, epilepsy, cancer, heart failure, rheumatoid arthritis, diabetes, and other major illnesses have certainly changed the lives of those afflicted. However, there is almost unbelievable misuse of medications because of our social rituals, patients' demands, doctors' encouragement, and massive advertising.

The vast majority of all medical problems resolve themselves without the use of any medication. These illnesses include common colds, influenza, diarrhea, rashes, upset stomachs, headaches, and most of the other problems discussed in Part IV. However, we are bombarded with advertisements implying that these problems can be cured only by, or much faster with, the use of some medication. (One out of every eight television advertisements is for an over-the-counter medication.) These claims are simply not true. For nearly every advertised drug, there is a cheaper alternative that is just as good or better. In many instances, the preferred alternative is nothing at all.

Finding a product on the shelf of a supermarket or pharmacy does not mean that it is either safe or effective. In 1966, the Food and Drug Administration (FDA) commissioned a study to evaluate 400 common over-the-counter (nonprescription) drugs. More than 75% of those drugs were found to be less than effective for some or most of their claims. Products that have been on the market since before 1938 have never been subject to requirements for demonstrating safety or efficacy. Therefore, most of the estimated 250,000 to 500,000 products available on the shelves are less than effective, and many are unsafe. Well-intentioned use of these products results in many deaths annually.

The FDA is currently taking steps to review over-the-counter products. But it will be many years before consumers can purchase medications with the knowledge that they are both safe and effective. And "safe" is a relative term. All medications can cause serious side effects. Aspirin, a potent and useful drug, causes more serious reactions and more deaths than any other medication. Be careful with every drug.

The previous two paragraphs have been included in all previous editions of this book since 1976. Finally, in the fall of 2007, following a lawsuit and several deaths from cold preparations, the FDA began to review cough and cold preparations. As a result many infant cough and cold preparations were voluntarily withdrawn by the manufacturers. A list of the withdrawn medications can be found on the American Academy of Pediatrics website (aap.org) and should be discarded if you have them at home. In addition, cough and cold preparations should **not** be given to children less than 2 years. We also stand by our position of more than thirty years; when it comes to children's colds, spending money on cough and cold preparations will have very little, if any benefit. It is better to put your money in your child's college fund.

Tincture of Time

Used prudently, time is the most important medicine. It is the only known cure for the common cold, as well as most of the other problems of everyday life. With time, things get better. In Part IV, we try to tell you how to use time and how long recovery from specific problems should take.

Why do we, as a society, use drugs rather than time, even though time usually works and the drugs usually don't? Sure, we are impatient, confused by the complexities of science, and hustled by the advertisers. But let's not ignore the biggest reason. We use drugs, and sometimes the doctor, to prove that we care for our children. The statements "I'll run down and get something from the drugstore" and "You're going to the doctor first thing in the morning" are part of our everyday life. We have equated the giving of drugs with caring.

Consider the consequences of such actions. A child receives a pill rather than a parent. He or she fails to learn that the body is strong and thinks instead that health is frail and only precariously maintained by an intake of chemicals. Colds, scrapes, headaches, and constipation are associated with the need to take a pill or imbibe some fluid. And although time will take the symptom away, the drug will take the credit. Later, the parent is disturbed when the child wants pills, shots, or fluids to cure boredom, unhappiness, or agitation, or just to interact socially with friends.

With a sick child, you can care by spending time instead of money. Nondrug treatments, such as encouraging the child to drink fluids, running the vaporizer, and cleaning and soaking the wound will give you plenty to do. Most medical problems are learning experiences. If you and your child react and interact appropriately, the lessons can be positive and can lead to emotional growth and physical confidence. The choice is yours—drug dependence or personal independence—and the consequences are immense. We hope that the guidelines in Part IV will help your family to achieve the goal of personal self-reliance and independent living.

Giving Children Medicine

Doctors frequently prescribe medicines for children. Parents often leave the doctor's office or pharmacy confused and with many unanswered questions. One study of patients leaving doctors' offices revealed that more than 50% made at least one error when describing what their doctors expected. This is not surprising, for recordings of the medical visits revealed that the doctors did not even discuss 20% of the medicines they prescribed. For 30% of these medications, the doctors gave no information about the name or purpose of the drug. Of all the patients in this study, 90% were not told by their doctors how long to take the medicines, and fewer than 5% of the prescription bottles contained this information. Clearly, then, there is a need for both better communication between doctors and patients and more information for young patients and their parents.

Here are some of the more important things to keep in mind whenever you give your child medicine.

▲ Understand the instructions. Make sure you understand before you leave the doctor's office. If the instructions on the medication bottle differ from what the doctor or pharmacist said, call your doctor immediately. If you are confused at all, call your doctor or the pharmacist.

▲ Be sure of the strength of the medication. Some common medications appear in many different concentrations, and the wrong strength may be dangerous.

▲ Be sure your child is not allergic to the medication. Even the most careful doctor occasionally forgets that a child is allergic to penicillin and may prescribe it. Do not give your child anything that you know he or she is allergic to.

▲ Be as precise as possible in your measurements. Tableware teaspoons vary greatly in size. When most doctors prescribe a teaspoon, they mean 5 cubic centimeters (cc) of medication. Measuring spoons are more accurate. Many pharmacies sell small plastic measuring devices or give them away.

▲ Never give a child medication intended for another person.

▲ Never give a child medication if the expiration date has passed.

See Table 3 for a list of questions you should ask yourself before giving your child any medicine.

Some of your most interesting moments with your children will be spent trying to give them medications. An average child seems able to spit an average medication a distance of 15 feet. Although this may be good practice for the annual North Carolina Watermelon Pit Spitting

Table 3: Parent Medication Checklist

BEFORE GIVING your child ANY medication, make sure that the following questions are answered and understood.

▲ What is the medicine's name?

▲ What does it do?

▲ How much do I give?

▲ How often must I give it?

▲ How long do I need to continue giving the medicine?

▲ Are there special preparation instructions—for example, do I need to shake it vigorously?

▲ Are there special times to take the medicine?

▲ Must I refrigerate the medicine?

▲ Are there common side effects I can expect?

▲ Are there rare adverse risks that I should be aware of?

▲ If my child has a particular allergy, might he or she also be allergic to this drug?

▲ How much does this medicine cost?

▲ Is a generic form of comparable quality available?

▲ Does my child really need this medicine? Do its benefits outweigh its risks and costs?

Contest, medication on the walls has seldom been known to do the child any good. Getting medication into your children will be a great test of your ingenuity. Remember, you are older, wiser, more clever, and ultimately bigger. But here are some hints so that you won't have to use force.

▲ Never tell a child that medication is candy. As soon as your back is turned, your child will try to get as many of these "candies" into his or her mouth as possible.

▲ Do not tell a child a medication tastes good when you know it doesn't. This will help get the first dose into the child, but you will have an impossible time with the second.

▲ For younger infants, you can mix some medications with applesauce or ice cream.

▲ Medications usually do not give a pleasant flavor to milk, and we discourage mixing them with milk. Most children are familiar with how their milk tastes and are suspicious of funny-tasting milk.

▲ Toddlers often prefer tablets ground up in ice cream to seemingly tasty syrup preparations. Cranberry juice is another good place to hide a medication.

▲ For infants younger than six months, use a syringe or calibrated eyedropper to administer medications.

Ultimately, every parent will participate in a knock-down, drag-out fight with a toddler or preschool-age child over taking medicine. The child in this situation, with his or her ability to spit, vomit, and clench teeth, will win every time. In fact, the more intense the struggle, the more the child will relish the fight. In these situations, it pays to draw back for a few minutes, let the struggle defuse itself, and try again. This method may provide the toddler with enough sense of control that he or she will agree to take the medicine the next time around. The truly recalcitrant child poses a difficult problem that you should discuss with your doctor, who may be able to suggest an easier way to deliver the medicine (for example, by syringe) or other approaches to giving it.

Finally, older children should be required to take medication as a matter of course. They should not need to be threatened or bribed any more than they need to be bribed or threatened when it is their bedtime. Children over the age of three and one-half can begin to be treated as adults with regard to taking medication. Development of proper respect for medication is important at this age. Start talking to them about the importance of medication to help them through their illnesses. Do not talk of medication as either magic or a reward. Ultimately, emphasize the importance of taking medication as directed, not more or less. Enlist the help of older children in keeping to a medication schedule.

Complementary and Alternative Medicine

Today's home remedy or folk medicine may be next year's scientific breakthrough. Over the years countless medical triumphs, from the development of vaccinations (smallpox) to life-saving cardiac medications (digoxin), began as folk wisdom. Most folk medicines, however, have little therapeutic benefit, although many may provide some comfort or taste good. A few can be harmful.

Complementary medicines are products used in addition to traditional medicine. Alternative medicines are used as substitutes for therapies with proven scientific benefit (for example, acupuncture instead of pain medicine). Integrative medicine combines traditional medical therapies with complementary and alternative medicine (CAM) therapies that have been shown scientifically to be safe and effective. The National Center for Complementary and Alternative Medicine currently recognizes five categories of therapy: **alternative medical systems** such as homeopathic medicine and traditional Chinese medicine;

mind-body interventions such as prayer or creative outlets such as music; **biologically based therapies** such as vitamins and herbs; **manipulative and body-based therapies** such as chiropractic and massage; **energy therapies** including biofield therapies such as therapeutic touch and bioelectromagnetic-based therapies.

Many families are turning to alternative therapies, particularly those who have children with severe conditions that are not being helped by our current therapies, such as autism. Sorting through the countless alternative remedies available on store shelves or through the Internet can be a daunting task. Fortunately, there has been increasing scientific interest in alternative remedies in recent years. The National Institutes of Health and many universities are conducting research and providing parents with timely information.

If you are considering the use of CAM, you can turn to one of several websites for current information, including the National Center for Complementary and Alternative Medicine of the National Institutes of Health (http://nccam.nih.gov) and sites developed by faculty at Columbia University (www.rosenthal.hs.columbia.edu) and the University of California, San Francisco (www.osher.ucsf.edu). Additional helpful websites include www.integrativepeds.org and www.childrensmn. org/Communities/IntegrativeMed.asp. The latter website includes helpful videos directed toward children. You should also discuss potential benefits and harms with your heath care provider. Take an active role by providing all pertinent information you may have concerning your child's condition and the CAM you are considering. The American Academy of Pediatrics has recommended pediatricians work closely with families in making decisions about CAM. Always tell your physician if you are using CAM.

Remember, time will heal most childhood illnesses, occasionally helped by prescription medications or commercial products that are designed to be safe for children.

Additional Reading

Be the Boss of Your Body series, Timothy Culbert and Rebecca Kajander. (Minneapolis: Free Spirit Publishing, 2007).

Be the Boss of Your Stress
Be the Boss of Your Pain
Be the Boss of Your Sleep

Integrative Pediatrics, Timothy Culbert and Karen Olness. (New York: Oxford University Press, 2009).

Hypnosis and Hypnotherapy with Children, 3rd ed., Karen Olness and Daniel P. Kohen (New York: Guilford Press, 1996).

Your Medicine Cabinet

No Aspirin

Only two medications are essential for the home pharmacy when children are in the home: **acetaminophen** (Tylenol), to relieve fever and pain (page 217), and **ibuprofen** (Advil, Motrin, Nuprin), which relieves fever and pain and also reduces inflammation. Even acetaminophen and ibuprofen are potentially fatal and should be kept out of the reach of children. (Very few childproof caps are childproof. Often the best way to open a childproof cap is to ask your child to open it for you.)

Also essential to have is the number for the national poison control center: 1-800-222-1222. Write this telephone number (or that of your local poison control center) on your telephone, on the second page of this book, and on page 251. Do it now.

In addition to these two medicines, have on hand the following items.

▲ Bandages, adhesive (Band-Aids) and elastic (page 221)
▲ Antiseptic cleanser (page 221)
▲ Thermometers (page 222)
▲ Vaporizer (page 223)
▲ Sunscreen (page 224)
▲ Antihistamines (page 224)

You probably do not need to keep the following medicines on hand, but you may wish to purchase them for special situations.

▲ Syrup of ipecac (page 220) can induce vomiting in children who have swallowed dangerous medications. It can be used immediately when a child has swallowed pills, liquid medications, or plants. For other poisonous substances, it may be dangerous to induce vomiting. Although no longer recommended by some organizations, syrup of ipecac may have a role **if other medical care is unavailable**.
▲ Decongestants (page 224)
▲ Cough and cold medicines (page 225)
▲ Nose drops (page 226)
▲ Soothing lotions (page 227)
▲ Constipation medicines
▲ Diarrhea medicines
▲ Eyedrops
▲ Vitamins

All drugs kept at home should be in childproof bottles. Because there are no totally childproof bottles, drugs should also be kept out of small children's reach.

Pain and Fever Relievers

Purpose

Pain. Children may experience pain following an injury such as a burn or trauma, during the course of an acute illness (sore throat) or chronic disease (arthritis), or even following a medical intervention such as immunization or surgery. For chronic conditions or after surgery, you, your child, and your physician will need to establish a pain management plan. For most everyday conditions, pain can be effectively managed at home.

Talk is often the best medicine. Most minor injuries will not even require a trip to the medicine cabinet. In fact, a parent who reaches for a pain reliever every time a tear accompanies a fall is teaching a child to rely on bottled solutions. For most injuries, distraction works well. Discussing plans for later in the day and talking about imaginary situations are often effective and have no side effects. Even children with chronic pain from serious medical conditions benefit enormously from verbal techniques such as guided imagery and hypnosis. Children who are about to undergo painful procedures in a medical setting will benefit from adequate preparation, including age-appropriate discussions of what will happen and opportunities to ask questions. The accompanying reduction in anxiety and pain has been well documented.

Fever. Fever with no other symptoms present is not necessarily a sign of illness. Normal body temperature varies from individual to individual and according to time of day. Furthermore, an elevated temperature sometimes signifies that the body's immune system is already responding to an illness—a positive sign.

Parents frequently ask us what temperature should be considered dangerous or at what temperature a child should be brought to the doctor if no other symptoms are present. Consult a doctor immediately for the following:

▲ Temperature of more than 100°F (37.7°C) in a child younger than one week
▲ Temperature of more than 100.4°F (38°C) in a child younger than three months
▲ Temperature of more than 103°F (39.4°C) in a child younger than two years
▲ Temperature of more than 105°F (40.5°C) if the home treatment measures described below fail to reduce the temperature at least partly
▲ Temperature of 106°F (41.1°C)
▲ Fever persisting for more than five days

With an extremely high fever, there is a danger of seizures. This is a special situation and not to be treated with oral medications. (See Fever, page 289.)

Recommendations

Pain. If medicine is necessary to relieve a child's pain, we recommend a three-tiered pain management plan that begins with adequate and timely doses of mild (and inexpensive) pain relievers such as ibuprophen. If pain continues, the next step is to move on to mild opioid (addictive) drugs such as codeine or moderate opioids such as meperidine (Demerol) or oxycodone (OxyContin, Vicodin). The final stage is to use drugs restricted to hospitals, such as morphine. All but the mildest pain relievers require physician contact and prescriptions.

Fever. Do not give medication by mouth to a child having a febrile seizure. (See Fever, page 288.) A child who has just had a seizure can be given a suppository. For a conscious, alert child, acetaminophen is an effective fever reducer. Ibuprofen is equally effective when given in appropriate doses. We do not recommend aspirin.

Acetaminophen

This is a mainstay of treatment for pain and fever. It is very safe and works by blocking the pain sensations carried through the nerves. It is available in a number of familiar brand names (Tylenol, Datril, Liquiprin, Phenaphen, Tempra, Tenlap, Valadol) as well as generically. Unfortunately, it is also available in many forms (drops, elixir, tablets, capsules) and concentrations. This is confusing and often leads to consistent underdosing and overdosing by parents, particularly with liquids. Always read the label.

A tablet or capsule contains 325 mg, more than a preschooler needs. A teaspoon (5 cc) of one preparation (drops) can contain four times as much drug as a teaspoon (5 cc) of another preparation (elixir). An unsuspecting person used to a different preparation can create a problem by using the wrong dose.

Each dose should give a child 10 mg for every 2.2 pounds (1 kg) of body weight. Therefore, a 20-pound (9 kg) child should receive 100 mg. A 65-pound (29 kg) child should receive 325 mg (one regular adult tablet). See Table 4 for recommended doses.

Acetaminophen is a very good pain reliever (analgesic) but lacks the ability of aspirin and other anti-inflammatory drugs to manage the inflammation that often occurs with joint or bone pain. It is the primary drug used for fever reduction in children because it is very effective, it is much safer than aspirin, and it is easy to administer as a liquid. Acetaminophen has sometimes been called "liquid aspirin," but it is a completely different medication from aspirin. It is also less expensive than ibuprofen. In extremely high doses, however, even acetaminophen can be fatal by causing massive liver damage.

Ibuprofen

Ibuprofen is an example of the relatively new and increasingly popular drugs known as nonsteroidal anti-inflammatory drugs (NSAIDs). It possesses many of the features characteristic of steroids for reducing pain from inflammation in the bones or joints. However, some of the side effects seen with aspirin (such as stomach upset) also occur, though less frequently. If your child has problems with stomach irritation, ibuprofen can be taken after a meal without adversely affecting its absorption.

Ibuprofen is increasingly favored over acetaminophen for pain, particularly from injuries or inflammation. It is available over the counter in tablet form under different brand names (Advil, Motrin, Nuprin) and appears in some other medications (such as Midol). It is also available in liquid form as concentrated infant drops or children's elixir. Liquid ibuprofen's concentration differs from the tablet form. Read the labels carefully.

Ibuprofen is safer for children than aspirin, but it is not available in as many

Table 4: Acetaminophen and Ibuprofen Dosages for Fever Relief*

Weight of Child	Acetaminophen Dosage	Ibuprofen Dosage		
		6 months–2 years (Temp. below 102.5°F)	6 months–2 years (Temp. at or above 102.5°F)	Over 2 years
Up to 12 pounds (infants)	40 mg			
13–17 pounds	80 mg	25 mg	50 mg	
18–23 pounds	120 mg	50 mg	100 mg	
24–35 pounds	160 mg	100 mg	100 mg	100 mg
36–47 pounds	240 mg			150 mg
48–59 pounds	325 mg **			200 mg
60–71 pounds	325 mg **			250 mg
72–95 pounds	325 mg **			300 mg
Adolescents	500 mg **			400 mg

*   The recommended dosage for acetaminophen is 10 mg for every 2.2 pounds (1 kg) of the child's weight every four hours, up to five times in one day. The amounts given here are **estimated** dosages.

The recommended dosage for ibuprofen depends on age, temperature, and weight, and is given every 6 to 8 hours. The amounts given here are **estimated** dosages for children over 6 months.

** 325 mg of acetaminophen equals 1 regular tablet or capsule; 500 mg of acetaminophen equals 1 "extra strength" tablet or capsule.

forms as acetaminophen. It is considered as effective as acetaminophen in treating fevers in children older than 6 months. The fever reduction is actually somewhat better, and a single dose lasts longer than a single dose of acetaminophen for children older than 2 years with temperatures over 102.5°F (39°C). Nevertheless, it is still considered a second line of defense after acetaminophen, because it has more side effects and is more expensive. It shares a positive feature with acetaminophen in that both reduce fever without reducing the production of interleukin-1, an impor-

tant body chemical that fights infections. See Table 4 for recommended dosages.

In some situations doctors may advise combining acetaminophen with ibuprofen. They can be given together or alternated. Do not give more than four doses of ibuprofen a day.

In addition to the types of acetaminophen and ibuprofen sold over the counter, there are higher strengths of these drugs (potentially more than twice the strength of the nonprescription formulas) available by prescription. If you have different strengths of one drug in the house, be careful not to mix them up. Medication prescribed for one person should never be given to another, especially a child.

Aspirin

We do not recommend aspirin for children because of its potential side effects. Among these are gastrointestinal disturbances, including bleeding; an allergic reaction that causes wheezing (this is very rare); and **Reye syndrome,** a very rare but serious condition of the brain and liver. Reye syndrome is a particular concern for children exposed to chicken pox or influenza (flu).

Aspirin suppositories can be given to a child who has just had a febrile seizure and cannot take any medicine by mouth. (See Fever, page 288.) These usually require a prescription and should be avoided if at all possible because of the risk of Reye syndrome. Most aspirin suppositories come in 5-grain sizes. Approximately 1¼ to 1½ grains per year of age can be given. The suppository can be cut lengthwise using a warm knife to give the proper dose.

Other Nonsteroidal Anti-inflammatory Drugs (NSAIDs)

NSAIDs other than ibuprofen abound. Aleve (naproxen) and Celebrex (celecoxib—expensive without extra benefits) are sometimes suggested. In general ibuprofen and acetaminophen will suffice unless your doctor recommends otherwise.

Codeine

This weak narcotic requires a prescription and instructions from your physician. It is effective for pain relief and is often com-bined with acetaminophen for increased relief. It is not used to treat fever.

Syrup of Ipecac

Purpose

Children often put things in their mouths. Inevitably, some of these things are swallowed. When there is a danger of poisoning or drug overdose, inducing vomiting may be the appropriate treatment. For any item other than medication, call the poison control center (1-800-222-1222) or your doctor before attempting to induce vomiting. (See Poisoning, page 250.) With medicines, call right after inducing vomiting. **Syrup of ipecac is no longer recommended for routine use. It may be appropriate in some situations, however, when medical care is not available.**

Recommendations

Anytime your child swallows a large number of pills or liquid medication, you can give the child syrup of ipecac to induce vomiting. The dose is 1 tablespoon (15 ml) for young children, 2 tablespoons (30 ml) for older children. Give the child a glass of water or milk immediately after administering a dose of syrup of ipecac to induce vomiting. If there is no vomiting after 20 minutes, repeat with another dose. If there is no vomiting after 40 minutes, the child must see the doctor to have his or her stomach emptied. Ipecac itself can produce problems if it is not vomited up.

Other methods of inducing vomiting in children include having them drink a mixture of mustard and warm water or touching the back of the child's throat. These are less "aesthetic" but sometimes just as effective as syrup of ipecac.

Bandages

Adhesive Bandages

Adhesive bandages (Band-Aids) are for children what medals are for adults. They are worn proudly as symbols of surviving major confrontations with the ground. As such, they may be awarded whenever the child feels they are necessary. Or you can encourage your child to make a decision about the application of a treatment. Wounds in areas likely to have heavy exposure to dirt may require a Band-Aid (and occasionally a gauze dressing) to prevent further contamination and the possibility of infection.

Elastic Bandages

Elastic bandages (Ace) are to treat strains and sprains. Their main function is to support an injured area, thereby reducing the chance of reinjury while the body heals itself.

When wrapping an elastic bandage, start at the far end of the injured area and wrap toward the trunk of the body. Wrap more loosely as you go. (See page 222.) The bandage should never be so tight that it hampers circulation.

If you have any doubt that an elastic bandage is the appropriate treatment for a particular injury, call your doctor.

Antiseptic Cleansers

The best way to clean a dirty wound is to rinse it with lots of water. You can also scrub it with soap and water or a medical antiseptic such as Betadine. There is no need to use a product such as hydrogen peroxide or mercurochrome.

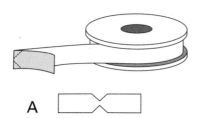

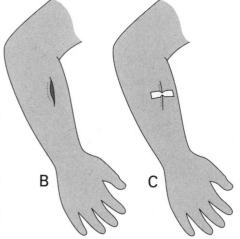

Butterfly bandage. This type of bandage allows a short, shallow wound to heal quickly.

(A) Fold a length of adhesive tape in two and snip off the folded corners.

(B) Make sure the wound is clean, and that one edge is not lying over the other.

(C) Tape the wound together so that its edges meet and the narrow part of the bandage lies over the cut.

Use this only in the first six hours after injury; otherwise bacteria may grow in the wound.

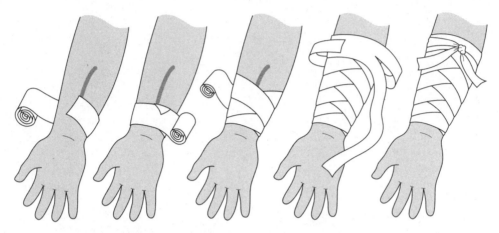

Wraparound bandage. This type of bandage makes a neat, long-lasting wrap for a large wound. It is easier to tape the end of the bandage, but if you have no tape you can tie the bandage as shown.

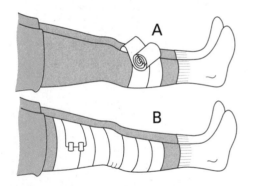

Wrapping an elastic bandage.
(A) Start wrapping the bandage on the far end of the joint (in this case, the knee). Don't stretch the bandage as you wrap.

(B) Wrap past the joint, firmly at first then more loosely the farther up you go. Use the clips that come with most elastic bandages to fasten the loose end.

Thermometers

Purpose

Fever is a common symptom of many childhood problems. Folk wisdom suggests that a parent's hand touched to a child's forehead is the quickest way to check for fever. For a more exact diagnosis, however, nearly every parent relies on a thermometer. We recommend digital thermometers for rectal, oral, and underarm use. Because of potential problems if broken, mercury thermometers should not be used.

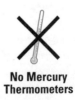

**No Mercury
Thermometers**

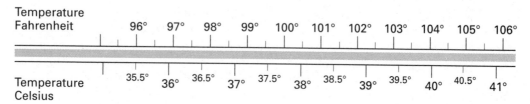

Temperature taking. The figure shows comparative temperatures for the Fahrenheit and Celsius (Centigrade) scales.

Recommendations

Rectal temperatures are usually more accurate and are about 0.5°F (0.25°C) higher than oral temperatures. Oral temperature can be affected by hot or cold foods, routine breathing, and smoking. Generally, oral thermometers can be recognized by the longer bulb at the business end of the thermometer. The length of the bulb is to provide for a greater surface area and a faster, more accurate reading. Rectal thermometers have a shorter, rounder bulb to facilitate entry into the rectum.

Rectal thermometers can be used to take oral temperatures, but they require a longer period in the mouth to achieve the same degree of accuracy as an oral thermometer. Oral thermometers can be used to take rectal temperatures, but their shape is not ideal for younger children, and we do not recommend their use in any children.

A lubricant can facilitate the placement of a rectal thermometer. You need not bury the thermometer. Only an inch or so need be inside the child's rectum. The mercury will rise within seconds on a rectal thermometer because the rectum comes in close contact with the thermometer. Remove the thermometer when the mercury is no longer rising, after a minute or two. Children should be placed on their stomachs when rectal temperatures are being taken. You should place a hand on their bottoms to prevent them from moving.

Underarm thermometers are reliable for young infants. The new electronic thermometers that take a measurement through the ear are fast, generally (though not always) reliable, and expensive. The disposable plastic skin patches that have been marketed as thermometers are not consistently reliable.

Either Fahrenheit or Celsius thermometers are acceptable.

Vaporizer

A vaporizer is a good investment. It efficiently provides the fog necessary for the relief of croup (see pages 352–353) and is soothing for many other coughs. A cold-mist vaporizer is preferable because there is no possibility of a child's being burned by hot steam. It is not necessary to add any medication to the vaporizer. These preparations make the room smell nice but do not add to the therapy offered by the fog alone. Some recent studies suggest that a vaporizer may not be as effective as previously believed. However, it will do no harm and may benefit some children.

Sunscreen

Products with a variety of ingredients effectively block out some of the sun's rays and can reduce the risk of sunburn and skin cancer. (See Sunburn, page 398.) Get a product with a sun protection factor (SPF) of at least 15, which blocks out 94% of ultraviolet (UV) light. SPF 30 blocks out 97% of UV light.

Antihistamines

Antihistamine compounds are useful in children who have well-documented cases of allergic skin reactions to insect bites, allergic rhinitis, hay fever, or chronic hives. The discomfort of hay fever should always be balanced against the risk of the side effects caused by antihistamines. Antihistamines are often dispensed in combination with a decongestant. (See Cough and Cold Medicines, on page 225.)

The most common antihistamines are chlorpheniramine (Chlor-Trimeton); brompheniramine (Dimetane); triprolidine (Actidil); diphenhydramine (Benadryl); and hydroxyzine (Atarax, Vistaril). Newer preparations, such as loratadine (Claritin) and cetirizine (Zyrtec), have fewer side effects.

Drowsiness is the most common side effect and can interfere with a child's schoolwork. Some parents feel that antihistamines are useful in helping children get to sleep at bedtime, but children really never go into the sleep stage that is most restful while on antihistamines. In fact, such children have an insufficient amount of the proper type of sleep. Antihistamines can occasionally cause hyperactivity in children. Follow package instructions for dosage.

Decongestants for Colds

A concern with colds is that the swelling and secretions associated with them may block either the sinus outlets or the eustachian tube. Because the sinuses are very poorly developed in very young children, there is not as much need to worry about sinusitis in these children. However, if the eustachian tube, which drains the normal secretions from the middle ear into the child's nasal cavity, remains plugged for a day or so, a middle ear infection may begin. It is easier for this tube to swell and close in younger children because it is shorter, narrower, and at a more horizontal angle than in older children.

Decongestants cause constriction of blood vessels in the nose and may reduce stuffiness. However, they have the same effect on many other blood vessels, which may not be desirable.

At this time, there is no convincing evidence that the use of these decongestants prevents the complications of sinusitis or middle ear infection. However, decongestants used in recommended doses are safe and may provide symptom relief for colds. They should **not** be given to infants and toddlers younger than two years old.

Cough and Cold Medicines

The most common type of cough medication is a **suppressant.** The cough reflex is a natural defense that helps clear the child's lungs of mucus that is accumulating because of infection. The reflex usually should be encouraged. But there are times when coughing seems to interfere with a child's getting better, such as when a cough keeps the child from getting to sleep. Occasionally during the daytime, children may have coughing that is so prolonged and so severe that it begins to cause chest pain. This may be another indication for suppressing the cough.

Studies do not support the effectiveness of cough suppressants such as dextromethorphan in children, they may potentially be of benefit. Dextromethorphan is sometimes sold in combination with other drugs, which have also not been shown to be effective against coughing. An antihistamine, diphenhydramine, has also been used occasionally for cough suppression, but it is associated with drowsiness. Until studies demonstrate some benefit to cough suppressants, we do not recommend them.

Although there are only two commonly available cough medications, these are prepared in dozens of ways. Many familiar products now come in a range of formulas. For instance, Robitussin, Vicks Formula 44, and PediaCare all have numerous preparations marketed with such terms as cough, cough and cold, decongestant, long-acting cough and cold, and allergy. Such variety can confuse parents. This is particularly troublesome as some preparations contain acetaminophen and parents may mistakenly be giving their children too much acetaminophen by combining a cold medicine with this product with a fever reducer such as Tylenol. Read the label carefully to be sure that a particular preparation contains the correct essential ingredient. Avoid preparations that combine acetaminophen with other cold relievers unless they have been specifically recommended by your doctor.

Although research has not shown cough or cold preparations to be effective, a study published in 2007 documented the effectiveness of buckwheat honey in reducing the frequency of cough. Buckwheat honey is difficult to find on store shelves but can be ordered on the Internet. It is unclear whether regular honey works. Honey should **never** be given to infants less than one year old because of the risk of botulism.

While we do not recommend cough and cold medicines, and national guidelines indicate they should **not** be given to children younger than two years, some parents and a few physicians may recommend them for older children. For this reason we are providing Table 5 on page 226.

In addition to cough suppressants there are cough expectorants.

Guaifenesin is an example of an **expectorant.** Its purpose is to help liquefy the secretions in the lungs and help the cough reflex to remove these secretions from the lungs. The principle of liquefaction is extremely important, especially in illnesses such as croup. However, there is little evidence to indicate that any cough syrup is very effective in producing this liquefaction. Vaporizers (see page 223) are far more useful for liquefying secretions.

Table 5: Ingredients in Some Common Brand-name Medicines

Medicine	Fever/ Pain Reducer	Antihistamine	Decongestant	Cough Suppressant
Tylenol	Acetaminophen			
Advil	Ibuprofen			
Motrin	Ibuprofen			
Robitussin Cough				Dextromethorphan
Robitussin Cough & Cold		Chlorpheniramine		Dextromethorphan
PediaCare Children's Allergy & Cold		Diphenhydramine	Phenylephrine	
PediaCare Children's Long-acting Cough			Pseudoephedrine	
Sudafed Nasal Decongestant			Pseudoephedrine	
Actifed		Chlorpheniramine	Phenylephrine	
Vicks Formula 44 Custom Care Congestion			Phenylephrine	Dextromethorphan
Vicks DayQuil Cold & Flu	Acetaminophen		Phenylephrine	Dextromethorphan
Vicks NyQuil Cold & Flu	Acetaminophen	Doxylamine	Phenylephrine	Dextromethorphan

Nose Drops

A runny nose is often the worst symptom of a cold or allergy. Although a runny nose is a nuisance and not very aesthetic, it is seldom a serious problem and does help to carry the virus outside the body.

Nose drops usually contain decongestants (see Decongestants, page 224) such as phenylephrine (Neo-Synephrine), or oxymetazoline (Afrin). These drugs work by causing the muscles in the walls of the blood vessels to constrict, decreasing blood flow. After many applications, these small muscles become fatigued and fail to respond. Finally, they are so fatigued that they relax entirely, and the situation becomes worse than it was in the beginning. Generally, this fatigue process does not occur in the first three days, so most doctors recommend the use of nose drops only for a short, temporary problem. The advantage of Afrin is that it is reputed to have a longer-lasting effect than Neo-Synephrine, but it is more expensive. For children with severe allergic rhinitis or hay fever, effective anti-inflammatory drugs such as nasal cromolyn (Nasalcrom) and nasal steroids (Flonase, Vancenase) are available by prescription.

Perhaps the cheapest and safest nose drops can be made by mixing ½ teaspoon (2.5 ml) of salt in a glass of water. Many doctors feel that these drops are as effective as medicated nose drops. Our favorite remedy for a runny nose is the tissue, used frequently and gently!

Soothing Lotions

These lotions, such as calamine, have a cooling effect and are useful in diminishing the itching of a variety of rashes, from poison ivy to chicken pox. They should not be applied to raw or weeping skin.

Other Medicines

Constipation Medicines

Constipation is very seldom a serious problem in children. (See Constipation, page 300.) Medication should be used only after dietary changes. Prune juice, every grandmother's favorite remedy, is still effective in relieving constipation. Prune juice acts by drawing a large amount of water into the intestines, thereby helping to soften hard stools. Food high in fiber or bran is also extremely effective. Drinking lots of water also will help. Although laxatives (Maltsupex, milk of magnesia, Ex-Lax, Colace, mineral oil, and Metamucil) are used commonly in children, they are only very rarely required. Mineral oil is perhaps the cheapest and most effective remedy but it is dangerous in infants and toddlers because of the potential problems it can

cause if vomited and inhaled into the lungs. A safe lubricant, MiraLAX, is now available over the counter.

There is virtually no indication for giving a child an enema. An enema can be extremely frightening, and serious complications can occur.

Diarrhea Medicines

The proper management of diarrhea is discussed elsewhere. (See Diarrhea, page 459.) Medication is of little use in the treatment of ordinary diarrhea. Compounds such as attapulgite (frequently found in preparations such as Kaopectate) or kaolin and pectin will help change a liquid stool into a more gelatinous stool. We do not see the necessity of using these types of preparations merely to change the form of the stool. They do not decrease the diarrhea or the amount of water lost. Some parents, however, find that leakage out of diapers is less of a problem with a more formed bowel movement.

In one study, bismuth subsalicylate (the active ingredient in Pepto-Bismol) was shown to reduce diarrhea if given in oral solutions every four hours over three days. However, the children in this study who were not given medicine for diarrhea had no greater weight loss than the children who were treated. Again, giving this medicine seems like a lot of effort for a minimal benefit.

Paregoric-containing preparations (such as Parepectolin and Parelixir) are not recommended for use in children. Paregoric is a narcotic that decreases the activity of the digestive tract. The increased activity of the digestive tract caused by diarrhea is a defense mechanism that usually should not be suppressed. In addition, a narcotic overdose can occur with paregoric, as can drowsiness and nausea. And, like most other narcotics, paregoric can produce constipation. Lomotil contains a narcotic-like compound that is also not recommended for children.

Certain solutions available in supermarkets and drugstores (Pedialyte, Ricelyte) are quite valuable in preventing or treating dehydration in a child with diarrhea. These solutions are not diarrhea treatments, however.

Eyedrops

Eye irritations in children seldom require the use of over-the-counter preparations such as Visine or Murine. Pinkeye and its treatment are discussed in Eye Redness, Burning, Itching, and Discharge, page 321.

Vitamins

We mention vitamins only to emphasize that vitamin supplementation is not required for most children. An ordinary diet, balanced with foods from each of the major groups, contains far more vitamins than a growing body requires. Vitamin D supplementation is recommended for infants who are breast-feeding, but that is all. Minerals are also abundantly present in common foods. (See Weakness and Fatigue, page 308), for a list of iron-containing foods.) For teens adopting a vegetarian or vegan diet, vitamins and iron are often necessary. Fluoride needs to be provided if the water supply is deficient (see page 186). An American child taking vitamin and mineral supplements secretes the most expensive urine in the world, because that is where these excess materials end up.

Chapter Twelve

Minimizing Risks in an Age of Uncertainty

Some days it is tempting to stop reading or listening to news. Keeping ourselves and our children safe and healthy can seem overwhelming. It is not only terrorist attacks that are alarming. The Institute of Medicine recently estimated that nearly 100,000 people die annually because of errors by their health care providers. Drugs that have been used for years are pulled off the market because they increase the risk of suicide, heart attack, or breast cancer. Nonsmokers die of lung cancer because they lived with a smoker or were exposed to smoke at their jobs. For all of these reasons, we advocate throughout this book that parents adopt a healthy lifestyle and be actively involved in decisions about their health and the health of their children.

Creating a Safer Environment

Our environment poses numerous threats. Some we can see: the reckless driver, the broken fence allowing children access to a drainage ditch, the child riding a bike without a helmet. Many hazards we cannot see, but we become aware of these invisible environmental dangers as they attract media attention in brief bursts throughout the year.

While we cannot live outside our environment, we can take actions to limit some of the risks.

Infants

Pregnant and nursing mothers should avoid mercury- and PCB-containing fish if breast-feeding. (Call 1-888-SAFEFOOD or check the following websites: www.cfsan.fda.gov/seafood1.html; www.epa.gov/ost/fish; www.epa.gov/mercury.) Avoid polycarbonate bottles with formula. Get rid of your mercury thermometer and buy a digital model. NO SMOKING anywhere in the baby's living area

Toddlers

Make sure your house does not contain lead pipes. Older paint may contain lead. If your home has these conditions, or other risks of lead exposure, your child should be checked for lead (see pages 154–155). If your home has lead pipes, let water run cold before using. Install carbon monoxide detectors if you have any open flames in the home.

Avoid using pesticides in areas with children. The sun can be toxic; don't forget sunscreen. NO SMOKING anywhere in the toddler's living area.

Children and Adolescents

As children get older, there are special issues in addition to the above precautions. You are the most important source of support and teaching in your children's lives. They will learn to do what you do. If you smoke, they will be more likely to smoke. If you drink excessively, they may develop a casual approach to alcohol and other substances. Your children are more likely to live healthy lives if they observe you being healthy. NO SMOKING anywhere in your child's living area. When adolescence approaches, alcohol, tobacco, and other toxins pose a particular danger. While adolescence is a time of experimentation, alcohol and other substances can turn into fatal experiments. If you are concerned, insist your physician provide or direct you to appropriate help. (The National Alcohol/Drug Abuse hotline is 1-800-662-HELP.)

Parenting in an Age of Bioterrorism

After the World Trade Center attacks of September 11, 2001, and the following mail-based anthrax attacks, many remarked that the world had changed forever and that we would, from now on, live in a climate of fear. Widespread emotional effects were reported in adults and children alike. The need for an expanded role for parenting was apparent—a need for calm appraisal, wise counsel, and planning for the future.

The world has changed forever before. Part of parental wisdom comes from our experiences with the past. The world changed after Hiroshima with the proliferation of nuclear weapons. It changed with the epidemic of HIV/AIDS. These were bad changes, yet at some point we stopped building bomb shelters. We adapted to these large but remote risks, and the positive aspects of life grew and flourished.

We have trouble understanding risks, and we fear risks that seem catastrophic and uncontrollable. We fear risks that are new to us, and those that have a high "dread factor." We live with little fear of riding in automobiles despite the fact that 35,000 people die in accidents each year. We buckle seat belts, drive with care, and avoid driving impaired or riding with an impaired driver, but the risks are still there and largely not under our control. So it is clear that we can be comfortable with substantial risk. Many still smoke cigarettes, apparently without fear, although smoking kills 400,000 people each year. Contradictory approaches to personal risks are the rule rather than the exception.

Terrorism risks have been much lower than our everyday risks, even though each terrorism death is an individual tragedy. Quite likely if we could put all of the effort against domestic terrorism into reducing cigarette smoking we could save hundreds of thousands of lives. The anti-terror campaign is of course justified, but we need at the same time to keep it in perspective.

The underlying fear of terrorism is that a massive attack with an agent such as anthrax could cause a large number of casualties. This scenario is possible, but unlikely. These agents are hard to deliver, and the casualties are largely preventable. The anthrax attacks in 2001 were dealt with quite efficiently even with an unprepared public health system, and future attacks will evoke a faster and better response.

Anthrax

Anthrax is the most likely bioterror agent, and accidental releases from facilities have documented the nature of the threat, although most attacks, including eight separate attacks in Japan, have fizzled. Anthrax spores are very small, and when milled even smaller they can get into the lungs. The spores can then germinate and the bacteria multiply, and after a few days they produce toxins that are usually fatal. It takes 5,000 or so spores to cause illness. Treatment is usually effective if begun before the toxins are formed. Prevention by use of antibiotics before actual infection occurs is highly effective. The public health response has been to begin antibiotics after exposure if the chance of infection developing is greater than about 1 in 1,000. None of the exposed postal workers put on antibiotics in late 2001 got the disease, but it is not known how many would have developed clinical illness without the antibiotics.

Other Bioterror Agents

Smallpox is usually considered the next most likely threat, since population immunity is low and smallpox is very contagious. However, there are many public health measures that could contain an epidemic, and risk for a given individual should be very low. Quarantine is the oldest method of controlling smallpox epidemics. Vaccination of exposed persons is effective in four days, and the disease's incubation period is twelve days, so you can successfully vaccinate even after exposure. Mass vaccination would eliminate the threat of smallpox, but at the cost of some vaccination reactions. In a smallpox epidemic, well-defined procedures will be explained by public health officials through the media.

Other bioterror agents, such as plague, tularemia, botulism toxin, and hemorrhagic fevers appear much less likely to be used and less likely to cause major problems.

Talking with Children

Children will hear about a threat or an attack, and will often have inaccurate information. They pick up clues that suggest fear in their parents. You need to talk with them, for reassurance and about preparation.

Children under five often pick up bits and pieces. There may be increased clinginess or changes in sleeping or eating patterns. Ask them what they have heard. Be aware of what they are seeing on television and avoid live broadcasts.

Children aged six to eight may also show regressive behavior, emotional disturbance, and firmly held opinions. "This food may have anthrax in it." Try not to directly confront such statements but offer solid facts. "Anthrax is not catching." Keep television to a minimum. Ask them what they can do to be safer. Make them part of the plan.

Children aged nine to eleven may become obsessed with details. They may wonder why someone would do a thing like that. They may have rigid opinions about risks that are not real. They may have nightmares. They are often receptive to reassurance. Keep television to a minimum.

Children twelve and over are likely to keep any thoughts to themselves. They may use a form of denial. You may need to introduce the subject as one for easy conversation, and you may need to do this every few days. Ask: "What is new?" "What does it mean?" "Do you think that this is a problem for us?"

The most important thing is to show control of your own fears. Parenting is experience, calmness, reassurance, and preparedness.

Perspective

As a parent you need to provide perspective for your children, an even and consistent approach to risks, a demeanor of confidence, and honest discussions aimed at what your child is capable of understanding. You need to have a family plan for a mass exposure scenario. As with other problems in this book you can have a certain level of personal control, decide on rational action, and use personal responsibility to reduce chances of illness.

It is good to know what to do. But the chances you will need the advice provided here are very small. Use your concern about threats to health to plan to avoid larger risks, such as smoking cigarettes, not exercising, poor diet, and taking risks while driving. Be consistent in how you approach risks; take care of the biggest ones first.

The Child and the Common Complaint

Interpreting Childhood Complaints

In this part of *Taking Care of Your Child,* you will find information and decision charts that show you how to deal with more than 100 common medical problems of children. The general information describes possible causes of the problems, methods for treating them at home, and what to expect at the doctor's office if you need to take your child there. The decision charts summarize this information, helping you decide whether to use home treatment or to consult a physician.

How to Use Part IV

Follow these steps to use these sections.

1. **Is emergency action necessary?**
    Usually the answer is obvious. The most common emergency signs are listed in the top left box on page 237. More advice on these emergency problems is found in Chapter A, "Emergencies," starting on page 242. Other signs of illness that might indicate the need to take your child to the doctor are discussed in "The Sick Child," starting on page 240.

    It is a good idea to read Chapter A now so that you're prepared if an emergency occurs. Fortunately, the great majority of children's complaints don't require emergency treatment.

2. **Find the section that covers your medical problem.**
    Determine your child's chief complaint or symptom—for example, a cough, an earache, dizziness. Use the decision chart on page 237 to find the appropriate chapter. The first page of each chapter lists the problems the chapter covers, organized by type of complaint or by area of the body: neck pain, chest pain, abdominal pain, and so on.

    The illustration on pages 238–239 will help you to find the right section for problems that are localized in one part of the child's body. You can also look up a symptom in the table of contents or the index.

3. **Find the section for your child's worst problem first.**
    Your child may have more than one problem, such as abdominal pain, nausea, and diarrhea. In such cases, look up the most serious complaint first, then the next most serious, and so on.

You may notice some duplication of questions in the decision charts, especially when the symptoms are closely related. If you use more than one chart, use the most "conservative" outcome: If one chart recommends home treatment and the other advises a call to the doctor, call the doctor.

4. **Read all the general information in the section.**
The general material gives you important information about interpreting the decision chart. If you ignore it, you may inadvertently select the wrong course of action.

5. **Go through the decision chart.**
Start at the top. Answer every question, following the arrows indicated by your answers. Don't skip around; that may result in errors. Each question assumes that you've answered the previous question.

6. **Follow the treatment indicated.**
Sometimes there will be an instruction to go to another section, or a description or diagram of the action to take. More often you will find one of the instruction icons shown on the next page.

Don't assume that an instruction to use home treatment guarantees that the problem is trivial and may be ignored. Home therapy must be used conscientiously if it is to work. Also, as with all treatments, the home therapy may not be effective in a particular case, so don't hesitate to visit the doctor if the problem doesn't improve.

Similarly, if the chart indicates that you should consult the doctor, it does not necessarily mean that the illness is serious or dangerous. Often a physical examination is necessary to diagnose the cause of the problem, or you will benefit from certain facilities at the doctor's office.

The charts usually recommend one of the following actions.

▲ **Use Home Treatment**
Follow the instructions for home treatment closely and keep it up. Most doctors recommend these steps as a first approach to these problems.

If over-the-counter medications are suggested, look them up in the index and read about dosage and side effects in Chapter 11, "The Home Pharmacy," before you use them.

There are times when home treatment is not effective despite conscientious application. Think the problem through again, using the decision chart. The length of time you should wait before calling the doctor can be found in the general information in most sections. If you become seriously worried about your child's condition, call the doctor.

▲ **Seek Medical Care Now**

Go to your doctor or health care facility right away. In the general information, we try to give you the medical terminology related to each problem so that you can "translate" the terms your doctor may use during your conversation.

▲ **Seek Medical Care Today**

Call your pediatrician's office and say that you are bringing your child in. Describe your child's problem over the phone as clearly as you can.

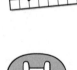

▲ **Make Medical Appointment**

Schedule a visit to your doctor's office anytime during the next few days.

▲ **Call Medical Advisor**

Call your child's doctor or nurse as a way to avoid unnecessary visits and to use medical care more wisely. Remember that most doctors do not charge for telephone advice but regard it as part of their service to regular patients. Don't abuse this service in an attempt to avoid paying for necessary medical care.

If every call results in a recommendation for a visit, your pediatrician is probably sending you a message: Come and don't call. This is unfortunate, and you may want to look for a doctor willing to put the telephone to good use.

With these guidelines, you will be able to use the following sections to locate quickly the information you need while not burdening yourself with information you don't require. Examine some of the charts now; you will swiftly learn how to find the answers to health problems.

On the following pages, we list several indications that your child may be ill. Noticing most of these signs depends on your knowledge of how your child usually behaves. Above all, trust your own judgment. Remember that you know your child best. If your child appears quite sick, be sure to get the necessary help. Common sense is your best guide in such matters.

Common Injuries
Chapter B

Common Concerns
Chapter C

How to Use
the Decision Charts

Does the child show any of
these emergency signs?
▲ Major injury
▲ No pulse or breath
▲ Unconsciousness
▲ Active bleeding
▲ Stupor or drowsiness
▲ Disorientation
▲ Shortness of breath
while resting
▲ Severe pain

Yes

Emergency
Call for help (911) or
go to the emergency
room immediately.
Turn to page 243 in
the black-edged
pages in the center
of this book for
more instructions.

Eye Problems
Chapter D

Ear, Nose, and
Throat Problems
Chapter E

No

Is the child choking and
unable to speak or cry out?

Yes *Emergency*
Turn to page 246.

Skin Problems
Chapter F

No

Has the child swallowed
poison?

Yes *Emergency*
Turn to page 250.

Childhood Diseases
Chapter G

No

Identify the type of problem
and turn to the appropriate
chapter. Use the blue tabs
to help you locate the
section. You may also look
up the problem in the index
or the table of contents.

Bones, Muscles,
and Joints
Chapter H

Chest and Digestive
Tract Problems
Chapter I

The Urinary Tract
and the Genitals
Chapter J

Adolescent Sexuality
Chapter K

KEY TO LOCALIZED PROBLEMS
See table of contents for a complete listing of problems

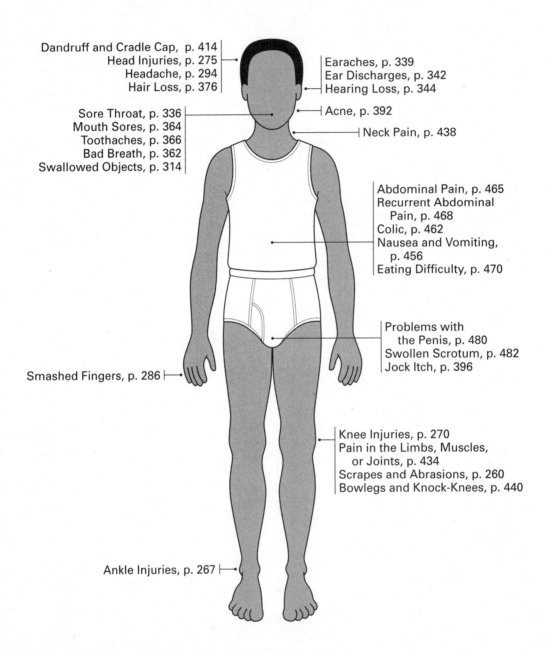

Dandruff and Cradle Cap, p. 414
Head Injuries, p. 275
Headache, p. 294
Hair Loss, p. 376

Earaches, p. 339
Ear Discharges, p. 342
Hearing Loss, p. 344

Sore Throat, p. 336
Mouth Sores, p. 364
Toothaches, p. 366
Bad Breath, p. 362
Swallowed Objects, p. 314

Acne, p. 392

Neck Pain, p. 438

Abdominal Pain, p. 465
Recurrent Abdominal
    Pain, p. 468
Colic, p. 462
Nausea and Vomiting,
    p. 456
Eating Difficulty, p. 470

Problems with
    the Penis, p. 480
Swollen Scrotum, p. 482
Jock Itch, p. 396

Smashed Fingers, p. 286

Knee Injuries, p. 270
Pain in the Limbs, Muscles,
    or Joints, p. 434
Scrapes and Abrasions, p. 260
Bowlegs and Knock-Knees, p. 440

Ankle Injuries, p. 267

KEY TO LOCALIZED PROBLEMS
See table of contents for a complete listing of problems

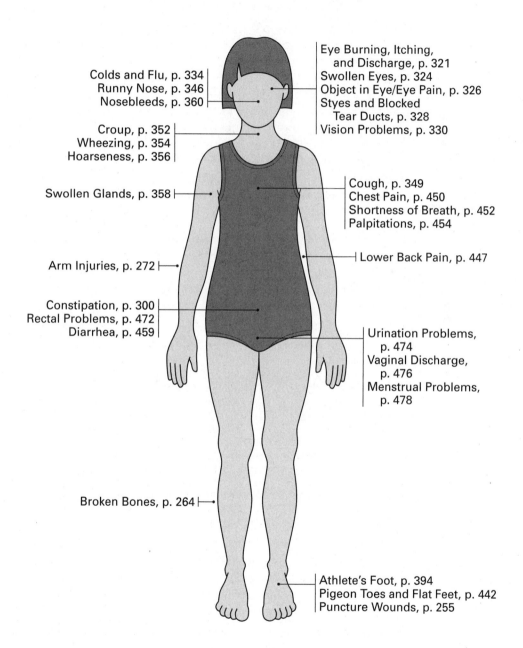

Colds and Flu, p. 334
Runny Nose, p. 346
Nosebleeds, p. 360

Croup, p. 352
Wheezing, p. 354
Hoarseness, p. 356

Swollen Glands, p. 358

Arm Injuries, p. 272

Constipation, p. 300
Rectal Problems, p. 472
Diarrhea, p. 459

Broken Bones, p. 264

Eye Burning, Itching,
    and Discharge, p. 321
Swollen Eyes, p. 324
Object in Eye/Eye Pain, p. 326
Styes and Blocked
    Tear Ducts, p. 328
Vision Problems, p. 330

Cough, p. 349
Chest Pain, p. 450
Shortness of Breath, p. 452
Palpitations, p. 454

Lower Back Pain, p. 447

Urination Problems,
    p. 474
Vaginal Discharge,
    p. 476
Menstrual Problems,
    p. 478

Athlete's Foot, p. 394
Pigeon Toes and Flat Feet, p. 442
Puncture Wounds, p. 255

The Sick Child

Sudden illness in a child can be very frightening. Children who are playing and well one minute may appear completely devoid of energy the next. It is a testimony to the strength of children that they have the resiliency to recover as quickly as they become ill.

All experienced parents can recognize the early signs of illness in their children. For some it is a dazed or glassy-eyed look; for others it is lethargy or bags under the eyes; for still others it is a pale or "pre-vomit white" color. In general, observation and common sense will tell you how sick your child is. An extremely active child who begins to slow down may be showing early signs of an illness, whereas a quiet child who becomes fussy or irritable should be suspected of having an illness. You should assess the following areas whenever you're considering illness in your child.

▲ **How old is your child?** As a general rule, all ill children under the age of six weeks should be brought to the doctor immediately. Illness in the first three to four months generally warrants a phone call. Illness in this age group is potentially more serious because it may progress far more rapidly than in older children.

▲ **What is your child's activity compared to usual at this time of day?** Is your child's sleep pattern disturbed? Is your child playing the way he or she usually plays?

▲ **How does your child respond to pleasant or unpleasant stimulation?** If he or she usually squirms or protests during a procedure such as temperature taking or swallowing medicine, the absence of this protest can signal a serious illness.

▲ **Is your child eating normally?** All children have some food finickiness, but severely ill children will refuse almost all food.

▲ **If vomiting or diarrhea is present, what is its nature?** If a child loses an excessive amount of fluid from vomiting or diarrhea, dehydration can result. The larger the amount of fluid lost in the vomitus or diarrhea, the greater is the likelihood of dehydration. Not only the frequency but also the amount is important to consider in your evaluation. If there is blood in either the vomitus or diarrhea, contact your doctor. If the vomiting is extremely violent, this is another indication for contacting your doctor.

▲ **Has your child urinated?** Infrequent urination and dark yellow urine are signs that your child is becoming dehydrated.

▲ **What is your child's skin turgor like?** Gather the skin on your child's stomach together using your five fingers. When you release it, it should spring back immediately. Dehydrated skin does not have the elasticity of normal skin. If there is a question in your mind, compare the sick child's skin with another child's or your own. The skin of a dangerously dehydrated child is like the skin of a very old person.

▲ **What is your child's skin color?** Children often become flushed or may even look pale, but a bluish color should prompt an immediate consultation with your doctor.

▲ **How do your child's eyes and mouth appear?** A dry mouth and eyes that appear sunken are signs of dehydration that require immediate attention by your doctor.

▲ **What is your child's temperature?** Fever is discussed extensively in its own section (page 288). A high fever can make your child feel quite uncomfortable and increase fluid requirements. A fever not associated with physical exertion is a sign of illness in a child.

▲ **What is your child's heart rate?** Children have a higher heart rate than adults, and the heart rate increases further with fever. It may decrease after severe head injury. In general, pulse rates over 130 or under 60 when a child is resting warrant an immediate doctor visit.

▲ **How fast is your child breathing?** The rate at which a child breathes decreases as the child becomes older. Breathing rates are far higher after activity. When evaluating your child's breathing rate, the child should be resting. Whereas many newborns have breathing rates of 50 to 60, by age 1 resting rates are usually between 25 and 35. A resting rate over 40 is of concern except in children under 1 year old. By age 6, resting respiratory rates should be below 30, and by age 10 below 25. Fever is a common cause of an elevated breathing rate, so assess your child's breathing rate at rest after you have attempted to reduce the fever. If rapid breathing is accompanied by labored breathing or shortness of breath, see the doctor immediately.

As you become more experienced with illnesses in your children, these observations and many of your own that are far more subtle will become intuitive. You will soon learn that you are the best judge of illness in your child. Doctors can help only in diagnosing the specific causes of an illness. The purpose of Part IV of this book is to assist you in managing many of the more commonly recognized illnesses on your own.

Emergencies

What Action Is Appropriate?

Emergencies require prompt action, not panic. What action you should take depends on the nature of the problem and the facilities available.

If there are massive injuries or your child is unconscious, you must get help immediately. Usually a 911 call brings the quickest response. However, if there is no 911 service in your area and if the emergency room is close by, go there. Have someone call ahead if you can.

If you can't get to the emergency room quickly, you can often obtain help over the phone by calling the emergency room. Calling for help is especially important if you think that your child has swallowed poison. Poison control centers and emergency rooms can often tell you over the phone how to counteract the poison, thus beginning treatment as early as possible. (See Poisoning, page 250.)

The most important thing is to be prepared. Use the spaces in the front of this book and on page 251 to record the phone numbers of the nearest emergency room, poison control center, and, if 911 service is not available, ambulance or paramedic rescue squad. Know the best way to reach the emergency room by car. Develop these procedures *before* an actual emergency arises.

Plan for Emergencies

Work out a procedure for medical emergencies. Develop and test it before an actual emergency arises. If you plan your actions ahead of time, you will decrease the likelihood of panic and increase the probability of your child receiving the proper care quickly.

Emergency Signs

The decision charts in the rest of this book assume that no emergency signs are present. Emergency signs "overrule" the charts and dictate that medical help should be sought immediately. Be familiar with the following emergency signs.

Major Injury

Common sense tells us that a child with an obviously broken leg or a large chest wound deserves immediate attention. Emergency facilities exist to take care of major injuries. They should be used promptly.

No Pulse or Breath

Again, a child whose heart or lungs are not working needs help right away. Call 911 for help. If you know cardiopulmonary resuscitation (CPR), start it after you call for help.

Unconsciousness

Obviously, any child in a state of coma or semiconsciousness should be brought immediately to the nearest medical facility. Coma is most often due to a medication or other toxic product taken by mouth, a seizure, drowning, severe head trauma, or a severe allergic reaction. Bring with you to the medical facility any medication or other material that you suspect might have been taken. Children breathing with difficulty should have their mouths cleared. You can give artificial respiration at the rate of 10 breaths per minute through the mouth or nose.

Active Bleeding

Most cuts will stop bleeding if pressure is applied to the wound. Unless the bleeding is obviously minor, a wound that continues to bleed despite the application of pressure requires attention to prevent unnecessary loss of blood. The average adult can tolerate the loss of several cups of blood with little ill effect, but children can tolerate only smaller amounts, proportional to their body size. Remember that active and vigorous bleeding can almost always be controlled by the application of pressure directly to the wound. This is the most important part of first aid for such wounds.

Stupor, Drowsiness, or Lethargy

A decreased level of mental activity, short of unconsciousness, is termed "stupor." A practical way of telling whether the severity of stupor, drowsiness, or lethargy warrants urgent treatment is to note the child's ability to answer questions. If he or she is not sufficiently awake to answer questions concerning what has happened, urgent action is necessary. Children are difficult to judge, but a child who cannot be aroused needs immediate attention.

Disorientation

In medicine, disorientation is described in terms of time, place, and person. This simply means that a disoriented child cannot tell the date, the location, or who he or she is. A child who does not know his or her own identity is in a more difficult state than one who cannot give the correct date. Disorientation may be part of a variety of illnesses and is especially common when a high fever is present. A child who becomes disoriented and confused needs immediate medical attention.

Shortness of Breath

Shortness of breath is described more extensively on page 452. As a general rule, a child deserves immediate attention if he or she exhibits shortness of breath while resting. However, in young adults the most frequent cause of shortness of breath at rest is the hyperventilation syndrome, which is not a serious concern. (See Stress, Anxiety, and Depression, page 306.) Nevertheless, if you cannot confidently determine that shortness of breath is due to the hyperventilation syndrome, the only reasonable course of action is to seek immediate aid.

Severe Pain

Surprisingly enough, severe pain is rarely the symptom that determines whether a problem is serious or urgent. Most often pain is associated with other symptoms that indicate the real problem. The most obvious example is pain associated with a major injury, such as a broken leg, which itself clearly requires urgent care.

The severity of pain is subjective and depends on the particular child. Emotional and psychological factors may make a child's pain worse. Nevertheless, severe pain demands urgent medical attention, if for no other reason than to relieve the pain.

Much of the art and science of medicine is directed at the relief of pain, and the use of emergency procedures to secure this relief is justified even if the cause of the pain eventually proves to be inconsequential. However, the person who frequently complains of severe pain from minor causes is in much the same situation as the boy who cried wolf. Calls for help will inevitably be taken less and less seriously by the doctor. This situation is a dangerous one, for a parent may have more difficulty obtaining help when it is most needed.

Poisoning

Seldom does the delay of a few minutes make any difference in the eventual outcome of poisoning. However, making a hasty *wrong* decision can be dangerous. Many poisons do their damage while being swallowed (acids, strong alkalis, drain and oven cleaners), and vomiting should *not* be induced. Other poisons

Ambulance and 911 Calls

Usually, the slowest way to reach a medical facility is by ambulance. It must go both ways and is not twice as fast as a private car. If your child can readily move or be moved and a private car is available, use the car and have someone call ahead.

The ambulance brings with it a trained crew who know how to lift a patient to minimize the chances of further injury. Oxygen is usually available, splints and bandages are carried in the ambulance, and, in some instances, lifesaving resuscitation may be used en route to the hospital. The care afforded by the ambulance attendants may most benefit a child who:
▲ Is gravely ill
▲ Has a back, neck, or head injury
▲ Is severely short of breath

Ambulances are too expensive to use as taxis. The type of accident or illness, the facilities available, and the distance involved are all important factors in deciding whether an ambulance should be used.

(turpentine, gasoline, furniture polish) cause damage from their vapors, and again vomiting should *not* be induced. Medication can be safely vomited. *Always bring the poison with you to the doctor or emergency room.* (For more on poisoning, see page 250.)

Seizures (Convulsions)

During a seizure, it is most important to protect the child from injury. Except for children known to have recurrent seizures, a prompt medical visit is required. See Seizures, page 312, for more information.

Choking

If an object has become lodged in your child's windpipe, choking may ensue. A child who can still speak or cry out is still breathing. In this case, it is best to have the object removed in the emergency room. Do not try to dislodge the object yourself if the child can breathe, because you might inadvertently cause complete obstruction. Violent coughing will often dislodge the object naturally.

If the child is choking on an object and not breathing, see Choking, page 246, for advice.

Choking

Choking is an emergency situation, but emergency medical services—doctors, emergency medical technicians (EMTs), ambulances, emergency rooms, hospitals—play virtually no role in its treatment. In almost every case, the child's fate will be decided by the time these sources respond. Someone must step forward and relieve the choking.

Reading the advice in this book is not the best preparation for a real choking emergency. Learn how to deal with choking by taking a CPR course.

Home Treatment

The most effective way to relieve choking in adults, adolescents, and older children is with the abdominal-thrust, or Heimlich, maneuver. Pushing on the lungs from below rapidly raises the air pressure inside the lungs and behind the foreign object causing the choking. This results in the forceful expulsion of the object—most often food—from the throat back into the mouth. Done properly, an abdominal-thrust maneuver does not pose a great risk of harm. Still, it's not the kind of thing that you want to do to a child who will not benefit from it. If the child in difficulty can speak, forget about the abdominal-thrust maneuver.

For Adolescents and Older Children

1. Stand behind the child and place your arms around him or her. Make a fist and place it against the child's abdomen, thumb side in, between the navel and the breastbone.

2. Hold the fist with your other hand, and push upward and inward, four times quickly.

If the victim is a pregnant or obese adolescent, place your arms around his or her chest and your hands over the middle of the breastbone. Give four quick chest thrusts.

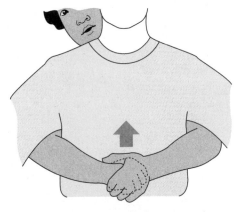

Abdominal-thrust (Heimlich) maneuver for adolescent or older child. The figures show the proper hand positions.

Above: standing position
Facing page: prone position.

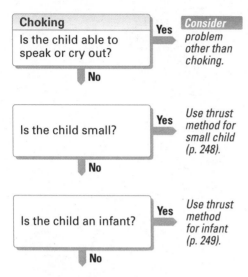

Choking		
Is the child able to speak or cry out?	**Yes** →	*Consider* problem other than choking.

No ↓

| Is the child small? | **Yes** → | *Use thrust method for small child (p. 248).* |

No ↓

| Is the child an infant? | **Yes** → | *Use thrust method for infant (p. 249).* |

No ↓

Use thrust method for adolescent or older child (facing page and this page).

Prevent Choking

The best approach to choking is preventive. Keep latex balloons away from children—they are a common cause of choking. Don't feed hard or large pieces of food to small children. Be especially careful with hot dogs, grapes, peanuts, and hard candy. Unfortunately, infants seem to put everything in their mouths.

If the child is lying down, roll the child over onto his or her back. Place your hands on the abdomen and push in the same direction on the body as you would if the victim were standing (inward and toward the upper body).

3. If the child does not start to breathe, open the mouth by moving the jaw and tongue, and look for the swallowed object. *If you can see the object, sweep it out with your little finger. If you try to remove an object you can't see, you may push it in farther.*

4. If the victim does not begin to breathe after the object has been removed, use mouth-to-mouth resuscitation.

5. Call for help, and repeat these steps until the object is dislodged and the victim is breathing normally.

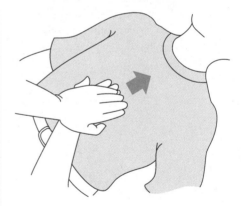

For Small Children

1. Kneel next to the child, who should be lying on his or her back.

2. Position the heel of one hand on the child's abdomen between the navel and the breastbone. Deliver 6 to 10 thrusts inward and toward the upper body.

3. If this doesn't work, open the mouth by moving the jaw and tongue and look for the swallowed object. *If you can see the object,* sweep it out of the throat using your little finger. If you try to remove an object you can't see, you may push it in farther.

4. If the child does not begin to breathe after the object has been removed, use mouth-to-mouth resuscitation.

5. Call for assistance, and repeat these steps until the object is dislodged and the child is breathing normally or until help arrives.

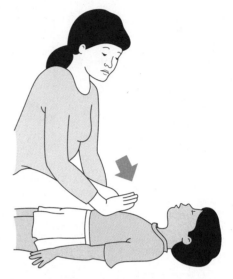

Abdominal-thrust for small child. Place the heel of your hand between the child's navel and breastbone. Deliver 6 to 10 quick thrusts. If this doesn't work, go to step 3.

For Infants

1. Hold the infant along your forearm, facedown, so that the head is lower than the feet.

2. Deliver four rapid blows to the back, between the shoulder blades, with the heel of your hand.

3. If this doesn't work, turn the baby over and, using two fingers, give four quick thrusts to the chest.

4. If you're still not successful, look for the swallowed object in the throat the same way you would for an older child. *If you can see it*, try to sweep it out gently with your little finger. If you try to remove an object you can't see, you may push it in farther.

5. If the infant doesn't begin to breathe after the object has been removed, use mouth-to-nose-and-mouth resuscitation.

6. Call for assistance, and repeat these steps until the object is dislodged and the infant is breathing normally.

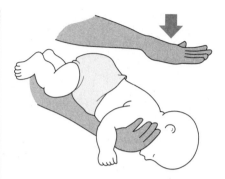

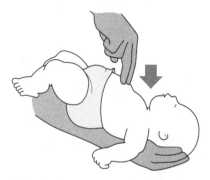

Abdominal-thrust for infant. If 4 rapid blows to the infant's back don't work, deliver 4 quick thrusts to the infant's chest, as shown above.

Infant CPR

Most communities now offer courses in infant CPR. Costs are usually minimal, and this may be a valuable investment of time for your child and your peace of mind.

Poisoning

Although poisons may be inhaled or absorbed through the skin, for the most part they are swallowed. The term *ingestion* refers to oral poisoning.

Most poisoning can be prevented. Children almost always swallow poison accidentally.

Don't allow children to reach potentially harmful substances such as the following:

▲ Medications
▲ Insecticides
▲ Caustic cleansers
▲ Organic solvents
▲ Fuels
▲ Furniture polish
▲ Antifreeze
▲ Drain cleaners

The last item is the most damaging. Drain cleaners such as Drano are strong alkali solutions that can destroy any tissue they touch.

Identifying the Problem

Treatment must be prompt to be effective, but identifying the poison is as important as speed. Don't panic. Try to identify the swallowed substance without taking up too much time. If you cannot, or if the victim is unconscious, go to the emergency room right away.

If you can identify the poison, call the doctor or poison control center immediately and get advice on what to do. Always bring the container of poison with you to the hospital. Life-support measures come first in the case of an unconscious victim, but the ingested substance must be identified before proper therapy can begin.

Many suicide attempts by teenagers involve significant medication overdoses. Any suicide attempt is an indication that the child needs help. Such help is not optional, even if the patient has "recovered" and is in no immediate danger. Most successful suicides are preceded by unsuccessful attempts.

Home Treatment

All cases of poisoning require professional help. Someone should call for help immediately. If the child is conscious and alert and the ingredients swallowed are known, there are two types of treatment: those in which vomiting should be induced and those in which it should not. Call 1-800-222-1222 for advice on poisonings and vomiting.

Do *not* induce vomiting if the child has swallowed any of the following:

▲ *Acids*—battery acid, sulfuric acid, hydrochloric acid, hair straightener, bleach
▲ *Alkalis*—drain cleaners, oven cleaners
▲ *Petroleum products*—gasoline, furniture polish, kerosene, lighter fluid

These substances can destroy the esophagus or damage the lungs as they are vomited. Neutralize them with milk while contacting the physician. If you don't have any milk, give the child water or milk of magnesia.

Vomiting is a safe way to remove medications or plant materials from the stomach and does not require a doctor's help. Vomiting can sometimes be achieved immediately by touching the back of the throat with a finger. Don't be squeamish!

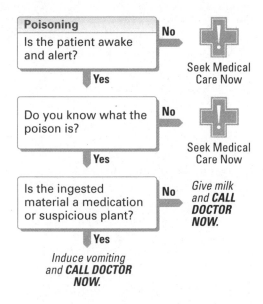

Poisoning

Is the patient awake and alert? — No → Seek Medical Care Now

Yes ↓

Do you know what the poison is? — No → Seek Medical Care Now

Yes ↓

Is the ingested material a medication or suspicious plant? — No → *Give milk and* **CALL DOCTOR NOW.**

Yes ↓

Induce vomiting and **CALL DOCTOR NOW.**

Emergency Numbers

Write these numbers down now, here and in the front of this book, and keep them by your phone.

National Poison Control

1-800-222-1222

Local Poison Control Center

_____

Emergency Room

_____

Many communities have established poison control centers to identify poisons and give advice. These are often located in emergency rooms. Find out if such a center exists in your community. If so, record the telephone number here and in the front of this book. Quick first aid and fast professional advice are your best chances to avoid a tragedy.

This is usually the fastest way to induce vomiting, and time is important.

Although no longer routinely recommended, another way to induce vomiting is to give the child 2 to 4 teaspoons (10 to 20 ml) of syrup (not extract) of ipecac (page 210), followed by as much liquid as the child can drink. Vomiting usually follows within 20 minutes. Mustard mixed with warm water also works. If vomiting occurs, collect what comes up so that the doctor can examine it.

Before, during, and after first aid for poisoning, contact the doctor.

If an accidental poisoning has occurred, make sure it doesn't happen again. Refer to pages 185–188 for information on "childproofing" your house.

What to Expect

Significant poisoning is best managed in the emergency room. Treatment of a conscious child depends on the particular poison and whether vomiting has been achieved. Activated charcoal is often used to remove poison from the stomach. If indicated, the stomach will be evacuated by vomiting or by the use of a stomach pump. Children who are unconscious or have swallowed a strong acid or alkali will require admission to the hospital. For those who are not admitted to the hospital, observation at home is important.

Common Injuries

Cuts (Lacerations)

Most cuts affect only the skin and the fatty tissue beneath it. Usually, they heal without permanent damage. However, injury to internal structures such as muscles, tendons, blood vessels, ligaments, or nerves presents the possibility of permanent damage. Your doctor can decrease the likelihood of this occurring.

Deeper Damage
You may find it difficult to determine whether major blood vessels, nerves, or arteries have been damaged. The following signs call for examination by the doctor.

▲ Numbness
▲ Bleeding that cannot be controlled with pressure
▲ Tingling
▲ Weakness in the affected limb

Signs of an infection—such as pus oozing from the wound, fever, or extensive redness and swelling—will not appear for at least 24 hours. Bacteria need time to grow and multiply. If these signs do appear, consult the doctor.

Stitches
Stitching (suturing) a laceration is a ritual in our society. The only purpose in suturing a wound is to pull the edges together to hasten healing and minimize scarring. If the wound can be held closed without the use of stitches, they are not recommended because they themselves injure tissue to some extent. A recently licensed skin glue can replace stitches in many situations. The glue works well in parts of the body with little stress on the skin and is used for small lacerations.

Stitching must take place within eight hours of the injury, because germs begin to grow in the wound and can be trapped under the skin to fester. Decide immediately whether to see the doctor or treat at home. Also refer to Does My Child Need a Tetanus Shot?, page 262.

Difficult Cuts
A cut on the face, chest, abdomen, or back is potentially more serious than one on the legs or arms (extremities). Luckily, most lacerations do occur on the extremities. Cuts on the trunk or face should be examined by the doctor unless the injury is very small or extremely shallow. If you see fat protruding from the wound, see the doctor.

In a young child who drools, facial wounds are often too wet to treat with bandages, so the doctor's help is usually needed. Because of potential disfigurement, all but minor facial wounds should

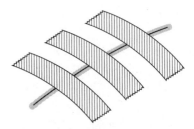

Steri-Strips. These sterile paper tape strips are the preferred bandage for closing and holding together the edges of clean, minor cuts.

Cuts (Lacerations)

Is there a possibility of damage to major blood vessels or nerves, or is there fever, pus, or extensive redness and swelling?

Yes →

Seek Medical Care Now

No ↓

Can the edges of the wound be brought together easily?

No →

Seek Medical Care Now

Yes ↓

Is the cut shallow (skin only), and is the laceration located on an arm or leg, on the scalp, or under the chin?

No →

Seek Medical Care Now

Yes ↓

Use Home Treatment

See:
Does My Child Need a Tetanus Shot?, p. 262

Removing Stitches

Your doctor will tell you when stitches are to be removed. While most stitches are removed in physicians' offices, you can perform this simple procedure yourself; ask your doctor if this is appropriate.

1. Clean the skin and the stitches. Sometimes a scab must be removed by soaking.

2. Gently lift the stitch away from the skin by grasping a loose end of the knot.

3. Cut the stitch at the far end as close to the skin as possible and pull it out. Small, sharp scissors or fingernail clippers work well. It is important to get close to the skin so that a minimum amount of the stitch that was outside the skin is pulled through. This reduces the chances of contamination and infection.

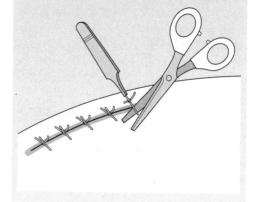

be treated professionally. Often stitching is required in young children, who are apt to pull off bandages, or in areas that are subject to a great deal of motion, such as the fingers or joints. Cuts in the palm are also prone to infection, so do not attempt home treatment unless the cut is shallow.

See Pain and Fever Relievers, page 217, for advice on pain medication.

Home Treatment

Cleanse the wound. The best method is to use lots of water. Soap is not needed, and hydrogen peroxide is no longer recommended. Make sure no dirt, glass, or other foreign material remains in the wound. This is very important. Antiseptics such as mercurochrome and Merthiolate are unlikely to help, and some are painful. Iodine will kill germs, but it is not really needed and also is painful. (Betadine is a modified iodine preparation that is painless but costly.)

The edges of a clean, minor cut can usually be held together by "butterfly" bandages or "Steri-Strips" (strips of sterile paper tape—preferred). Apply either of these bandages so that the edges of the wound join without "rolling under." See Bandages, page 221.

See the doctor if the edges of the wound cannot be kept together, if signs of infection appear (pus, fever, or extensive redness and swelling), or if the cut is not healing well within two weeks.

What to Expect

The doctor will thoroughly cleanse and explore the wound to be sure that no foreign particles are left inside and that blood vessels, nerves, and tendons are undamaged. If stitches are needed, the doctor may use an anesthetic to deaden the area. Be aware of any allergy to lidocaine (Xylocaine) or other local anesthetics; report any possible allergy to the doctor. The doctor will determine whether a tetanus shot or antibiotics are needed (usually not). Frequently doctors will close a clean, minor laceration with either Steri-Strips or a medical glue known as Dermabond.

Lacerations that may require a surgical specialist include those with injury to tendons or major blood vessels, especially when this damage has occurred in the hand. Facial cuts may also require a surgical specialist if a good cosmetic result is in question.

Puncture Wounds

Puncture wounds are those caused by nails, pins, tacks, and other sharp objects. The most important question is whether a tetanus shot is needed. See Does My Child Need a Tetanus Shot?, page 262, to determine this. Occasionally, puncture wounds do occur in which further medical attention is required.

Signs to Call the Doctor

Most minor puncture wounds are located in the extremities, particularly in the feet. If the puncture wound is located on the head, abdomen, or chest, a hidden internal injury may have occurred. Unless a wound in these areas is obviously minor, see the doctor.

Many doctors feel that puncture wounds of the hand, if not very minor, should be treated with antibiotics. Once started, infections deep in the hand are difficult to treat, and many lead to loss of function. Call the doctor.

Injury to a nerve or major blood vessel is rare but can be serious.

▲ Injury to an **artery** may be indicated by blood pumping vigorously from the wound.

▲ Injury to a **nerve** usually causes numbness or tingling in the wounded limb beyond the site of the wound.

▲ Injury to a **tendon** causes difficulty in moving the limb (usually finger or toe) beyond the wound.

Major injuries such as these occur rarely with a small object such as a sewing needle. They are more likely with a nail, ice pick, or larger object.

Unfortunately, because drug abuse remains common in our society, children encounter discarded hypodermic needles in playgrounds and on buses and beaches. A puncture wound from a discarded needle requires prompt medical care.

Infection

To avoid infection, be absolutely sure that nothing has been left in the wound. Sometimes, for example, part of a needle will break off and remain in the foot. If there is any question of a foreign body remaining in the wound, see the doctor.

Signs of infection do not occur immediately at the time of injury. They usually take at least 24 hours to develop. The formation of pus, a fever, or severe swelling and redness are indications that you should see the doctor.

Home Treatment

Cleanse the wound thoroughly with warm water. Let it bleed as much as possible to carry foreign material to the outside, because you cannot scrub the inside of a puncture wound. Do not apply pressure to stop the bleeding unless there is a large amount of blood loss and a "pumping," squirting bleeding.

Soak the wound in warm water several times a day for four or five days. The object of the soaking is to keep the skin puncture open as long as possible, so that any germs or foreign debris can drain from the wound. If the wound is allowed to close, an infection may form beneath the skin but not become apparent for several days.

See Pain and Fever Relievers, page 217, for advice on pain medication.

See the doctor if there are signs of infection or if the wound has not healed within two weeks.

What to Expect

The doctor will take the patient's history and examine the wound. He or she will explore the wound surgically if necessary. More frequently, the doctor will instruct you to watch for a reaction to a foreign body over the next few days. If the doctor suspects a metallic foreign body, he or she may order X rays. Be prepared to tell the doctor the date of the child's last tetanus shot.

Most doctors will recommend home treatment and only rarely prescribe antibiotics. In puncture wounds caused by buckshot, the shot may be left in the skin. Occasionally, glass or wood may be left in for a period of time to give the body time to push it to the surface.

In the unlikely event of an injury with a needle used for injections, the doctor may consider measures to protect your child from acquiring hepatitis. Risks of hepatitis and AIDS also will be discussed. Infants who have received hepatitis B immunization will not be at risk for this infection.

Puncture Wounds

Are any of the following present?

▲ Injury to a major nerve or blood vessel

▲ Any foreign material in the wound

▲ Fever, pus, or extensive redness and swelling

▲ Injury due to a needle used for injections

Yes → Seek Medical Care Now

No ↓

Is this a puncture wound of the hand, foot, face, or genitalia?

Yes → Seek Medical Care Today

No ↓

Are tetanus shots current?

No → *See:* Does My Child Need a Tetanus Shot, p. 262, and . . .

Seek Medical Care Today

Yes ↓

Is wound clean and minor?

No → Seek Medical Care Today

Yes ↓

Use Home Treatment

Animal Bites

The question of rabies is uppermost following an animal bite. Although 3,000 to 4,000 animals are found each year with rabies, only 1 or 2 humans contract the disease annually in the United States.

The main carriers of rabies are wild animals, especially skunks, foxes, bats, raccoons, and opossums. Raccoon rabies has been increasing in the Northeast and Mid-Atlantic States. Bats are increasingly implicated in rabies; children should keep out of caves in areas with bats. Rabies is also carried, though rarely, by cattle, dogs, and cats, and it is extremely rare in squirrels, chipmunks, rats, and mice.

Rabid animals act strangely, attack without provocation, and may foam at the mouth. Be concerned if the attacking animal has any of these characteristics.

Any bite by an animal other than a pet dog or cat requires consultation with the doctor as to whether the use of antirabies vaccine will be required. If the bite is by a dog or cat, if the animal is being reliably observed for sickness by its owner, and if its immunizations are up-to-date, consultation with the doctor is not required.

If the bite has left a wound that might require stitching or other treatment, see Cuts (Lacerations), page 252, or Puncture Wounds, page 255. Also see Does My Child Need a Tetanus Shot?, page 262. Facial wounds should be checked by the doctor because of potential disfigurement.

Home Treatment

An animal whose immunizations are up-to-date is, of course, unlikely to have rabies. However, arrange for the animal to be observed for the next 15 days to make sure that it does not develop rabies. Most often, the animal's owner can be relied on to observe it. If the owner cannot be trusted, the animal must be kept for observation by the local animal control agency. Many localities require that animal bites be reported to the health department. If the animal should develop rabies during this time, a serious situation exists, and your child must be treated by the doctor immediately.

For the wound itself, use soap and water. Treat bites as cuts (page 252) or puncture wounds (page 255), depending on their appearance. The best approach to animal bites is to avoid getting them. On pages 196–197, we suggest some ways in which parents can teach their children to get along with dogs and avoid bites.

See Pain and Fever Relievers, page 217, for advice on pain medication.

What to Expect

The doctor must balance the usually remote possibility of exposure to rabies against the hazards of rabies vaccine or antirabies serum. An unprovoked attack by a wild animal or a bite from an animal that appears to have rabies may require both the rabies vaccine and the rabies immune globulin. The extent and locality of the wounds also play a part in this decision. Severe wounds of the head are the most dangerous.

A bite caused by an animal that escapes after the bite will often require the rabies vaccine. Public health officials can

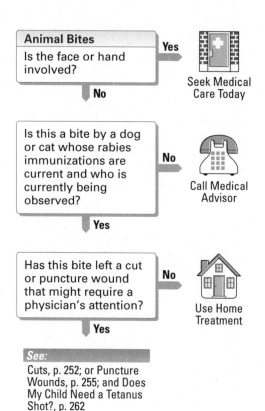

Animal Bites

Is the face or hand involved? — **Yes** → Seek Medical Care Today

No ↓

Is this a bite by a dog or cat whose rabies immunizations are current and who is currently being observed? — **No** → Call Medical Advisor

Yes ↓

Has this bite left a cut or puncture wound that might require a physician's attention? — **No** → Use Home Treatment

Yes ↓

See:
Cuts, p. 252; or Puncture Wounds, p. 255; and Does My Child Need a Tetanus Shot?, p. 262

be helpful by providing information on local patterns of rabies in animals.

Many doctors give a tetanus shot if the child is not up-to-date, because tetanus bacteria can (rarely) be introduced by an animal bite. Be sure you know when your child last received a tetanus shot.

Antibiotics usually will be given, especially for cat bites on the extremities.

Scrapes and Abrasions

Scrapes and abrasions are shallow. Several layers of the skin may be torn or even totally scraped off, but the wound does not go far beneath the surface. Abrasions are usually caused by falls onto the hands, elbows, or knees, but skateboard and bicycle riders frequently get abrasions on just about any part of their bodies. Because abrasions expose millions of nerve endings, all of which send pain impulses to the brain, they are usually much more painful than cuts.

Home Treatment

Remove all dirt and foreign matter. Washing the wound thoroughly with lots of warm water is the most important step in treatment. Hydrogen peroxide is no longer recommended. We recommend covering scrapes with an ointment to promote healing. Petroleum jelly works fine. Most antibiotics are no better than petroleum jelly for healing and cost more. Using mercurochrome, iodine, and other antiseptics does little good and is usually painful.

Adhesive bandages (page 221) help keep dirt out. Remove or replace bandages if they get wet.

Loose skin flaps, if they are not dirty, can be left to form a natural dressing. If the skin flap is dirty, cut it off carefully with nail scissors. (If it hurts, stop! You're cutting the wrong tissue.)

Watch the wound for signs of infection—pus, a fever, or severe swelling or redness—but don't be concerned about redness around the edges; this indicates normal healing. Infection will not be obvious in the first 24 hours. Serious infection without fever is rare.

Pain can be treated for the first few minutes with an ice pack in a plastic bag or towel. The worst pain will subside fairly quickly, and pain medication (page 217) can be used if necessary.

See the doctor if the scrape does not heal within two weeks.

What to Expect

The doctor will make sure that the wound is free of dirt and foreign matter. He or she will often use sterile solutions to wash out particles. Sometimes a local anesthetic is required to reduce the pain of the cleansing process.

The doctor may apply an antibacterial ointment after cleansing the wound. Mupirocin is especially effective. Betadine is a painless iodine preparation that also may be used.

A tetanus shot is not required for minor scrapes, but if your child is overdue for a shot, this is a good time to get caught up.

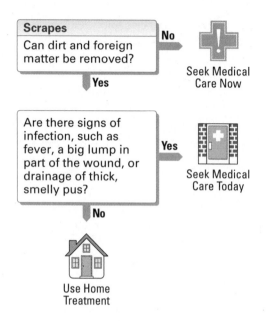

Scrapes

Can dirt and foreign matter be removed?

No → Seek Medical Care Now

Yes

Are there signs of infection, such as fever, a big lump in part of the wound, or drainage of thick, smelly pus?

Yes → Seek Medical Care Today

No

Use Home Treatment

Does My Child Need a Tetanus Shot?

Parents often wonder if a tetanus shot is needed after a child is injured. Often the wound is minor and needs only some soap and water. If the shot is not needed, you don't need a doctor. The decision chart illustrates the essential recommendations. It can save you and your children several visits to the doctor.

The question of whether a wound is minor may be troublesome. Wounds caused by sharp, clean objects, such as knives or razor blades, have less chance of becoming infected than those into which dirt or foreign bodies have penetrated. Abrasions and minor burns will not result in tetanus. The tetanus germ cannot grow in the presence of air; the skin must be cut or punctured for the germ to reach an airless location.

Immunization

If your child has never had a basic series of three tetanus shots, then you should see the doctor. Sometimes a different kind of tetanus shot is required if you have not been adequately immunized. This shot is called **tetanus immune globulin** and is used when immunization is not complete and there is a significant risk of tetanus. This shot is more expensive, more painful, and more likely to cause an allergic reaction than is the tetanus booster. So keep a record of your family's immunizations in the back of this book and know the dates.

During the first tetanus shots (usually a series of three injections given in early childhood), immunity to tetanus develops over a 3-week period. This immunity then slowly declines over many months. After each booster, immunity develops more rapidly and lasts longer. If your child has had an initial series of five tetanus injections, immunity will usually last at least 10 years after every booster injection. Nevertheless, if a wound has left contaminated material beneath the skin and not exposed to the air, and if your child has not had a tetanus shot within the past 5 years, a booster shot is advised to keep the level of immunity as high as possible.

Tetanus immunization remains very important, because the tetanus germ is quite common and the disease (lockjaw) is so severe. Be absolutely sure that your child has had the basic series of three injections and appropriate boosters. Because the immunity lasts so long, adults usually get away with a long period between boosters, but with children it should be "by the book." (See pages 165 and 173.)

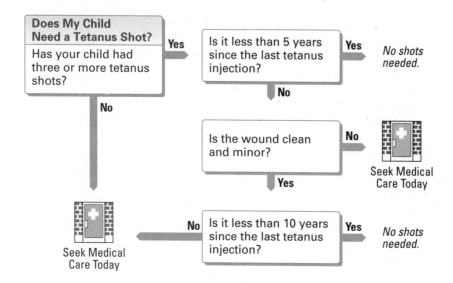

Does My Child Need a Tetanus Shot?

Has your child had three or more tetanus shots?

Yes → Is it less than 5 years since the last tetanus injection?

Yes → *No shots needed.*

No ↓

Is the wound clean and minor?

No → Seek Medical Care Today

Yes ↓

No ← Is it less than 10 years since the last tetanus injection?

Yes → *No shots needed.*

Seek Medical Care Today

No ↓ (from first question)

Seek Medical Care Today

Broken Bones

Neither parent nor doctor can always see whether a bone is broken. You often need an X ray if there is a reasonable suspicion of a fracture. The decision chart provides a guide to "reasonable suspicion."

In most fractures, the bone fragments are already aligned for good healing, and prompt manipulation of the fragments is not necessary. If the injured part is protected and resting, a delay of several days before casting does no harm. Remember that the cast does not have healing properties; it just keeps the fragments from getting joggled too much during the healing period. Possible fractures are discussed further in Ankle Injuries, page 267; Knee Injuries, page 270; and Arm Injuries, page 272.

Serious Fractures

A fracture can injure nearby nerves and arteries. If the limb is cold, blue, or numb, see the doctor now. Fractures of the pelvis or thigh are particularly serious. Fortunately, these fractures are relatively rare, except when great force is involved, as in automobile accidents. In these situations, the need for immediate help is obvious. For head injuries, see page 275.

Paleness, sweating, dizziness, and thirst can indicate shock, and immediate attention is needed.

A crooked limb is an obvious reason to check for a fracture. Pain that prevents use of the injured limb suggests the need for an X ray. Soft-tissue injuries (skin, muscle, fat, tendons) usually allow some use of the limb.

Although large bruises under the skin may be caused by soft-tissue injuries alone, marked bruising in a limb that may have a fracture means that you should see the doctor.

Common sense tells us that when great force is involved, such as in an auto accident, the possibility of a broken bone increases. A child who has fallen 20 feet out of a tree is much more likely to have a broken limb than a child who has stumbled and fallen.

Children's bones are more flexible and resilient than adults' bones. Instead of outright breaks, young bones often bend or splinter like young tree limbs; these breaks are called **greenstick fractures.** Young bones are also still growing. The growth plates of bones are near the ends. As a result, an injury to a bone near the end must be treated more cautiously because damage may stop limb growth.

Home Treatment

Apply ice packs. The immediate application of cold will help decrease swelling and inflammation. If a broken bone is suspected, the involved limb should be protected and rested for at least 48 hours. Here are some guidelines.

▲ The joint above and below the bone should be immobilized. For example, if you suspect a fracture of the lower arm, the splint should prevent the wrist and elbow from moving.

▲ For splinting, you can use magazines, cardboard, or a rolled-up newspaper.

▲ Do not wrap the arm tightly, or you will cut off circulation.

Do not forget pain control with ibuprofen or acetaminophen.

Broken Bones

Are any of the following conditions present?

- ▲ The limb is cold, blue, or numb.
- ▲ The fracture is in the pelvis or thigh.
- ▲ The child is sweaty, pale, dizzy, or thirsty.

Yes → Seek Medical Care Now

No ↓

Is the limb crooked?

Yes → Seek Medical Care Now

No ↓

Is the limb not usable or unable to bear weight?

Yes → Seek Medical Care Today

No ↓

Is there a great deal of bleeding and bruising in the area, was the injury the result of a severe blow, or is the possible fracture near a joint?

Yes → Seek Medical Care Today

No ↓

Use Home Treatment

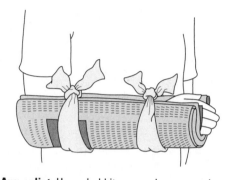

Arm splint. Household items such as magazines and cardboard can be used to make a splint. The forearm splint in the figure is made of rolled newspapers and cloths. Be careful not to cut off circulation by wrapping too tightly.

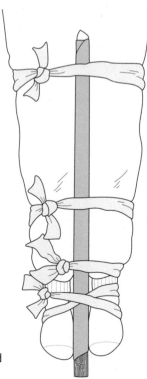

Leg splint. If a person may have a broken limb, it is important to keep that limb from shifting as you apply home treatment or go to the hospital. In the figure at right, a splint for one leg is anchored by the other leg and by a board wrapped with a towel.

Any injury that is still painful after 48 hours should be examined by a doctor. Minutes and hours are *not* crucial unless there is misalignment or injury to arteries or nerves. A limb that is adequately protected and rested is likely to have a good outcome even if casting is delayed. See Pain and Fever Relievers, page 217, for advice on pain medication.

What to Expect

Usually, an X ray will be required. In a small number of cases, it is possible to be relatively sure that an X ray is not needed from the history and physical examination. A crooked limb must be "set." Plastic splints are rapidly replacing plaster casts. Prescription pain medications may be used. Sometimes sedation or general anesthesia is required to realign a bone. Pinning the fragments together surgically is required for certain fractures, such as elbow fractures.

Ankle Injuries

Ligaments are tissues that connect the bones of a joint to provide stability during the joint's action. When the ankle is twisted severely, either the ligaments or the bones must give way. If the ligaments give, they may be stretched (strained), partially torn (sprained), or completely torn (torn ligaments). If the ligaments do not give, one of the bones around the ankle must break (fracture).

Strains, sprains, and even some minor fractures of the ankle will heal well with home treatment. Even some torn ligaments may do well without a great deal of medical care. Immediate attention is necessary when the injury has been severe enough to fracture a bone or tear a ligament. This is indicated by a deformed joint with abnormal motion. Fractures are more likely in a fall from a considerable height or in automobile or bicycle accidents. They are *not* likely to happen when the ankle is twisted while walking or running.

Swelling
The typical ankle sprain swells either around the bony bump at the outside of the ankle or about two inches in front of and below it. The usual sprain does not need prolonged rest, casting, or an X ray. Home treatment should be started promptly. Detection of damage to the ligaments is difficult immediately after the injury because of the amount of swelling that may be present. Because it is easier to do an adequate examination of the foot after the swelling has gone down and because no damage is done by resting a mild

fracture or torn ligament, there is no need to rush to the doctor.

Sprains and torn ligaments usually swell quickly, because there is bleeding into the tissue around the ankle. The skin will turn blue-black in the area as the body breaks down the blood. The amount of swelling will not help you differentiate between a sprain, a tear, and a fracture.

Pain
Pain tells you what to do with ankle injuries. If what the child is doing hurts, have him or her refrain from doing it. If pain prevents standing on the ankle after 24 hours, see the doctor. If pain still makes weight bearing difficult after 72 hours, see the doctor.

Home Treatment
Home treatment is adequate for all ankle injuries except for some fractures and complete ligament tears. Even if a fracture is present, if the ankle is rested and protected, no harm will result from waiting and watching.

Wrapping the ankle with an elastic bandage (page 221) may prevent some swelling and damage. Have the child elevate the ankle and keep it elevated. Do *not* let the child return to play as soon as the pain becomes bearable. Apply ice in a towel to the injured area and leave it there for at least 30 minutes. If there is any evidence of swelling after the first 30 minutes, apply ice for 30 minutes on and 15 minutes off during the next few hours. If the pain subsides completely when the ankle is in the elevated position, have the child cautiously attempt to stand. If pain is present, weight bearing should be avoided for the first 24 hours.

If at the end of the first 24 hours the pain prevents weight bearing, see the doctor. If pain is present but not severe, use crutches until walking can be accomplished with little discomfort, usually 2 to 3 days. During this time, you may apply an elastic bandage, but this will not prevent reinjury if full activity is resumed. Do not stretch the bandage so that it is very tight and interferes with circulation. The ankle should feel relatively normal by about 10 days. Full healing will not take place for 4 to 6 weeks.

See Pain and Fever Relievers, page 217, for advice on pain medication.

What to Expect

The doctor will examine the motions of the ankle to see if they are abnormal and may order an X ray. If there is no fracture, it is likely that the doctor will recommend a continuation of home treatment. He or she also may recommend home treatment if a minor chip fracture is noted. For other fractures, a cast, and perhaps an operation (rarely), will be necessary. Depending on the nature and extent of a ligament injury, an operation may be required to repair a completely torn ligament.

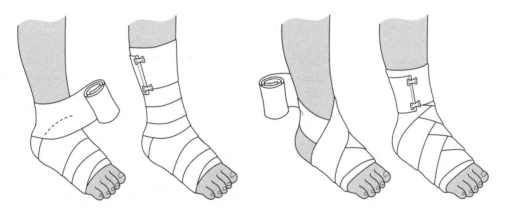

Ankle wraps. An elastic bandage, after an initial treatment of ice, may reduce swelling and damage in an ankle injury. Two wrapping styles are shown. Either should be effective if done properly. The bandage should not be too tight and should not cover the toes.

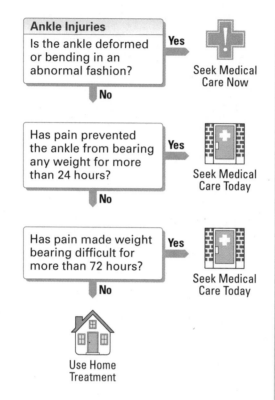

Ankle Injuries

Is the ankle deformed or bending in an abnormal fashion?

Yes → Seek Medical Care Now

No ↓

Has pain prevented the ankle from bearing any weight for more than 24 hours?

Yes → Seek Medical Care Today

No ↓

Has pain made weight bearing difficult for more than 72 hours?

Yes → Seek Medical Care Today

No ↓

Use Home Treatment

Crutches

Adjust crutches so that the shoulder support is two finger-widths short of the armpit. The hand, not the armpit, should bear the weight.

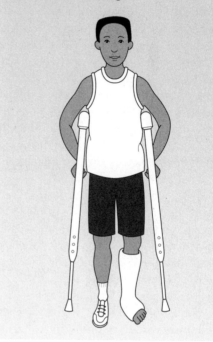

Knee Injuries

The ligaments of the knee may be injured in several ways. They may be stretched (strained), partially torn (sprained), or completely torn (torn ligament). Unlike in the ankle, torn ligaments in the knee need to be repaired surgically as soon as possible after the injury occurs. If surgery is delayed, the operation is more difficult and less likely to be successful. For this reason, the approach to knee injuries is more cautious than to ankle injuries. If there is any possibility of a torn ligament, go to the doctor.

Fractures in the area of the knee are less common than around the ankle, and all need to be cared for by the doctor.

Knee injuries usually occur during sports, when the knee is more likely to experience twisting and side contact. (Deep knee bends stretch knee ligaments and may contribute to knee injuries. They should be avoided.) Serious knee injuries occur when the leg is planted on the ground and a blow is received to the knee from the side. If the foot cannot give, the knee will. There is no way to avoid this possibility totally in athletics. The use of shorter spikes and cleats helps, but elastic knee supports and wraps give virtually no protection.

Abnormal Motion

When ligaments are completely torn, the lower leg can be wiggled from side to side when the leg is straight. Compare the injured knee to the other knee to get some idea of what amount of side-to-side motion is normal. Your examination will not be as skilled as that of a doctor, but if you think that the motion may be abnormally loose, see the doctor.

If the cartilage within the knee has been torn, the normal motion of the knee may be blocked, preventing it from being straightened. Although a torn cartilage does not require immediate surgery, it deserves prompt medical attention.

Pain and Swelling

The amount of pain and swelling does not necessarily indicate the severity of the injury. The ability to bear weight, to move the knee through the normal range of motion, and to keep the knee stable when wiggled is more important.

Typically, strains and sprains hurt immediately and continue to hurt for hours and even days after the injury. Swelling in strains and sprains tends to come on rather slowly over a period of hours, but it may reach rather large proportions. When a ligament is completely torn, there is intense pain immediately, which subsides until the knee may hurt only a little or not at all for a while. Usually, there is significant bleeding into the tissues around the joint when a ligament is torn, so major swelling tends to come on quickly.

The best policy when there is a potential injury to the ligament is to have the child avoid any major activity until it is clear that this strain or sprain is minor. Home treatment is intended only for minor strains and sprains.

Home Treatment
"RIPE" is your memory key.

▲ Rest
▲ Ice
▲ Protection
▲ Elevation

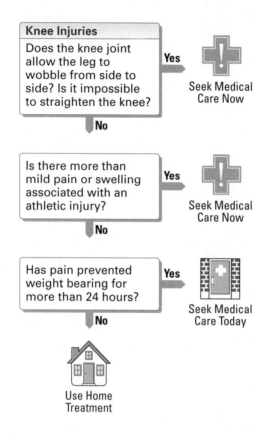

Knee Injuries

Does the knee joint allow the leg to wobble from side to side? Is it impossible to straighten the knee?

Yes → Seek Medical Care Now

No ↓

Is there more than mild pain or swelling associated with an athletic injury?

Yes → Seek Medical Care Now

No ↓

Has pain prevented weight bearing for more than 24 hours?

Yes → Seek Medical Care Today

No ↓

Use Home Treatment

Get the child off the knee and have him or her elevate it. Apply ice in a towel for at least 30 minutes to minimize swelling. If there is more than slight swelling or pain, see the doctor. If not, apply ice for 30 minutes on and 15 minutes off during the next several hours. Wrapping the knee with an elastic bandage (page 221) may prevent some swelling and damage. Limited weight bearing may be attempted during this time, with a close watch for increased swelling and pain.

Heat may be applied after 24 hours. By 24 hours, the knee should look and feel relatively normal. By 72 hours, this definitely should be the case. Remember, however, that a strain or sprain will not be completely healed for 4 to 6 weeks and that it requires protection during this healing period. An elastic bandage will not give adequate support but will ease symptoms a bit and remind the child to be careful with the knee.

See Pain and Fever Relievers, page 217, for advice on pain medication.

What to Expect

The doctor will examine the knee for range of motion and test the lateral stability by stressing the knee from side to side. With a massively swollen knee, he or she may remove blood from the joint with a needle. Torn ligaments need surgical repair. X rays may be taken but are not always helpful. For injuries that appear minor, the doctor will usually advise home treatment. Pain medications are sometimes, but not often, required.

Arm Injuries

The ligaments of the wrist, elbow, and shoulder joints may be stretched (strained) or partially torn (sprained), but complete tears are rare in children. This is because the weakest points of long bones in children are the soft cartilage growth plates at the bone ends. Trauma will often result in injury to these growth plates. Injuries to bone ends must be treated cautiously. Fractures may occur at the wrist, are less frequent around the elbow, and are uncommon around the shoulder. Injuries to the wrist and elbow occur most often as a result of a fall, when the outstretched arm catches the weight of the body.

Wrist

The wrist is the most frequently injured of these joints. Strains and sprains are common, and the small bones in the wrist may be fractured. Fractures of these small bones may be difficult to see on an X ray. The most frequent fracture of the wrist involves the ends of the long bones of the forearm and is easily recognized because it causes an unnatural bend near the wrist. Doctors refer to this as the **silver fork deformity.**

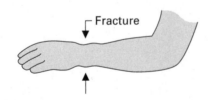

Elbow

The most frequent elbow injury is the **pulled elbow,** or nursemaid's elbow, which is often not even suspected. A young child (usually younger than five years old) is noted cradling one arm in the other and holding the arm or elbow. Parents often think that the arm is paralyzed because the child cannot lift it. Parents may not remember that the toddler was pulled along by the arm an hour before, although this is probably what caused the injury.

In the case of a pulled elbow, the palm of the hand faces down toward the floor or inward toward the belly. The cure for a pulled elbow is to turn the palm upward. The parent, nurse, or X-ray technician may perform this cure unknowingly before the child is seen by the doctor. A pulled elbow does not show up on an X ray.

Shoulder

Injuries to the shoulder usually result from a direct blow. The collarbone (clavicle) is a frequently fractured bone in children. Fortunately, it has remarkable healing powers. Parents will often notice the fracture because of the child's inability to raise the arm on the affected side. The shoulders also may appear uneven. This fracture occurs in newborns as well as in older children. Bandaging and a sling for comfort are the only treatment required.

The **shoulder separation** often seen in high school athletes is perhaps the most common injury of the shoulder. It is a stretching or tearing of the ligament that attaches the collarbone to one of the bones that forms the shoulder joint. It causes a slight deformity and extreme tenderness at the end of the collarbone. Sprains and strains of other ligaments occur, but complete tearing is rare, as are fractures. Dislocations of the shoulder are rare outside of high school athletics, but they are best treated early when they do occur.

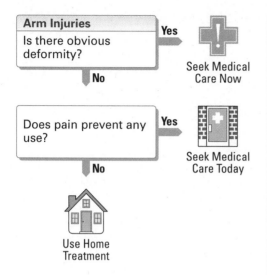

Arm Injuries
Is there obvious deformity?

Yes → Seek Medical Care Now

No ↓

Does pain prevent any use?

Yes → Seek Medical Care Today

No ↓

Use Home Treatment

In summary, severe fractures and dislocations of the arm are best treated early. These usually cause deformity, severe pain, and limitation of movement. Other fractures will not be exacerbated if the injured limb is rested and protected for a time before treatment. Complete tears of ligaments are rare. Strains and sprains will heal with home treatment.

Home Treatment

Pulled Elbow

Bend the elbow so that the forearm and upper arm form a right angle. With one hand, hold the elbow so it cannot move. With the other hand, grasp the child's hand and wrist and turn the palm upward, while gently pulling away from the body at the elbow. Some doctors prefer a quick, forceful twist, but we think a gentle turn works just as well. Initially, this turning will cause discomfort. You may feel, or even hear, a click. Repeating this maneuver, followed by bringing your child's palm up to the shoulder (bending the elbow), may enhance your chances of success. Stop the procedure if your child complains of severe pain.

If treatment occurs soon after the injury, immediate relief of pain is usual. If treatment is delayed, some soreness usually remains for a short period. Great force is not required for this treatment. If success does not come easily, see your doctor.

Sprains and Strains

"RIPE" is the memory key.

▲ Rest
▲ Ice
▲ Protection
▲ Elevation

Rest and elevate the arm and apply ice for at least 30 minutes. If the pain is gone and there is no swelling at the end of this time, the ice may be discontinued. A sling for shoulder and elbow injuries and a partial splint for wrist injuries will give protection and rest to the injury while allowing the child to move around.

If swelling occurs, ice wrapped in a towel applied for 30 minutes on and 15 minutes off may be continued through the first 8 hours. Heat may be applied *after* 24 hours. The injured joint should be usable with little pain within 24 hours and should be almost normal by 72 hours. If this is not the case, see the doctor.

Complete healing takes four to six weeks. If possible, the child should avoid activities with a likelihood of reinjury during this time.

See Pain and Fever Relievers, page 217, for advice on pain medication.

What to Expect

The doctor will perform an examination and sometimes call for X rays. He or she will fix a pulled elbow if you haven't already done so. A broken bone may require a cast. A sling may be devised. Strong pain medication is sometimes given, but acetaminophen and ibuprofen are often effective and safer.

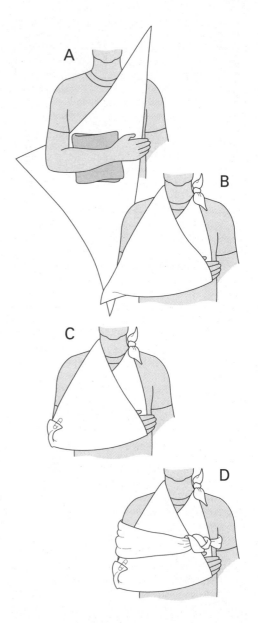

Tying an arm sling. (A) Use a triangular piece of cloth (or a folded square sheet). A small folded towel adds support.

(B) Tie as shown.

(C) A safety pin will hold it securely.

(D) To add even greater security, tie another strip of cloth around the chest and arm as shown.

Head Injuries

Every child will experience a bump on the head sometime in life, and many children seem to bump their heads every few days. Many of these injuries will be minor, such as those from walking into a table or falling from the couch.

A serious head injury is more likely to occur with more severe trauma, such as falling from a roof, being hit by a baseball, or being involved in an automobile accident. Injuries from such accidents are usually preventable.

▲ Bicyclists, skateboarders, roller skaters, scooter riders, and baseball players should always wear helmets.
▲ Children riding in a car should always wear seat belts or, if younger, be protected by car seats (see pages 192–193).
▲ Parents should educate their children about safety.

All head injuries are potentially serious, but few lead to problems. The major concern in a head injury in which the skull is not obviously damaged is bleeding inside the skull. The accumulation of blood will eventually compress the brain and cause damage. Fortunately, nature has carefully cushioned the valuable contents of the skull. In infants, the fontanel, or soft spot, serves as a safety valve to help diminish the severity of head injuries.

Signs of Serious Injury
Careful observation is the most valuable tool for diagnosing a serious head injury. Observation of your child begins with the accident. If the child was knocked unconscious or cannot remember the events immediately before or after the accident, he or she has a concussion, and you should take the child to the doctor.

The initial observation period is crucial. Bleeding into the head can be very rapid within the first 24 hours (this type of bleeding is potentially very serious and is called an **epidural hematoma**) and may continue for 72 hours or more. Some very slow bleeding may occur. This is called a **subdural hematoma** and may produce chronic headache, persistent vomiting, or personality changes months after the injury.

How does your child act? Increased lethargy (laziness), alternating alert and drowsy periods during the day, and unresponsiveness are all signs of possible bleeding within the skull. The child may be lethargic, seem to recover, and then become lethargic again.

Vomiting usually occurs at least once after any significant head injury. If *repeated* vomiting occurs, see the doctor. A seriously affected child also cannot be easily aroused.

How does your child look? Bring the child to the doctor if he or she appears persistently pale, sweaty, or weak. Look for unequal pupil size, which can be caused by pressure on the brain created by blood within the skull. Some children have pupils that are unequal all the time; this is normal for them. If the pupils become unequal after an injury, however, it is a sign of serious injury.

A slow pulse (less than 60) or an irregular pulse may be a sign of internal bleeding in the head.

In a typical minor head injury, a bump may develop immediately. The child will remain conscious and cry immediately.

For a few minutes, the child will be inconsolable, and he or she may vomit once or
twice over the first few hours. You may notice some sleepiness from the excitement,
but the child will be easily aroused from a
nap. Neither pupil will be enlarged, and
the vomiting will cease shortly. The child
will not appear pale, and the pulse will be
strong and regular. Within eight hours,
the child will be back to normal, except
for the tender and often prominent
"goose egg."

Home Treatment

For minor injuries, ice applied to a
bruised area may minimize swelling, but
children often develop "goose eggs" anyway. The size of the bump does not necessarily indicate the severity of the injury.

In serious accidents, also look for injury to the chest, abdomen, or extremities.

Reassess your child's condition frequently. If there are any suspicious signs,
consult the doctor by phone at once. Because most accidents occur in the evening,
the child may be asleep for several hours
after the accident. If you are concerned
about the injury, look in on the child periodically to check his or her pulse, pupils,
and arousability. Nighttime checking is
usually not necessary with minor bumps.

What to Expect

The doctor will take an extensive history
on the nature of the accident, assess the
child's general appearance, and repeatedly check blood pressure and pulse rate.
In addition, the doctor will examine the
head, eyes, ears, nose, throat, neck, and
nervous system. He or she also will check
for other possible sites of injury, such as
the chest, abdomen, and arms and legs.

A diagnosis of bleeding within the
skull cannot be made with great accuracy.
Skull X rays are seldom helpful, except in
detecting whether a fragment of bone has
been pushed into the brain, but this situation is rare. With severe injuries, neck
X rays may occasionally be required.

Where internal bleeding is of concern,
the doctor may order special radiological tests (computerized tomography, or
CT, scans), or the child may be hospitalized for observation. During this observation period, the child's pulse, pupils, and
blood pressure will be checked periodically. Use of medications, which may ob-
scure the situation, will be avoided.

Head Injuries

Have any of the following occurred?

▲ Moderate to severe injury

▲ Child was knocked unconscious

▲ Child cannot remember injury

▲ Seizure

Yes →

Seek Medical Care Now

↓ **No**

Are any of the following present?

▲ Visual problems

▲ Bleeding from other than scalp

▲ Black eyes or blackness behind ears

▲ Change in child's behavior (irritability, sleepiness, laziness)

▲ Fluid draining from nose

▲ More than 2 episodes of vomiting

▲ Irregular breathing or heartbeat

Yes →

Seek Medical Care Now

↓ **No**

Is child younger than one year?

Yes →

Call Medical Advisor

↓ **No**

Is there a cut?

Yes →

See:
Cuts, p. 253, and Does My Child Need a Tetanus Shot?, p. 262

↓ **No**

Use Home Treatment

Burns

How bad is your child's burn? Burns are classified according to depth.

First-degree burns are superficial and cause the skin to turn red. A sunburn is usually a first-degree burn. (See Sunburn, page 398.) First-degree burns may cause a lot of pain but are not major medical problems. Even when they are extensive, they seldom give rise to lasting problems or need a doctor's attention.

Second-degree burns are deeper and result in splitting of the skin layers or blistering. Scalding with hot water and a very severe sunburn with blisters are common instances of second-degree burns. Second-degree burns are painful, and extensive second-degree burns may cause significant fluid loss. Scarring, however, is usually minimal, and infection usually is not a problem.

Second-degree burns can be treated at home if they are not extensive. See the doctor for any second-degree burn that involves an area larger than the child's hand. Also see the doctor for a second-degree burn that involves the face or hands. These might result in cosmetic problems or loss of function.

Third-degree burns destroy all layers of the skin and extend into the deeper tissues. They are *painless,* because nerve endings have been destroyed. Charring of the burned tissue is usually present. Third-degree burns result in scarring and present frequent problems with infection and fluid loss. The more extensive the burn, the more difficult these problems. See the doctor for all third-degree burns, because not only can they lead to scarring and

infection, but skin grafts also are often needed.

Home Treatment

Apply cold water immediately. This reduces the amount of skin damage caused by the burn and also eases the pain. Keep the skin cold for at least five minutes and continue until the pain is relieved or up to one hour, whichever comes first. Ice packs are excellent in this situation. Be careful not to apply cold so long that the burned area turns numb, because frostbite can occur. Reapply cold if the pain returns.

Acetaminophen can be used to reduce pain. Blisters should not be broken. If they burst by themselves, as they often do, the overlying skin should be allowed to remain as a wet dressing. The use of local anesthetic creams or sprays is not recommended, because they may slow healing. Also, some patients develop an irritation or allergy to these drugs. Do not use butter, cream, or petroleum jelly; they may slow healing and increase the possibility of infection. Certain antibiotic creams (such as Neosporin and Bacitracin) probably neither help nor hurt minor burns and are expensive.

See the doctor for any burn that continues to be painful for more than 48 hours.

What to Expect

The doctor will establish the extent and degree of the burn and will determine the need for antibiotics and further treatment. He or she will often recommend an antibacterial ointment and dressing, with frequent changes and checks for infections. Extensive burns may require hospitalization, and third-degree burns may eventually require skin grafts.

Burns

Is this a third-degree burn with painless or charred areas?

Yes →

Seek Medical Care Now

No ↓

Is this a second-degree burn that is:
- ▲ Extensive?
- ▲ On the face or hands?
- ▲ Encircling the arm or leg?
- ▲ On the genital areas?

Yes →

Seek Medical Care Now

No ↓

Use Home Treatment

Prevention

Most burns are avoidable. Review potential fire hazards in your home with the help of Chapter 10. Set your hot water thermostat to 120°F. Teach your older child what to do if burned. Be sure your child knows not to run if his or her clothing catches on fire, as this will fan the flames. A child should **stop, drop, and roll** on the ground to put out flames.

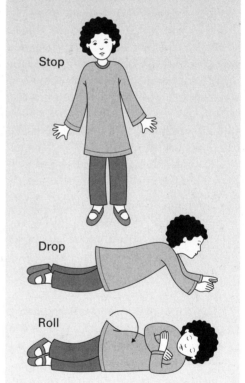

Stop

Drop

Roll

Infected Wounds

An infected wound usually festers beneath the surface of the skin, resulting in redness, pain, and swelling. A bacterial infection requires at least a day, and usually two to three days, to develop. Therefore, a delayed increase in pain or swelling is a legitimate cause for concern. A growing area of redness signifies a cellulitis, or infection of the skin tissue, while an area of redness that feels soft in the center may indicate an abscess, a collection of pus. If the festering wound bursts open, pus will drain out. This is good, and the wound will usually heal well. Still, this demonstrates that an infection is present, and the doctor should evaluate the situation, unless it is clearly minor.

An explanation of normal wound healing will be helpful.

1. The body pours out serum into a wound area. Serum is yellowish and clear and later turns into a scab. *Serum is frequently mistaken for pus. Pus is thick, cheesy, smelly, and never seen in the first day or so.*

2. The edges of a wound will be pink or red, and the wound area may be warm. Such inflammation around a wound is normal.

3. Pain along lymph channels or in the lymph nodes themselves may be present. This is because the lymphatic system is actively involved in debris clearance. Such pain can occur *without* infection.

Home Treatment

Keep a wound clean. If it is unsightly or in a location where it will get dirty easily, bandage it, changing the bandage daily (see Bandages, page 221). If not, leave it open to the air. Soak and clean it gently with warm water for short periods—three or four times daily to remove debris and to keep the scab soft. Children like to pick at scabs and often will fall on them. In these instances, bandages are useful and appreciated by most children.

The simplest wound of the face requires three to five days to heal. The healing period is five to seven days for the chest and arms and seven to nine days for the legs. Larger wounds, or those that are gaping and must heal across a space, take correspondingly longer to heal. Children heal more rapidly than adults do.

What to Expect

The doctor will examine the wound and regional lymph nodes and take the child's temperature. Sometimes the doctor will take cultures of the blood or wound. He or she also may prescribe a topical (mupirocin) or oral antibiotic.

If a wound is festering, the doctor may drain it with a needle or scalpel. This procedure is not very painful and actually relieves discomfort. For severe infections, an antibiotic injection or hospitalization may be required.

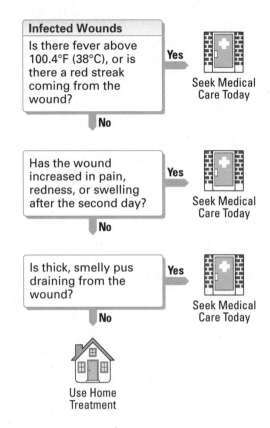

Infected Wounds

Is there fever above 100.4°F (38°C), or is there a red streak coming from the wound?

Yes → Seek Medical Care Today

No ↓

Has the wound increased in pain, redness, or swelling after the second day?

Yes → Seek Medical Care Today

No ↓

Is thick, smelly pus draining from the wound?

Yes → Seek Medical Care Today

No ↓

Use Home Treatment

Blood Poisoning

To a doctor, blood poisoning means bacterial infection in the bloodstream and is termed **septicemia**. Fever is a more reliable guide to this rare occurrence than red streaks. A local wound should cause only a very minor temperature elevation unless it is infected. If your child has a fever, see the doctor.

Traditionally, people believed that red streaks running up the arm or leg from a wound were blood poisoning and that the patient would die when the streaks reached the heart. In fact, such streaks are an inflammation of the lymph channels carrying the debris away from the wound. They will stop when they reach the local lymph nodes in the armpit or groin and do not, by themselves, indicate blood poisoning. However, they usually are worth checking with your doctor.

Insect Bites or Stings

Most insect bites are trivial, but some insect bites or stings, particularly bee stings, may cause reactions either locally or in the basic body systems. **Local reactions** may be uncomfortable but do not pose a serious hazard. By contrast, **systemic reactions** occasionally may be serious and may require emergency treatment.

There are three types of systemic reactions. All are rare.

▲ The most common is an attack causing difficulty breathing and perhaps audible wheezing.

▲ **Hives** or extensive skin rashes following insect bites are less serious but indicate that a reaction has occurred and a more severe reaction might occur if the child is bitten or stung again.

▲ Very rarely, **fainting** or loss of consciousness may occur. If a child has lost consciousness, you must assume that the collapse is due to an allergic reaction. This is an emergency.

If a child has had any of these reactions in the past, you should take the child immediately to a medical facility if he or she is stung or bitten again. If the local reaction to a bite or sting is severe or a deep sore is developing, consult the doctor by telephone. Children often have more severe reactions than adults.

Spider Bites

Bites from poisonous spiders are rare. The female **black widow spider** accounts for many of them. This spider is glossy black, with a body of approximately

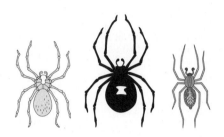

Poisonous spiders. *Left:* Brown recluse, shown from above. *Center:* Black widow, shown from below. *Right:* Hobo, shown from above. All appear at approximate actual size.

½ inch (13 mm) in diameter and a characteristic red hourglass mark on the underside of the abdomen.

The black widow spider is found in woodpiles, sheds, basements, and outhouses. The spider's bite is often painless, and the first sign of such a bite may be cramping abdominal pain. The abdomen will become hard as the waves of pain become severe. Breathing will be difficult and accompanied by grunting. There may be nausea, vomiting, headache, sweating, twitching, shaking, and tingling sensations in the hand. The bite itself may not be prominent and may be overshadowed by the systemic reaction.

Brown recluse spiders cause painful bites and serious local reactions but are not nearly as dangerous as black widows. They are slightly smaller than black widows and have a white violin pattern on their backs. Brown recluse spiders are found in the South, Southeast, and Midwest. **Hobo spiders** are similar in size and consequences to the brown recluse but are found mainly in the Northwest.

Tick Bites

Tick bites are common. Ticks live in tall grass or low shrubs and hop on and off of

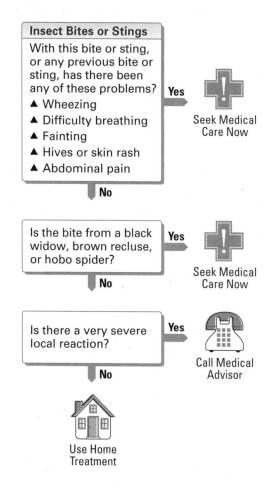

Insect Bites or Stings

With this bite or sting, or any previous bite or sting, has there been any of these problems?
- ▲ Wheezing
- ▲ Difficulty breathing
- ▲ Fainting
- ▲ Hives or skin rash
- ▲ Abdominal pain

Yes → Seek Medical Care Now

No ↓

Is the bite from a black widow, brown recluse, or hobo spider?

Yes → Seek Medical Care Now

No ↓

Is there a very severe local reaction?

Yes → Call Medical Advisor

No ↓

Use Home Treatment

passing mammals, such as deer and dogs. In some localities, ticks may carry Rocky Mountain spotted fever or Lyme disease (page 406), but most tick bites are not complicated by subsequent illness. Ticks are commonly found in the scalp. (See Ticks, page 404.)

Home Treatment

Apply something cold promptly. Ice or cold packs can be used. Delay in the appli-

cation of cold results in a more severe local reaction.

Acetaminophen or ibuprofen can be used (page 218). Antihistamines, such as diphenhydramine (Benadryl), can reduce the allergic response somewhat (page 224). If the reaction is severe, consult the doctor by telephone.

A bee sting is usually a good, though painful, reminder of preventive strategies. Many stings occur on bare feet when children disturb bees or other insects feeding on flowers in the lawn. Always have children wear shoes outside. If your child has an allergic reaction, especially to a bee sting, ask your doctor to prescribe an EpiPen Jr. for emergency use.

What to Expect

The doctor will ask what sort of insect or spider has inflicted the wound and will search for signs of a systemic reaction. If a systemic reaction is present, an injection of epinephrine or steroids may be needed. Rarely, measures to support breathing or blood pressure will be needed. These measures require the facilities of an emergency room or hospital.

If the problem is a local reaction, the doctor will examine the wound for signs of tissue death or infection. Occasionally, surgical drainage of the wound will be needed. In some cases, pain relievers or antihistamines may make the patient more comfortable. Epinephrine injections are occasionally used for very severe local reactions.

If there has been a severe allergic reaction, desensitization shots may be initiated (see pages 182–183). In addition, you may consider purchasing an emergency kit containing injectable epinephrine to help a child with a serious allergy.

Fishhooks

The problem, of course, is the barb. Whereas fish seem to get loose easily enough, children may stay hooked. If you and your child can keep calm, you can remove the fishhook, unless it is in the eye. Do *not* attempt to remove a hook that has penetrated the eyeball; this is a job for the doctor. A hook in the face also should be taken more seriously, because of cosmetic issues.

You will need your child's confidence and cooperation to avoid a visit to the doctor. The advantage of the doctor's office is a local anesthetic and extra hands to help hold the child. Remember that the injection of the anesthetic will hurt some, so this is not a clear-cut choice between pain and no pain. You also can save a lot of time by removing the hook at home.

Home Treatment

Occasionally, a hook will have come all the way around, so that it lies just beneath the surface of the skin. If this is the case, often the best technique is simply to push the hook through the skin, cut it off just behind the barb with wire cutters, and remove it by pulling it back through the way it entered. This may be painful, and some children may not tolerate it.

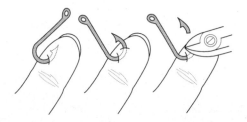

Note that a pair of needle-nosed pliers with a wire-cutting blade should be part of your fishing equipment.

Sometimes a hook will be embedded only slightly and can be removed by simply grasping the shank (pliers help), pushing slightly forward and away from the barb, and then pulling it out.

If neither of these maneuvers does the trick, try the method illustrated below.

If you cannot remove the fishhook easily, you may prefer to take the child to the doctor.

1. Put a loop of fishing line through the bend of the fishhook so that at the appropriate time you can apply a quick jerk and pull the hook out directly in line with the shaft.

2. Holding on to the shaft, push the hook slightly in and away from the barb to disengage it.

3. Maintaining this pressure to keep the barb disengaged, give a quick jerk on the line, and the hook will pop out.

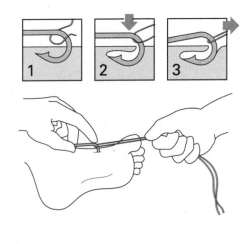

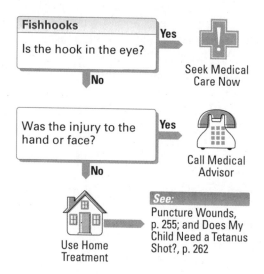

Fishhooks

Is the hook in the eye? — **Yes** → Seek Medical Care Now

↓ **No**

Was the injury to the hand or face? — **Yes** → Call Medical Advisor

↓ **No**

Use Home Treatment

See: Puncture Wounds, p. 255; and Does My Child Need a Tetanus Shot?, p. 262

If you are successful, be sure the child's tetanus shots are up-to-date (see Does My Child Need a Tetanus Shot?, page 262). Treat the wound as described in the home treatment section for puncture wounds (page 255). If all else fails, see the doctor.

What to Expect

The doctor will use one of the methods described above to remove the hook. He or she may use a local anesthetic to numb the area around the hook before removing it.

If the hook is in the eye, it is likely that you will need to see an ophthalmologist (eye specialist), and the hook may need to be removed in the operating room.

Splinters

You can often use tweezers to remove a splinter under the skin. If some material remains, you can usually dislodge it by picking away at the overlying skin with a clean needle. Sterilize the needle by dipping it in rubbing alcohol or holding it in a match flame. Another option is to soak the area twice a day in a cup of very warm, not hot, water mixed with a teaspoon of baking soda. The splinter will probably come out by itself in a day or two. Don't let a splinter wound become infected.

Smashed Fingers

Children always seem to be getting their fingers smashed in car doors or desk drawers or with hammers or baseballs. If the injury involves only the end segment of the finger *(terminal phalanx)* and does not involve a significant cut (see Cuts [Lacerations], page 252), these injuries seldom need the help of a doctor. Blood under the fingernail *(subungual hematoma)* is painful but treatable.

Joint Fractures

Fractures of the bone in the end segment of the finger are not treated unless they involve the joint. Many doctors feel that it is unwise to splint the finger even if there is a fracture of the joint. Although the splint will decrease the pain, it may increase the stiffness of the joint after healing. If the fracture is not splinted, the pain may persist, and your child may end up with a stiff joint anyway. Discuss the advantages and disadvantages of splinting with your doctor.

Dislocated Nails

Fingernails are often dislocated in these injuries. Except in extraordinarily unusual accidents—injuring and destroying a nail's growth plate—fingernails always grow back. Some nails that are attached precariously may need to be clipped off to avoid catching painfully on other objects. Nail regrowth will take four to six weeks. Dangling fingernails can be replaced over a clean nail bed and a bandage applied. The new nail will grow underneath and lift the old nail.

Home Treatment

If the injury does not involve other parts of the finger and the child can move the finger easily, apply an ice pack for the swelling and use acetaminophen (page 218) for the pain.

Blood Under a Nail

If a large amount of blood under a fingernail is causing pain, you can relieve the problem with the following procedure. This procedure is potentially dangerous, however, because it can introduce infection to the finger. If your child is diabetic, do not try this technique. We also recommend that you not use it on younger children and that you reserve it for situations where pain is severe and medical help not accessible. Care must be taken to employ a sterile technique.

1. Bend open a paper clip, holding the clip with a pair of pliers. (Do not use a plastic-coated paper clip.)

2. Heat one end using a candle or match.

3. When the tip is very hot, touch it to the nail. It will melt its way right through the nail, leaving a small, clean hole. Steady the hand holding the pliers with the opposite hand so that the paper clip will go only through the nail and not into the flesh below.

The blood trapped beneath the nail can now escape through the small hole, and the pain will be relieved as the pressure is released. If the hole closes and the blood reaccumulates, repeat the procedure, using the same hole.

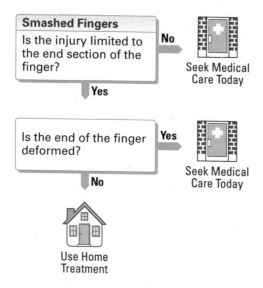

Smashed Fingers

Is the injury limited to the end section of the finger?

No → Seek Medical Care Today

Yes ↓

Is the end of the finger deformed?

Yes → Seek Medical Care Today

No ↓

Use Home Treatment

What to Expect

The doctor will examine the finger and usually call for an X ray if it appears that more than the end segment is involved. If there is a fracture of the joint nearest the fingertip, expect a discussion of the advantages and disadvantages of splinting the finger. Often splinting of one finger is accomplished by bandaging it together with the adjacent finger. If the finger is splinted, the child should exercise the finger periodically to preserve its mobility. Severe finger injuries may occasionally require surgery to preserve function.

For blood trapped beneath the nail, a more elegant device than a paper clip will be utilized to relieve the pressure.

Ingrown Nails

Ingrown nails can be treated at home, if there is no redness, swelling, or pain in the nail. Cut the nail straight across so that its corner can grow outside the skin. Let the nail grow free by firmly pushing the skin back from the corner with a cotton swab twice a day. Keep the area clean. For **hangnails**, keep them clean. Encourage your child not to chew on them.

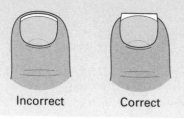

Incorrect   Correct

Common Concerns

Fever

Many people, including doctors, speak of fever and illness as if they were one and the same. Surprisingly, an elevated temperature is not necessarily a sign of illness. Normal body temperature varies from individual to individual. If we measured a large number of healthy children's body temperatures while they were resting, we would find a difference between the lowest and highest child of about 1.5°F (about 1°C). This is another reminder that children are individuals and that there is nothing magical about the average temperature 98.6°F (37°C).

Normal body temperature varies greatly during the day. Temperature is generally lowest in the morning upon awakening. Many things will elevate body temperature, including food, excess clothing, room temperature, excitement, and anxiety.

Vigorous exercise can raise body temperature to as much as 103°F (39°C). Severe exercise, without water or salt, can result in a condition known as **heatstroke**, with temperatures above 106°F (41°C). Other mechanisms also influence body temperature. Hormones, for example, account for a monthly variation of body temperature in ovulating women.

In general, children have higher body temperatures than adults and seem to have greater daily variation because of their greater amounts of excitement and activity. Fevers are easier to control as your child gets older. The child's temperature regulatory center matures. In addition, the child loses a layer of brown fat, located between the backbones, that is responsible for a great deal of heat insulation in infants.

If no other symptoms are present, consult a doctor immediately for the following:

▲ Temperature of more than 100°F (37.7°C) in a child younger than one week
▲ Temperature of more than 100.4°F (38°C) in a child younger than three months
▲ Temperature of more than 103°F (39.4°C) in a child younger than two years
▲ Temperature of more than 105°F (40.5°C) if the home treatment measures described below fail to reduce the temperature at least partly
▲ Temperature of 106°F (41.1°C)
▲ Fever persisting for more than five days

Causes of Fever

The most common causes of persistent fevers in children are viral and bacterial infections such as colds, sore throats, earaches, diarrhea, roseola, occasionally pneumonia and urinary tract infections, and rarely appendicitis and meningitis.

A viral infection can result in a normal temperature or a temperature of 105°F (40.5°C). Although the height of the temperature is *not* a reliable indicator of the seriousness of the underlying infection, higher temperatures do bring a slightly higher risk of serious problems, especially in children younger than two years.

Taking Your Child's Temperature

Either Fahrenheit or Celsius thermometers are acceptable. Rectal temperatures are usually more accurate and are about 0.5°F (0.25°C) higher than oral or axillary (underarm) temperatures. For a detailed discussion of temperature taking, see Thermometers, page 222.

Febrile Seizures (Fever Fits)

The danger of an extremely high temperature is the possibility that the fever will cause a seizure (convulsion). All of us are capable of "seizing" if our body temperatures become too high. Febrile seizures are relatively common in normal, healthy children; about 3 to 5% will experience such a seizure. Although common, the significance of seizures should not be minimized, and they must be treated with respect.

Febrile seizures occur most often in children between the ages of six months and four years. Illnesses that cause a rapid elevation in temperature, such as roseola, have frequently been associated with febrile seizures. Rarely, a seizure is the first sign of a serious underlying problem such as meningitis.

During a seizure, the brain, which is normally transmitting electrical impulses at a fairly regular rhythm, begins misfiring because of the overheating and causes involuntary muscular responses, termed a seizure, convulsion, fit, or "falling-out spell." The first sign may be a stiffening of the entire body. Children may have rhythmic beating of their hands and feet. The eyes may roll back, and the head may jerk. Urine and feces may pass involuntarily.

Most seizures last only a few seconds to a few minutes. There is very little evidence that such a short seizure is of any long-term consequence. Prolonged seizures of more than 30 minutes, however, are often a sign of a more serious underlying problem.

Fewer than half of all children who have one short febrile seizure will ever experience a second, and fewer than half who experience a second will ever have a third.

Although a "seizing" child is a terrifying sight, the dangers to the child are small. You should follow these common-sense rules during a seizure.

▲ Protect your child's head from hitting anything hard. Place the child on a bed.

▲ Considerable damage can be done by forcing an object into the child's mouth to prevent biting of the tongue. Surprisingly, bitten tongues are both uncommon and quick to heal.

▲ If there is vomiting, place the child on his or her side.

▲ Make sure the child's breathing passage is open. Forcing a stick in your child's mouth does not ensure an open airway. To facilitate breathing, (1) clear the nose and mouth of vomitus or other material, then (2) pull the head backward slightly to "hyperextend" the neck. Artificial respiration is almost never necessary. These techniques are best learned in demonstrations. In a true emergency, hyperextend the neck and breathe at least 10 times each minute through the child's nose while

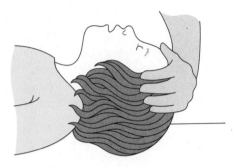

Open airway. If a child is having a febrile seizure, pull the head back slightly. Do not force anything into the mouth.

keeping the mouth covered (or through the child's mouth while keeping the nose pinched with your fingers). Only blow air in; the child will blow the air out naturally.

▲ Begin fever reduction (discussed below) and seek medical attention immediately. Do *not* give medicine by mouth to a seizing or unconscious child. Fortunately, once the seizure has stopped, the child is usually temporarily resistant to a second seizure. Because there are exceptions to this rule, however, medical attention is critical.

After the seizure has subsided, the child may be very groggy and have no recollection of what has occurred. Some children may show signs of extreme weakness and even paralysis of an arm or leg. This paralysis is almost always temporary but must be carefully evaluated.

A good doctor will do a careful evaluation to determine the cause of a febrile seizure. For the first febrile seizure, this may include a spinal tap (lumbar puncture) and fluid analysis if the child appears ill, to make certain that the seizure was not caused by meningitis. Following the termination of the fever, the doctor will stress the importance of fever control for the next few days. For further discussion, see Seizures, page 312.

The Meaning of a Chill

A chill is another symptom of a fever. The feeling of being hot or cold is maintained by a complex system of nerve receptors in our skin and in a part of our brain known as the hypothalamus. This system is sensitive to the difference between the body temperature and the temperature outside. Cold can be sensed in two different ways, either by lowering the environmental temperature or by raising the body temperature.

The body responds to a fever in a manner similar to the way it responds to a drop in the outside temperature. All the normal systems that increase heat production, such as shivering, become active. Food has already been mentioned as one factor that can raise body temperature, and a person experiencing a chill may feel hungry. The body tries to conserve heat by causing constriction of the blood vessels near the skin. Children will sometimes curl up in a ball to conserve heat. Goose bumps are intended to raise the hairs on our body to form a layer of insulation.

Don't bundle your child up in blankets if he or she shivers or becomes chilled; this will only cause the fever to go higher. Use home treatment as described below.

Home Treatment

Remember that a fever is the body's way of responding to a variety of conditions, including infection. A fever may signify the response of the body's immune system to an infection and thus be evidence of a beneficial process. Nonetheless, fevers can make children uncomfortable. Controlling a fever that is high enough to interfere with a child's eating, drinking, sleeping, or other important activities will make the child feel better. In short, if your child seems to be suffering from the fever, treat it. If the fever is mild and the child shows no effects, it may be unnecessary to treat.

There are two ways to reduce a fever: sponging and medication. If a fever remains above 103°F (39°C) after an hour or so of home treatment, call the doctor.

Sponging

Evaporation has a cooling effect on the skin and hence on the body temperature. Evaporation can be enhanced by sponging the skin with water. Do not use cold water; it can cause shivering and increase body temperature. Do *not* use alcohol! Although alcohol evaporates more rapidly, it is somewhat uncomfortable for the child, and the vapors can be dangerous. Generally, sponging with tepid water (water that is comfortable to the touch) will be sufficient.

Heat is also lost by conduction if a child is sponged or sitting in a tub. Conduction is the process by which heat is lost to a cooler environment (the bathwater or air) from the warmer environment of the body. A comfortable tub of water (70°F, or 21°C) will be sufficiently lower than the body temperature to encourage conduction. Although cold water will work somewhat faster, the discomfort of the procedure makes this less desirable. The child will tolerate cold bathing and sponging for a much shorter period.

Some doctors believe that sponging is unnecessary and a potential for ultimately

---

Starve a Fever?

This folk remedy probably came from individuals clever enough to notice the relationship between food and temperature elevation. However, there are many reasons why a child should be fed during a fever. The increased heat increases caloric requirements, because calories are being consumed rapidly at the higher body temperature. More important, there is an increased demand for fluid.

Liquids should never be withheld from a feverish child. If a child will not eat because of the discomfort caused by a fever, it is essential that he or she continue to drink fluids.

---

raising the body's temperature. Others disagree. For most fevers, sponging is not required. For very high fevers, your doctor may suggest sponging.

Medication

Medication should *not* be given by mouth to a seizing or unconscious child. A child who has just had a seizure can be given an acetaminophen suppository. Temperature can be controlled in the conscious, alert child with acetaminophen (Tylenol, Liquiprin, Feverall). Ibuprofen (Advil, Motrin) is equally effective in reducing fever when given in the appropriate dosage. See Table 6 on page 292 for recommended dosages. Also see Pain and Fever Relievers, page 217.

Dangers of Fever Medications

We do not recommend aspirin. Children and teenagers who take aspirin when they

Table 6: Acetaminophen and Ibuprofen Dosages for Fever Relief *

Weight of Child	Acetaminophen Dosage	Ibuprofen Dosage		
		6 months–2 years (Temp. below 102.5°F)	6 months–2 years (Temp. at or above 102.5°F)	Over 2 years
Up to 12 pounds (infants)	40 mg			
13–17 pounds	80 mg	25 mg	50 mg	
18–23 pounds	120 mg	50 mg	100 mg	
24–35 pounds	160 mg	100 mg	100 mg	100 mg
36–47 pounds	240 mg			150 mg
48–59 pounds	325 mg **			200 mg
60–71 pounds	325 mg **			250 mg
72–95 pounds	325 mg **			300 mg
Adolescents	500 mg **			400 mg

*   The recommended dosage for acetaminophen is 10 mg for every 2.2 pounds (1 kg) of the child's weight every four hours, up to five times in one day. The amounts given here are **estimated** dosages.

The recommended dosage for ibuprofen depends on age, temperature, and weight, and is given every 6 to 8 hours. The amounts given here are **estimated** dosages for children over 6 months.

** 325 mg of acetaminophen equals 1 regular tablet or capsule; 500 mg of acetaminophen equals 1 "extra strength" tablet or capsule.

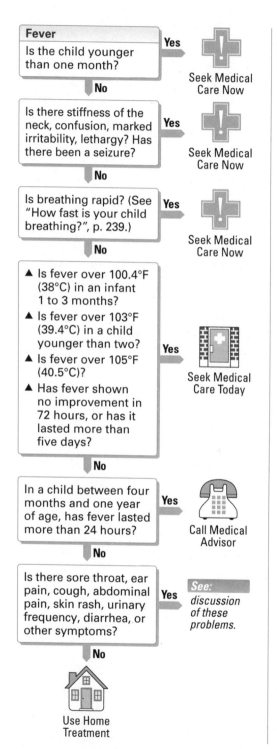

Fever

| Is the child younger than one month? | **Yes** | Seek Medical Care Now |

No

| Is there stiffness of the neck, confusion, marked irritability, lethargy? Has there been a seizure? | **Yes** | Seek Medical Care Now |

No

| Is breathing rapid? (See "How fast is your child breathing?", p. 239.) | **Yes** | Seek Medical Care Now |

No

| ▲ Is fever over 100.4°F (38°C) in an infant 1 to 3 months?
 ▲ Is fever over 103°F (39.4°C) in a child younger than two?
 ▲ Is fever over 105°F (40.5°C)?
 ▲ Has fever shown no improvement in 72 hours, or has it lasted more than five days? | **Yes** | Seek Medical Care Today |

No

| In a child between four months and one year of age, has fever lasted more than 24 hours? | **Yes** | Call Medical Advisor |

No

| Is there sore throat, ear pain, cough, abdominal pain, skin rash, urinary frequency, diarrhea, or other symptoms? | **Yes** | *See:* discussion of these problems. |

No

Use Home Treatment

have chicken pox or the flu stand a higher chance of developing Reye syndrome, a rare but serious problem of the brain and liver. Because it is hard to recognize chicken pox and the flu in their early stages, we recommend that parents always give children and teenagers acetaminophen or ibuprofen instead of aspirin. It does not carry the risk of Reye syndrome.

What to Expect

This will depend on how long your child has had a fever and how sick the child appears. The doctor will examine the child's skin, eyes, ears, nose, throat, neck, chest, and belly to determine whether an infection is present. If no other symptoms are present and the exam does not reveal an infection, the doctor may recommend watchful waiting. In girls and uncircumcised boys younger than one year old, urine is often required for analysis. If the fever has been prolonged, the child appears ill, or the child is very young, tests of the blood and urine may be done. A chest X ray or spinal tap may be needed. Specific infections will be treated appropriately. Fever will be treated as discussed under "Home Treatment."

Headache

More than 40% of children have had a headache by the age of 7, and 4% of 7-year-olds are troubled by frequent headaches. By the age of 15, 75% of children have had a headache, and 20% experience frequent headaches.

In younger children, the cause of head pain is frequently stress. In older children, most headaches are due to stress. Stress and tension can cause headaches even in 5-year-olds. Muscle spasms in the neck and scalp cause these pains, possibly aggravated by a widening of blood vessels inside the brain. Tension headaches can occur in any part of the head, produce a dull or swollen feeling, and usually come on slowly. Headaches are often the first symptom of stressful problems at school, at home, or with friends. A child who is functioning poorly in any of these areas needs help.

Many medications, including decongestants (page 224) and antihistamines (page 224), can cause headaches. Headaches are also common just before menstruation (see Menstrual Problems, page 478). Eyestrain is often blamed but is seldom the cause of headaches.

Migraines

Migraines may start in childhood. Some toddlers who vomit frequently have migraines. As they become older, they can tell you that their head aches. Children with classic migraines usually have at least two of the following symptoms.

▲ Headache on one side of the head
▲ Nausea
▲ Visual disturbance before an attack
▲ Other family members with migraines

Migraines often begin suddenly and are throbbing in character. There are also other forms of migraines that do not have all the above characteristics.

Other Causes

An isolated headache is often due to an earache, sore throat, toothache, or eye infection. Suspect **meningitis** when a child has a headache combined with a stiff neck, irritability, a soft spot (fontanel) that is bulging, or vomiting with a fever.

Occasionally, headaches are the only sign of a **seizure disorder** (page 312). These headaches usually begin suddenly and are followed by a period of drowsiness or sleep.

Many parents are concerned about **brain tumors**. Headaches associated with brain tumors are often persistent and progressive, present in the morning, and accompanied by other problems such as difficulty walking, personality changes, vomiting, visual problems, limb weakness, and speech difficulties. Fortunately, brain tumors are very rarely the cause of headaches. Only 1 in 40,000 children has a tumor of the brain or nervous system.

Home Treatment

Headaches due to ear infections, toothaches, strep throats, acute sinusitis, or other serious infections require medical help.

For headaches associated with colds, flu, or stress, acetaminophen may be effective. Headaches also may be relieved by massage or heat to the back of the neck. Children with hay fever often have headaches during the pollen season, and antihistamines and decongestants may help. But remember that these drugs *cause* headaches in some children!

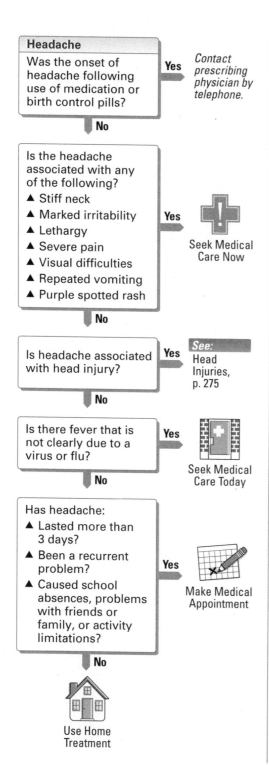

Headache

Was the onset of headache following use of medication or birth control pills?

Yes → *Contact prescribing physician by telephone.*

No ↓

Is the headache associated with any of the following?
▲ Stiff neck
▲ Marked irritability
▲ Lethargy
▲ Severe pain
▲ Visual difficulties
▲ Repeated vomiting
▲ Purple spotted rash

Yes → Seek Medical Care Now

No ↓

Is headache associated with head injury?

Yes → *See:* Head Injuries, p. 275

No ↓

Is there fever that is not clearly due to a virus or flu?

Yes → Seek Medical Care Today

No ↓

Has headache:
▲ Lasted more than 3 days?
▲ Been a recurrent problem?
▲ Caused school absences, problems with friends or family, or activity limitations?

Yes → Make Medical Appointment

No ↓

Use Home Treatment

For migraines, a combination of acetaminophen (Tylenol, Tempra) and ibuprofen (Motrin, Advil) is an effective approach.

Persistent headaches that do not respond to such measures should be called to the attention of a doctor. Headaches associated with weakness of the arms or legs or with slurring of speech, as well as those that are rapidly increasing in frequency and severity, also require a visit to the doctor.

Remember, tension is the usual cause of head pain. Whenever possible, identify the causes of stress and work with your children to relieve them.

What to Expect

The doctor will check the child's temperature, blood pressure, head, eyes, ears, nose, throat, and neck and also test nerve function. Laboratory tests will depend on what the doctor finds in the history and physical examination; usually none are needed. With an acute headache, a source of infection may be found. Even with most recurring headaches, a history and physical examination are probably all that is required. Occasionally, the doctor may order brain wave tests (electroencephalogram, or EEG) if he or she suspects a seizure disorder. If migraines are interfering with your child's functioning, the doctor may prescribe medication. Complementary and alternative therapies, including hypnosis, may be recommended for severe or persistent headaches.

Hyperactivity and ADHD

Hyperactivity can be a symptom of attention deficit disorder (ADD), also called attention deficit hyperactivity disorder (ADHD). However, it has other causes as well. Indeed, controversy and confusion are the rule when it comes to hyperactivity. The word means "more than normal activity." The problem here is in knowing what is "normal."

Children's activity levels change as they become older, as they are placed in new situations, or when they are excited or overtired. In addition, activity that is considered normal in the school yard may be considered abnormal in the classroom or dining room. Hyperactivity merely indicates someone's *perception* of the child's activity in relationship to the activities of other children of the same age.

Hyperactivity is a symptom, not a disease. It may be found in most normal children (especially ages two to four) and in the following children.

▲ Older children of above-average intelligence with inquisitive behavior
▲ Children reacting to problems in school, at home, or with friends or siblings
▲ Children unable to adjust to different standards of behavior and performance at home and in school
▲ Children who do not speak English in schools that are not bilingual
▲ Children with hearing difficulties, drug reactions, or visual difficulties

Causes
Medical causes of hyperactivity include hyperthyroidism and psychiatric disorders.

Common **drugs** may cause hyperactivity. These include Dimetapp, Actifed, Sudafed, Triaminic, and many other decongestants (page 224) and antihistamines (page 224).

Very often teachers will be the first ones to point out hyperactive behavior in a child. A **learning problem** may be the basis for hyperactive behavior in school. If a child is not able to comprehend what is going on in the classroom, boredom and ultimately hyperactive behavior may result. If there is a discrepancy between your child's behavior in school and at home, a learning problem should be suspected.

ADHD Syndrome
In medical terminology, a syndrome is a group of symptoms that occur together. Often there is no known cause for the syndrome. Hyperactivity is only one symptom of children classified with attention deficit hyperactivity disorder (ADHD) syndrome.

ADHD consists of greatly increased activity, easy distractibility, wide mood changes from moment to moment, poor impulse control, short attention span, explosive moods, and, often, learning problems. Some children with ADHD may be clumsy and have difficulty controlling fine movements.

The underlying cause of this syndrome is not known, although recent research suggests that some children with ADHD have atypical brain activity. ADHD may merely represent slower-than-usual maturation of attention. The decision chart lists some conditions you should watch for if you are concerned about ADHD. Recently, specific criteria have been developed. See www.cdc.gov/ncbddd/factsheets/ADHD_symptoms.pdf and www.aap.org/healthtopics/adhd.cfm.

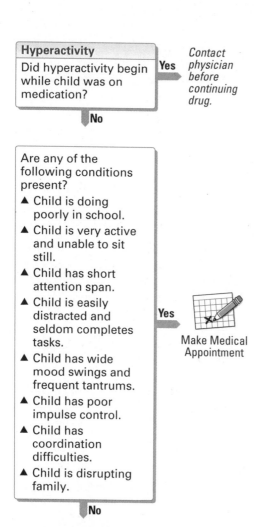

Hyperactivity

Did hyperactivity begin while child was on medication? — **Yes** → *Contact physician before continuing drug.*

No ↓

Are any of the following conditions present?
▲ Child is doing poorly in school.
▲ Child is very active and unable to sit still.
▲ Child has short attention span.
▲ Child is easily distracted and seldom completes tasks.
▲ Child has wide mood swings and frequent tantrums.
▲ Child has poor impulse control.
▲ Child has coordination difficulties.
▲ Child is disrupting family.

— **Yes** → **Make Medical Appointment**

No ↓

Consult
with physician during routine visit.

Home Treatment

Observation of other children is a good guide to your own child's activity. You will notice that there are many extremely active children of all ages. Some seem to be on constant "seek-and-destroy" missions.

If problems develop in school, request a conference with the teacher to deter-mine the precise nature of the problem. Medical assistance in dealing with this type of problem can be helpful.

If your child's hyperactivity began following the use of a medication, discontinue using this medication immediately and contact the prescribing doctor.

What to Expect

You may initiate a discussion with your doctor during your child's health-supervision visit. If the doctor suspects a problem, he or she will schedule a lengthy evaluation. Most doctors will wish to review a copy of the child's school records (you can save time by having these available at the time of the visit) and may wish to talk with the teacher. Teachers will usually be asked to complete a checklist of school behaviors.

The history and physical examination will emphasize the child's nervous system. Your observations with respect to the child's behavior are important. Tests of muscle coordination, reading, spelling, and so on may be conducted. Hearing and vision will be tested. If a seizure disorder is suspected, brain wave tests (EEG) may be performed.

Behavioral techniques will be used in an attempt to manage the problem. You should reach a decision to begin any form of therapy (such as the drug Ritalin or a special diet) only after careful consideration. A proper therapeutic approach requires coordination between doctor, parents, school, and child.

Bed-Wetting

Achieving nighttime bladder control has already been discussed on pages 76–77. A number of maturational factors determine when a child will become dry. Many children are dry at night by the age of four, but others are not. With each successive year, many more children will naturally develop control.

Children who have been dry for many months or even years may suddenly wet the bed, often in response to a stressful event. Children may regress because of the arrival of a new brother or sister, a move, or a severe illness. Only occasionally is a urinary tract infection the cause, and then there are usually other symptoms such as increased frequency of urination, burning, abdominal pain, or fever. When such symptoms occur, see the doctor.

Home Treatment

Most important is your attitude. First, you must expect bed-wetting to happen. It should not be considered unusual until after age six, and it is still normal for children to lose control occasionally during stressful events for the next year or so. A reaction of disgust or anger may make it more difficult for the child to gain control. Second, the child often cannot help it. Bladder control is a complex developmental and neurological task that requires a mature child. Making the child feel guilty about bed-wetting will only delay resolution of the problem. You should think in terms of supporting rather than punishing the child.

Because constant sheet changing is often tiresome for parents, placing a short sheet on top of a rubber pad placed on top of the regular sheet will cut down on laundry.

Most of the time, your best course is to ignore the problem and wait it out. After age six, you and your child may want to make a "team effort" to solve this problem.

1. Encourage the child to drink in the morning and early afternoon, not in the several hours before bedtime.

2. Have the child void (urinate) just before going to bed. Fluids during the day help ensure that the bladder is big enough, and voiding ensures that it is as empty as possible at bedtime.

3. Develop a chart or use a calendar to indicate when the child has achieved control by awarding a gold star. When your child gets tired of gold stars, you may try drawing smiling faces or sad faces on your calendar. Try these measures for several weeks or months.

4. If the child doesn't make progress, consider getting him or her up within the first three hours of sleep to empty the bladder again. If the child is already wet, awaken him or her a little sooner.

Older children can participate in the laundering process to learn that they are responsible for their actions and some of the consequences.

Nighttime alarms that sound when the child begins to void in bed are effective. Your doctor may want to include an alarm as *part* of a treatment program. If a child continues to wet the bed after age six, a consultation with the doctor may be helpful.

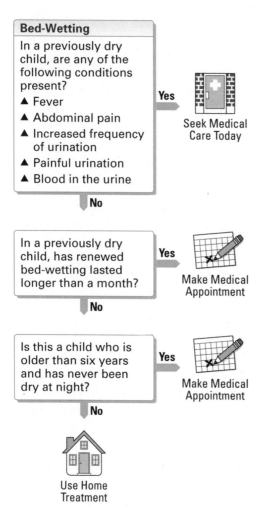

Bed-Wetting

In a previously dry child, are any of the following conditions present?
- ▲ Fever
- ▲ Abdominal pain
- ▲ Increased frequency of urination
- ▲ Painful urination
- ▲ Blood in the urine

Yes → Seek Medical Care Today

No ↓

In a previously dry child, has renewed bed-wetting lasted longer than a month?

Yes → Make Medical Appointment

No ↓

Is this a child who is older than six years and has never been dry at night?

Yes → Make Medical Appointment

No ↓

Use Home Treatment

What to Expect

The medical history is the most important part of the office visit. The doctor will inquire at what time of night the child wets the bed, as well as how often and under what circumstances. He or she will perform a physical examination with special attention to the genitals and call for a urinalysis. You should think of this visit as adding the doctor to the "team." Avoid the implication that the child is being punished.

The doctor will need to get to know your child; this may best be accomplished without your presence. Don't be offended.

Nighttime alarms are usually suggested first, before drugs. In some instances, the drug imipramine (Tofranil) will be added to the regimen of home treatment. Another drug used for nighttime bed-wetting is desmopressin (DDAVP).

Extensive tests such as X rays of the kidneys and bladder are seldom necessary. Bed-wetting almost never requires a surgical solution, and you should consult several doctors if surgery is suggested.

Constipation

It is not necessary to have a bowel movement every day. Many children have bowel movements only once every three or four days, and they are perfectly normal.

Stool consistency is important; a child with three hard stools daily is constipated; a breast-fed baby with one soft stool a week is not. Most parents are concerned about constipation when the stool (feces) is very hard or when a child experiences pain when passing stool. Sometimes the pain is due to a tear in the rectum (rectal fissure). It is often unclear whether the hard fecal matter is responsible for the tear or whether the tear is responsible for the child's holding back the bowel movement to avoid the pain. In any event, treatment is directed toward softening the stool.

Sometimes, infants with a severe diaper rash will withhold bowel movements to avoid pain. If this is the case, work to clear up the rash rather than to soften the stool. (See Diaper Rash, page 374.)

Infants and older children will frequently be constipated during illnesses. Adequate fluid intake is very important in such cases.

Constipation can have emotional causes. For example, it may begin at the time of toilet training. In the struggle of wills between child and parent, the child may decide to retain control by holding on to a bowel movement.

If a child retains stool for long enough, liquid material will escape around the hardened bowel plug. This liquid material is apt to leak and soil the child's underpants—hence the term **soiling**. Soiling in an older child is a sign of long-standing constipation and should be treated by a doctor.

Home Treatment

Dietary changes are usually all that is necessary and are superior to medicines. Prune juice is remarkably efficient. You might eliminate rice cereal for a while, because it tends to be constipating. In older children, encouraging them to eat bran products and other foods high in fiber (celery, whole oranges) often helps. Adequate fluid intake is essential; water is fine.

On rare occasions, your child may need a laxative. Metamucil and Maltsupex add fiber. Colace softens the stool by allowing water to more easily enter the stool, and MiraLAX lubricates the stool. Glycerin suppositories are safe and effective. Never give infants mineral oil, because it can cause serious pneumonia if it finds its way to the lungs. However, it is quite effective in older children. Enemas are virtually never needed and are potentially dangerous.

What to Expect

In some instances, the doctor will examine the abdomen and rectum. In the case of soiling, the doctor will assess whether the child has developed to the point where bowel control can be expected, and if so, whether stress might be causing the problem. The child will need your support if a serious soiling problem is to be treated successfully. Rarely, X rays of the lower bowel are necessary.

For constipation, the best doctor may well do few or no tests and perform little or no examination. A stool lubricant such as MiraLAX may be recommended. Soiling is a more serious problem and should be investigated more thoroughly.

Constipation

Are any of the following conditions present?

▲ Child is in pain when having a bowel movement.

▲ Blood is noticed on stool.

▲ Child has no bowel movement for four days.

▲ A crack or fissure is noticed in child's rectum.

Yes →

Call Medical Advisor

No

Has the problem persisted for more than four weeks?

Yes →

Make Medical Appointment

No

Has the problem recurred three or more times unaccompanied by an illness?

Yes →

Make Medical Appointment

No

Is your child soiling clothes, or is the problem interfering with school, friends, or family functioning?

Yes →

Make Medical Appointment

No

Use Home Treatment

Overweight/Obesity

The tendency of infants to be overweight is influenced by parents' genes and behavior. The discovery of a gene responsible for obesity in some individuals is not the basis for the considerable number of overweight individuals. The likelihood of being overweight (or underweight) is in part due to inheritance, but parents have tremendous power to influence whether children actually become fat. Although theories about obesity are being constantly developed and debated, one fact remains: A proper balance of diet and exercise will control weight. If the entire family eats and exercises properly, it is unlikely your child will become overweight.

There are a number of ways to detect obesity, but none beats the human eye. Fat is easy to see if you don't try to fool yourself. Weight and height charts often have such a wide range of "normal" weights that there is ample opportunity for self-deception.

Obesity is almost always due to too many calories and not enough exercise. Trying to find a way around this simple truth is one of America's favorite pastimes. The problem is complicated by the peculiar notion that a fat baby is happy and healthy. This, along with our traditional attitudes toward cleaning the plate ("Think of the starving orphans in Africa"), can lead to social problems and premature death as an adult.

There are certain hormonal disorders that cause what appears to be obesity, but glands get blamed for a lot more problems than they actually cause. Even to the untrained eye, children with glandular problems do not appear the same as a typical chubby child. For instance, children with thyroid problems usually have retarded growth, meaning they are short. Often they gain weight in a relatively short period, and this is associated with other symptoms. Glandular problems are not common and account for fewer than 1% of obese children.

Steroid medications can also be responsible for weight gain.

Home Treatment

With an infant, you must overcome the feeling that too much is better than not enough and that a fat baby is a healthy baby. Forcing food is not necessary. Infants have a pretty good idea of how much they need; they will not starve in the presence of food. Remember, a crying infant is not always hungry; comforting may be all that is called for. Also, start rewarding children with words, not foods, at an early age.

Older children and adolescents are a different story. As youngsters become adults, they take on adult patterns of obesity. Although older children may initially become discouraged when trying to slim down after years of being overweight, they should realize that proper nutrition and exercise at any age will eventually be rewarded.

Because eating is one way of handling stress and is enjoyable, the psychology of obesity is complex. Unhappiness is sometimes used as an excuse for not doing anything about obesity, but working on the obesity may help with the unhappiness. With one in three adults now obese, considerable national and state efforts are focused on both preventing and treating obesity in children. Substantial resources

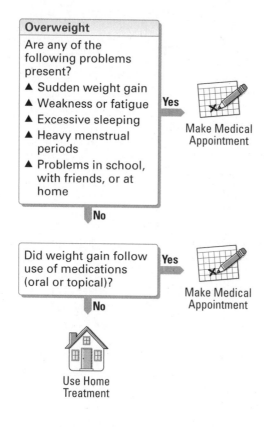

Overweight

Are any of the following problems present?

▲ Sudden weight gain
▲ Weakness or fatigue
▲ Excessive sleeping
▲ Heavy menstrual periods
▲ Problems in school, with friends, or at home

Yes → Make Medical Appointment

No ↓

Did weight gain follow use of medications (oral or topical)?

Yes → Make Medical Appointment

No ↓

Use Home Treatment

are available at www.cdc.gov/nccdphp/dnpa/obesity.

To help with the basics of losing weight, try these tips.

▲ Monitor portion size (see the food pyramid on page 200 and tips on page 58).
▲ Limit TV viewing.
▲ Encourage exercise.
▲ Encourage fruits, vegetables, lean meats, fish, poultry.
▲ Limit processed food.
▲ Limit soda intake.
▲ Limit juice intake.
▲ Limit snacks. Eat meals only at the table. The battle of the bulge is most often lost snacking at the refrigerator.
▲ Reward even minor weight loss.

Weight reduction is a family problem. Children's eating patterns are determined largely by those of their parents. Teenagers can participate in group programs for weight control; these methods are often helpful. Overweight parents may benefit from weight control programs such as Weight Watchers. Whatever method is used, success will depend on both you and your child. Do not expect the doctor to solve the problem for you.

If all else fails, a visit to the doctor or nutritionist may be needed. Don't go to the doctor for diet pills. These do not work and can hurt.

What to Expect

The doctor will take an extensive dietary history and perform a physical examination. Weight will be recorded on a Body Mass Index chart (see pages 500–501). Children between the 85th and 95th percentiles are at risk for becoming overweight. Children above than the 95th percentile are overweight. Blood tests may be done, but, as in adults, tests for thyroid function as a cause of obesity are usually not needed. The doctor may know of a group approach to weight control and be willing to refer your child to that group. Nutritional or behavioral counseling is often recommended. Most often the doctor will elaborate on the principles of controlling food intake and increasing exercise as a home treatment. (See also pages 199–201.)

Underweight

Parents are naturally concerned that their children grow and put on weight. Proper growth and weight gain are determined by adequate nutrition as well as genetic factors. Of course, we have control only over nutrition.

Infants

Often parents of a breast-fed baby will be concerned that their child is not as fat as the baby next door or the baby in the food ads. This is because many breast-fed babies gain weight at a slower rate than bottle-fed babies.

There are, of course, feeding problems in both breast- and bottle-fed infants that can cause a child to be underweight. Inadequate intake, excessive vomiting, or long-lasting diarrhea can all lead to inadequate weight gain in infants. Children with underlying heart failure or long-standing urinary tract infections also may gain weight poorly. This may occur with other serious medical problems as well.

Malabsorption is an intestinal disturbance that produces terrible-smelling, greasy-looking bowel movements. Food is absorbed poorly, resulting in insufficient weight gain.

Doctors are as concerned about weight gain as are parents. They will take height and weight measurements in the office during well-baby visits. A child who is more than two "weight lines" away from the "height line" is seriously underweight. You can check your child on the charts in Part V. For example, if your daughter is one year old and is 29 inches (74 cm) tall, this is on the 50th percentile line. If her weight is only 17 pounds (8 kg), this is only the 5th percentile and is more than two lines away from the 50th percentile. The child is underweight and should see the doctor.

Young Children

In general, if nutrition is adequate and weight loss has not been marked, it is far better to be on the lean side than on the fat side. Children who are lean (but not markedly underweight) have many health advantages. They often feel better about themselves and find physical activities much easier. Unfortunately, "thin is in" has been popularized and is leading to increasing anorexia in teenage girls (see below).

Some infants and young children are picky eaters and sometimes refuse to eat. Other children never seem to sit still long enough to finish a meal and are so active that they seem to burn off their few ingested calories instantaneously. These children should have their meals presented as consistently as possible, meals should be at routine times, and there should be a specified time period for eating (for example, 20 minutes). Struggling with children over food is seldom a useful strategy. If your child is truly underweight, it may be advisable to choose one meal a day during which you make an extra effort to have the child take in an adequate number of calories.

Older Children

Sometimes older children will refuse to eat. Although a short diet with a few pounds of weight loss is fine, prolonged or excessive weight loss can be dangerous. Such children frequently will insist that they feel fat and don't wish to eat, even

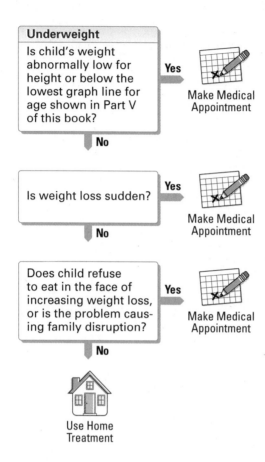

Underweight

Is child's weight abnormally low for height or below the lowest graph line for age shown in Part V of this book?

Yes → Make Medical Appointment

No ↓

Is weight loss sudden?

Yes → Make Medical Appointment

No ↓

Does child refuse to eat in the face of increasing weight loss, or is the problem causing family disruption?

Yes → Make Medical Appointment

No ↓

Use Home Treatment

after they have become emaciated and have developed other health problems. If prolonged, this problem, called **anorexia nervosa**, can be life threatening. Children with this problem have a real aversion to food and sometimes even induce vomiting (**bulimia**) after they eat. Anorexia nervosa requires medical help.

During periods of rapid growth, children often get gangly and "string out." This is not a cause for concern.

Home Treatment

Children will eat a sufficient amount if it is presented to them. Do not be concerned if your child refuses to eat a meal or two or is a picky eater. Children usually do not become underweight if adequate amounts of foods are available.

What to Expect

The doctor will take a complete history and perform a physical examination. He or she will pay special attention to the child's dietary and bowel patterns. The doctor also will carefully measure height and weight and record this on a Body Mass Index chart (pages 500–501). Children below the 5th percentile are underweight. Further investigations will depend on what the doctor finds. If he or she suspects an intestinal problem, stool analysis and possibly bowel X rays will follow. If the doctor suspects a heart problem, he or she will call for X rays or an electrocardiogram (EKG). If an infection is likely, the doctor will order a blood test and urinalysis. If anorexia nervosa is confirmed and the heart rate is slow, your doctor may recommend hospitalization for observation and counseling.

Stress, Anxiety, and Depression

Stress is a normal part of children's lives. Toddlers must learn to communicate. Preschoolers need to know how to interact in a socially acceptable fashion. School-age children have peer and teacher pressures. Adolescents must begin to think about future careers. In addition, they will find and often lose meaningful relations with members of the opposite sex. Leaving home is one of the greatest stresses children encounter.

Besides the daily stresses of their own lives, children absorb the stresses of their parents. It is difficult to shield a child from your own concerns about problems at work, problems with your spouse, and serious illness in relatives. In addition, we may be adding unnecessary burdens to the unavoidable stresses of growing up. In the decade of the "superbaby," increasing social and academic pressures on children are resulting in more and more children suffering from excess stress and fatigue.

With all these stresses, it is not unusual for children to show effects. Stress often appears as anxiety and may progress to depression. The degree of anxiety or depression is more a function of the individual than of the degree of stress. A child with a great deal of family support will be able to deal with minor stresses more easily. Major stresses, such as parental separation or a move, will affect all children.

The length of the recovery period will be a function of the child's strength and parental guidance during the stressful time. If the stress or its consequent anxiety or depression is severe enough, children may develop significant physical and emotional problems.

The following symptoms must be taken seriously if they persist for more than a few days.

▲ Failure to go to school
▲ Difficulty falling asleep
▲ Excessive sleeping
▲ Nightmares or night terrors
▲ Refusal to eat
▲ Significant weight loss or weight gain
▲ Constant sadness

Anxiety can often lead to the **hyperventilation syndrome**. Hyperventilation means excessive breathing. In this condition, an anxious older child or adolescent may rapidly develop the feeling that he or she is unable to get enough air into the lungs. Sometimes this is associated with chest pain or constriction. These sensations lead to further overbreathing and the lowering of the carbon dioxide level in the blood (carbon dioxide is present in exhaled air). The lower level of carbon dioxide may cause numbness and tingling of the hands, feet, and mouth, as well as dizziness. Any of these symptoms can predominate for a particular person.

Home Treatment

The best approach is to be open and to discuss stressful occurrences with your children as they are growing up. This teaches children that they can talk with their parents in working through their problems when they are young. And this support, hopefully, leads to a growing ability to work through stressful situations independently. Identification of the source of anxiety or depression can be difficult

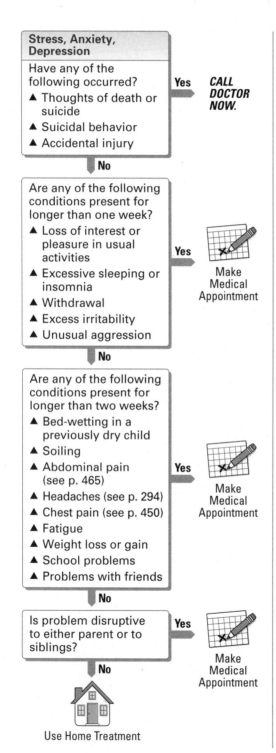

Stress, Anxiety, Depression

Have any of the following occurred?
▲ Thoughts of death or suicide
▲ Suicidal behavior
▲ Accidental injury

Yes → *CALL DOCTOR NOW.*

No ↓

Are any of the following conditions present for longer than one week?
▲ Loss of interest or pleasure in usual activities
▲ Excessive sleeping or insomnia
▲ Withdrawal
▲ Excess irritability
▲ Unusual aggression

Yes → Make Medical Appointment

No ↓

Are any of the following conditions present for longer than two weeks?
▲ Bed-wetting in a previously dry child
▲ Soiling
▲ Abdominal pain (see p. 465)
▲ Headaches (see p. 294)
▲ Chest pain (see p. 450)
▲ Fatigue
▲ Weight loss or gain
▲ School problems
▲ Problems with friends

Yes → Make Medical Appointment

No ↓

Is problem disruptive to either parent or to siblings?

Yes → Make Medical Appointment

No ↓

Use Home Treatment

and may require the help of a professional. Most communities have resources that can help.

With hyperventilation, recognition that this is a stress reaction is a first step. During an attack, a paper bag can be placed loosely over the nose and mouth so that the child can rebreathe the carbon dioxide in the expelled air. (Never use a plastic bag.) This will raise the blood level of carbon dioxide, and the attack will pass after 10 minutes or so. Alternatively, slow the child's breathing by having the child hold his or her breath repeatedly.

What to Expect

The doctor will attempt to identify the source of the problem. School records and records from other health professionals will help. Seldom can the problem be solved in one visit. Social workers, psychologists, or psychiatrists may help with the problem. A combination of therapy with the option to add medication is effective in improving anxiety and depression.

Many antidepressants previously recommended for adolescents have been associated with increased teenage suicide and are no longer in use. Some antidepressants such as fluoxetine (Prozac) have helped many adolescents, but we are concerned about their overuse and side effects. They should be used as part of a program of help and not as stand-alone quick fixes.

Weakness and Fatigue

Children often have periods of being extremely tired or feeling weak. These symptoms may appear quite suddenly. The sudden development of weakness often signifies the beginning of a cold or other infection. Weakness may precede a fever or occur simultaneously with the fever in the early stages of many infections. In younger children, colds, sore throats, earaches, and stomach flu are the most frequent reasons for weakness. In older children, infectious mononucleosis (a prolonged but seldom serious viral infection) or influenza is often the cause. Weakness is a signal that the body should rest.

The fatigue associated with an infection will usually develop quickly and last only for a short period. Exceptions are hepatitis and mononucleosis.

Lack of Sleep

Children have an extraordinary amount of energy, and it is unusual for them to complain of being tired for long. However, we often see young children who seem to have no energy during the day and can trace the problem to late-night television watching. It is not surprising that a young child who is awake until the wee hours of the morning will have little energy for usual daytime activities. Thin walls, noisy neighbors, and late-night talks with brothers or sisters are other factors that can interfere with sleep.

Normally, parents can let nature tell children when they need sleep. But if a child is droopy and sleepy late in the day, you may need to take some action to ensure that he or she is getting enough sleep.

Prolonged Weakness

Anemia (low blood) is a very occasional cause of chronic weakness or tiredness. The most common anemia is iron-deficiency anemia. Iron is abundant in meat products, cereals, nuts, lima beans, lentils, peas, soybeans, spinach, and many other products. Cow's milk is low in iron, and a diet consisting exclusively of cow's milk is dangerous because it can produce anemia in infants and young children. Exclusive ingestion of goat's milk can lead to another type of anemia in infants. Restrictive diets, such as the Zen macrobiotic diet, are inadequate for children. Variety of diet, including all the major food groups, is the most important principle, rather than a rigid set of rules. Given enough varied raw materials, the body is very good at selecting what is needed and eliminating the rest.

Hypoglycemia (low blood sugar) is another commonly discussed but rarely found medical problem. True hypoglycemia causes other symptoms, such as sweating, nervousness, headaches, and irritability, as well as fatigue.

Long-standing weakness and tiredness in children may result from **depression**. (See Stress, Anxiety, and Depression, page 306.) It is a common mistake to assume that only adults are capable of becoming depressed. Children may react severely—to a move, the loss of a pet or friend, difficulty in school, an inability to be successful with friends, or an inability to compete in sports—by withdrawing. Depressed children often have little energy or self-esteem, feel tired or sad all the time, refuse to eat or eat too much, have

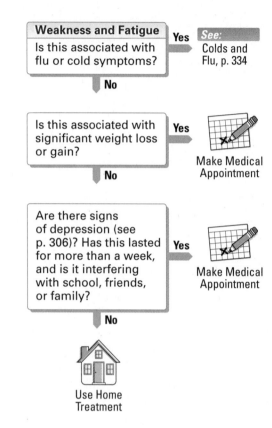

Weakness and Fatigue

Is this associated with flu or cold symptoms? — **Yes** → **See:** Colds and Flu, p. 334

No ↓

Is this associated with significant weight loss or gain? — **Yes** → Make Medical Appointment

No ↓

Are there signs of depression (see p. 306)? Has this lasted for more than a week, and is it interfering with school, friends, or family? — **Yes** → Make Medical Appointment

No ↓

Use Home Treatment

---

trouble falling asleep at night or sleep too much, and may complain of a number of physical ailments. These symptoms should be treated seriously. The longer a child spends away from school or from normal everyday activities, the harder it is to begin functioning normally again. If you are having difficulty dealing with a problem that is disturbing your child, you should seek professional help for the child.

Home Treatment

Watching and waiting are all that is called for in the case of weakness that accompanies a mild infection. As usual, adequate fluid intake and rest will help. If the problem persists for a week or more, consult the doctor.

What to Expect

The doctor will take a careful history and perform a physical examination, including measurement of height and weight. For some types of infections, he or she will order specific laboratory tests. For instance, infectious mononucleosis and hepatitis can be detected by a blood test. Most doctors will check for anemia and hypoglycemia only if the dietary history or symptoms suggest these problems.

Dizziness and Fainting

These complaints are frustrating to children, parents, and doctors alike. They are common, worrisome, and occasionally frightening, but most often they go unexplained. Defining the terms correctly will help you understand the problem.

Fainting

The term *fainting* may be used to describe a light-headed and woozy episode without loss of consciousness, or it may signify a complete collapse with loss of consciousness. Light-headedness frequently accompanies viral illnesses. It may also occur if a child suddenly stands up from a reclining or sitting position. It takes a few seconds for the body to adjust to this new position, so there is a temporary decrease in blood flow to the head. Low blood sugar and irregular heart rhythms occur rarely. A doctor's attention is needed if the light-headedness persists or recurs. If the child has lost consciousness completely, however, see the doctor without delay.

Breath-holding spells are described on page 85. Breath holding may lead to complete unconsciousness and even a seizure. Try to prevent injury from falling or from a seizure by observation and support. If you are certain that loss of consciousness occurred because of a breath-holding spell, apply home treatment and discuss the situation with your doctor on the phone.

Dizziness

Dizziness refers to a situation in which the room seems to spin about. This is also called vertigo and may be accompanied by nausea and vomiting. Except for the case when children spin themselves in a circle rapidly, vertigo indicates that the balance mechanism in the inner ear has been disturbed. This most often occurs because of minor viral infections called **labyrinthitis**. Sometimes it occurs with ear infections. If your child has an earache, see your doctor.

Some medications can cause vertigo. Call your doctor if this is a possibility.

Home Treatment

If light-headedness occurs upon arising suddenly from a sitting or reclining position, simply avoid such sudden changes in position. This problem is called **postural hypotension** and does not need the help of the doctor unless it has suddenly become worse. Encouraging increased fluids is important. Otherwise, you may wait to discuss the light-headedness at the next routine visit. If it is caused by a virus, it will go away within a few days.

Breath-holding spells are challenging problems. Drugs will not help. In the meantime, try to prevent damage from falls or seizures by alerting teachers and friends so that they may be aware of the possibility and ready to help. The child will outgrow them eventually.

What to Expect

The history of these episodes is the most important piece of information in deciding what to do. The physical examination will include examination of the eyes and ears and blood pressure measurements. An EKG will often be done to check on the heart's rhythm. Sometimes tests on the blood and the urine may be done. X rays

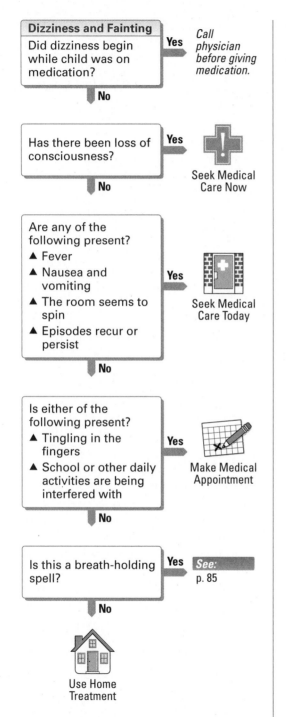

Dizziness and Fainting

Did dizziness begin while child was on medication? — **Yes** → *Call physician before giving medication.*

No ↓

Has there been loss of consciousness? — **Yes** → Seek Medical Care Now

No ↓

Are any of the following present?
▲ Fever
▲ Nausea and vomiting
▲ The room seems to spin
▲ Episodes recur or persist
— **Yes** → Seek Medical Care Today

No ↓

Is either of the following present?
▲ Tingling in the fingers
▲ School or other daily activities are being interfered with
— **Yes** → Make Medical Appointment

No ↓

Is this a breath-holding spell? — **Yes** → *See:* p. 85

No ↓

Use Home Treatment

and brain wave tests (EEG) are rarely of use. The doctor may perform tests of the inner ear. Vertigo may be treated with drugs.

Seizures

About 5% of all children will have a seizure (convulsion, fit, falling-out spell). Seizures occur because of a disruption of the normal electrical impulse pattern of the brain. This disruption can occur spontaneously; be triggered by fever, poison, or infection (meningitis); or occur after a breath-holding spell or immunization.

There are many types of seizures, but parents will have no trouble recognizing the abnormal condition in their child. Some children will become stiff and roll their eyes backward. Others will exhibit rhythmic jerking of their arms and legs. Some may have staring spells or suddenly collapse. All of these can cause great alarm. Fortunately, most seizures end in a few minutes without permanent damage to the child.

Fever Fits

The most common cause of seizures in children is a high fever. Such seizures are often referred to as "fever fits" or "febrile seizures." These occur most often in children between the ages of six months and four years. Anyone will have a seizure if his or her body temperature is sufficiently elevated, say to 107°F to 109°F (41°C to 42°C). Children are thought to have a lower threshold for seizing—as low as 103°F (39°C). Part of this lowered threshold may be due to the immaturity of the nervous system in young children.

More than half of the children who have a febrile seizure will never have a second. Yet in some children who have a febrile seizure, this is the first sign of the recurrent seizures of **epilepsy**, and later

seizures may be spontaneous and not associated with fever. Less than 0.5% of the population is diagnosed as having epilepsy. Almost all of these individuals are leading normal lives because of the remarkable effectiveness of medications.

Home Treatment

Home treatment consists of things to do before you see the doctor. Seizures are very frightening experiences, and it is easy to panic. You can avoid panic if you keep a few simple principles in mind.

▲ Most childhood seizures stop by themselves within a few minutes, and it is rare for a seizure to do any lasting harm to a child.

▲ While the seizure is occurring, you should be concerned with preventing injury to the child from a fall and preventing a blow to the head.

▲ Tongue chewing or swallowing does not often occur. Jamming an object into the child's mouth can do more harm than good.

▲ It is important for the child to have a good air passage. Extending the child's neck (chin as far from the chest as possible) while gently pulling on the jaw is the best way to accomplish this.

▲ If the seizure has stopped and the child has vomited, clear the mouth.

▲ Following a seizure, the child will be drowsy or may seem to be in a deep sleep. This is called the postictal state and is not harmful. You need not attempt to arouse the child from this state.

▲ If the seizure has stopped and your child has a fever, begin temperature-lowering procedures. You cannot give

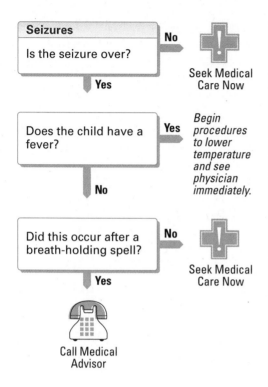

Seizures

Is the seizure over? — **No** → Seek Medical Care Now

↓ **Yes**

Does the child have a fever? — **Yes** → *Begin procedures to lower temperature and see physician immediately.*

↓ **No**

Did this occur after a breath-holding spell? — **No** → Seek Medical Care Now

↓ **Yes**

Call Medical Advisor

medicine by mouth, but you can use an acetaminophen suppository.

Sponging with tepid water will help lower the child's temperature. Beware of giving a bath to a semiconscious child; drowning is a danger. Sponging the child may continue during the trip to the doctor. Do not bundle the child up; both you and the child must keep cool. If there is a considerable distance to be traveled, temperature lowering en route becomes important. Remember that you can lower a fever as effectively as the doctor can.

Seizures resulting from breath-holding spells are seldom serious, but you should consult your doctor by phone.

What to Expect

If the seizure has not stopped, the doctor will give the child an injection to bring this about. Following control of the seizure, the doctor will perform a thorough physical examination and will want to talk to you in depth. If a fever is present, the doctor will search for the source of the infection. Most often the fever is due to one of the common viral infections of childhood.

The doctor may order a spinal tap to investigate the possibility of an infection in the brain or spinal cord. Hospitalization is sometimes required for observation, treatment, or further evaluation. The doctor also may order a brain wave test (electroencephalogram, or EEG). Often it is better to wait a week before doing an EEG. Brain wave tests do not necessarily require a hospital admission.

Swallowed Objects

Babies and small children delight in swallowing any and all things they can get their hands on and that are small enough to go down. In this section, we are concerned with things that will not dissolve in the stomach. Anything that *will* dissolve is a potential poison. See Poisoning, page 250, for more information.

A warning against traditional party balloons, which often wind up in a child's mouth, and even more tragically can block a child's breathing passage, with disastrous consequences. **Avoid latex balloons.**

Children's favorites among nondissolving objects are coins, buttons, the eyes from teddy bears and dolls, safety pins, and fruit pits. Nature seems to have prepared the digestive tract well, because even very sharp objects such as open safety pins, pieces of glass, needles, and straight pins regularly pass through the bowels with the greatest of ease. Coins often wind up in the trachea, however, and can be dangerous.

Swallowed objects can go into either the windpipe (trachea) or esophagus. Of immediate concern is the possibility that an object has become lodged in the windpipe. Violent coughing or difficulty breathing suggests this possibility. As long as the child is able to breathe, proceed immediately to the doctor or emergency room. Attempting to dislodge an object that is partially obstructing breathing may lead to complete obstruction. If the windpipe is completely obstructed, try the abdominal-thrust maneuver (see Choking, page 246) to force the object out.

Pain and/or vomiting indicate that help is needed for an abdominal problem. If the object swallowed is very sharp and could possibly puncture the intestine, you should call your doctor. The purpose of this call is to let the doctor know that assistance could be needed in the next few days on rather short notice. The doctor can make appropriate arrangements. If the object should perforate the intestine, surgery will be required, and these prior arrangements can make the surgery go more smoothly. Be prepared, but do not panic. Even razor blades have passed through the entire digestive system without noticeable effect.

Home Treatment

If the object is smooth, you may want to look at your child's bowel movements for the next few days to reassure yourself that it has passed. If you don't see it, it is a far better bet that you missed it than that it did not pass.

If the object is sharp, the doctor will likely ask you to look for the object to pass and to be on the alert for abdominal pain or vomiting. The doctor also should make sure that surgical help will be available if needed.

What to Expect

If the object is lodged in the throat, the doctor may be able to remove it in the office. Otherwise, a visit to the hospital may be necessary. If the problem is shortness of breath, wheezing, pain in the chest or abdomen, or vomiting, the doctor will take a history, perform a physical examination, and order X rays. Remember that nonmetallic objects may not be visible on an X ray. In this instance, special X rays

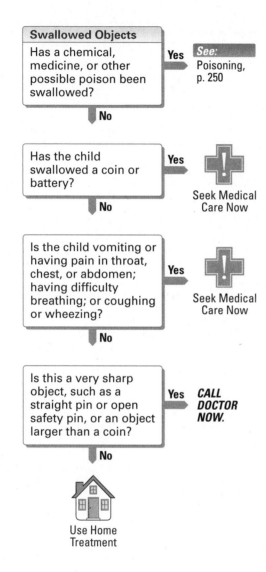

Swallowed Objects

Has a chemical, medicine, or other possible poison been swallowed? → **Yes** → *See:* Poisoning, p. 250

↓ **No**

Has the child swallowed a coin or battery? → **Yes** → Seek Medical Care Now

↓ **No**

Is the child vomiting or having pain in throat, chest, or abdomen; having difficulty breathing; or coughing or wheezing? → **Yes** → Seek Medical Care Now

↓ **No**

Is this a very sharp object, such as a straight pin or open safety pin, or an object larger than a coin? → **Yes** → *CALL DOCTOR NOW.*

↓ **No**

Use Home Treatment

(such as a barium swallow) may show the object, but these X rays may be unwise if the doctor suspects a puncture of the intestine.

If the intestine has been punctured, surgery will be necessary. If the object is in the respiratory tract, it must be removed. This can often be accomplished through an instrument known as a bronchoscope, which enables the doctor to visualize and remove foreign objects.

Frequent Illnesses

Frequent illnesses are the rule and not the exception for most children. Recent studies have revealed that the average child has between six and nine viral illnesses per year. In some children, these viral illnesses are so mild that the parent will not notice any symptoms. Other children will have a cough, a runny nose, or some other minor symptom. We do not think of these viral infections as illnesses but rather as immunizations that serve to protect children against the more serious consequences of these illnesses at a later age.

Besides the frequent minor colds that most children have, the majority of children will also experience one or more ear infections in a lifetime. Similarly, we expect most children to have several bouts of diarrhea while they are young and at least one or two strep throats in the school years. When you start adding up the number of illnesses we expect in children, it is a wonder that they spend so much time free of symptoms.

The younger children in a family often seem to have more colds than their older brothers and sisters did at the same age, but that doesn't mean that they're not as healthy. Younger children merely get many of the common viral illnesses at an earlier age because of their exposure to older siblings. Similarly, although some studies have shown that children in day care centers or nursery schools seem to get a few more colds early on than their peers who remain at home, there is no evidence that these children are any less healthy. There are at least 60 different viral strains against which most adults are partly immunized because of childhood illnesses. The sooner the child develops these immunities, the sooner the relatively illness-free years of adulthood can begin.

Immune Deficiencies

Abnormalities of the body's immune defense mechanisms, of concern to many parents, virtually never present themselves as frequent minor infections. Children with immune deficiencies often have repeated severe infections of the lungs or skin. These children seldom grow normally and are often quite underweight because of the repeated infections. For any of these problems, a medical evaluation is important. Similarly, if a relative died at a young age because of an overwhelming infection, you should discuss your concern with your doctor.

Children who received a blood transfusion before April 1985 had a very slight chance of acquiring the human immunodeficiency virus (HIV), which is responsible for AIDS. However, no new cases from transfusions have been seen for a number of years. Children can also acquire HIV while in the uterus. If the child's mother did not have an HIV test during pregnancy, discuss this situation with your doctor.

Allergies

Allergies are often confused with illnesses. Children with allergic rhinitis or hay fever will usually experience sneezing, itchy eyes, and runny noses at a particular time of year, normally in the spring and fall. These children will often rub their noses constantly.

Home Treatment

Home treatment of the minor problems of childhood are discussed throughout

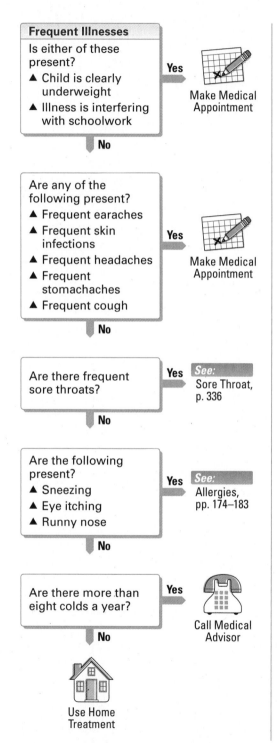

Frequent Illnesses

Is either of these present?
- ▲ Child is clearly underweight
- ▲ Illness is interfering with schoolwork

Yes → Make Medical Appointment

No ↓

Are any of the following present?
- ▲ Frequent earaches
- ▲ Frequent skin infections
- ▲ Frequent headaches
- ▲ Frequent stomachaches
- ▲ Frequent cough

Yes → Make Medical Appointment

No ↓

Are there frequent sore throats?

Yes → *See:* Sore Throat, p. 336

No ↓

Are the following present?
- ▲ Sneezing
- ▲ Eye itching
- ▲ Runny nose

Yes → *See:* Allergies, pp. 174–183

No ↓

Are there more than eight colds a year?

Yes → Call Medical Advisor

No ↓

Use Home Treatment

this book. Frequent illnesses that are troublesome enough to interfere with schoolwork should be evaluated by a doctor.

What to Expect

The doctor will take a careful history and perform a physical examination. He or she will record the nature and severity of the child's frequent illnesses. The doctor will pay particular attention to the child's height and weight development. Depending on the nature of the problem, the physician may order various laboratory tests.

True immune deficiency states in children are very rare, and children with this problem need special treatment. Frequent colds or recurrent earaches do *not* warrant the use of gamma globulin shots. Gamma globulin deficiency must be confirmed by blood tests.

Jaundice

The skin is often a good barometer of what's occurring in your child's body. Parents know this and often call the doctor with concerns that a child's complexion appears too pale, dusky, flushed, red, or occasionally yellow.

A yellow or orange tinge to a child's skin is not an immediate cause for alarm. Many infants and young children are large consumers of carrots or other foods containing carotenoids, which may cause a harmless and reversible discoloration of the skin. Yellowing of the skin also occurs in the area of a bruise. In distinction, the yellow coloring of the skin that occurs in jaundice will also be accompanied by a yellowing of the eyes.

Jaundice is a result of the body's inability to dispose of a normally occurring chemical called bilirubin. When red blood cells finally collapse because of old age (usually 120 days), they release bilirubin, which is processed by the liver and ultimately disposed of through the intestines. Problems that either cause red blood cells to dissolve more rapidly than normal (hemolysis) or interfere with the workings of the liver (hepatitis) or its outflow (obstruction) can produce jaundice.

Newborns

A majority of newborn babies will experience a slight amount of jaundice in the first few days of life while their livers are getting cranked up to produce the enzymes needed to break down bilirubin. As long as there is no problem with the baby's red blood cells stemming from incompatibility with the mother's blood (Rh or ABO problem), with an inherited blood problem (spherocytosis), or with an infection, the baby is considered to have a temporary problem known as **physiologic jaundice**.

If the baby appears quite yellow, blood measurements may be done to be certain bilirubin levels are not so high as to pose a risk to the baby's brain. We have seen too many parents terrorized by the bilirubin numbers game, and even brought to tears if a level of 12 goes to 13. Levels below 20 are generally considered safe, except in very small, very sick, or premature babies. Higher levels are currently being tolerated in infants without a hemolytic problem. Also, infants of Asian ancestry have higher levels.

A mild form of jaundice is seen in 1 to 2% of breast-fed infants whose mothers produce a substance in their breast milk that impedes the processing of bilirubin. This type of jaundice generally begins on day four and peaks at two weeks. Otherwise, there is no evidence that breast milk in the other 98 to 99% of infants is responsible for more jaundice than formula.

Older Children

Older children generally become jaundiced from a variety of liver infections, usually viral, that cause hepatitis. Despite the considerable anxiety evoked by the diagnosis of hepatitis, almost all children recover without any consequences. Many children have such mild cases that parents are unaware of the infection. The liver also can be damaged by toxins and too much acetaminophen.

Currently two vaccines are available to prevent hepatitis. Hepatitis B vaccination has been routine since the early 1990s; hepatitis A is recommended in certain states.

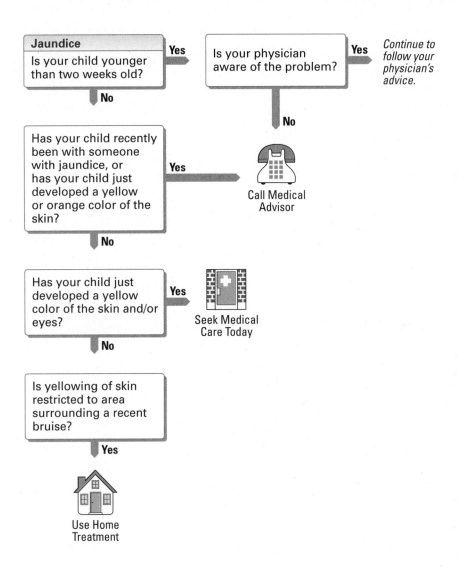

Jaundice

Is your child younger than two weeks old? — **Yes** → Is your physician aware of the problem? — **Yes** → *Continue to follow your physician's advice.*

No ↓

Has your child recently been with someone with jaundice, or has your child just developed a yellow or orange color of the skin? — **Yes** → Call Medical Advisor

Is your physician aware of the problem? — **No** ↓ Call Medical Advisor

No ↓

Has your child just developed a yellow color of the skin and/or eyes? — **Yes** → Seek Medical Care Today

No ↓

Is yellowing of skin restricted to area surrounding a recent bruise?

Yes ↓

Use Home Treatment

Home Treatment

For newborn infants, although sunlight appears to be helpful in promoting the proper decomposition of bilirubin, too much sun is harmful. We do not recommend sun exposure to treat jaundice. Instead, frequent feedings are encouraged. Breast-feeding mothers are encouraged to increase feedings; substituting formula or additional formula to guarantee adequate hydration is also acceptable.

What to Expect

After your doctor takes a careful history focusing on how your child might have acquired hepatitis and on other family members who were jaundiced (which might suggest an inherited blood problem), he or she will order blood tests to look at how effectively the liver is functioning and to identify the particular type of infection.

Depending on the type of hepatitis identified, the doctor may recommend that other family members or playmates receive a protective dose of a type of immune/gamma globulin. For certain types of viral hepatitis, several follow-up visits may be necessary to ensure that the body has mounted the appropriate response and that the child has not become a carrier of the infection.

Newborn infants with jaundice are often treated with blue fluorescent lights, which cause an increased processing and elimination of bilirubin. This procedure is relatively safe as long as care is taken to shield the infant's eyes from the light. Many communities have home bilirubin light services that can be far superior to having your infant return to the hospital. For very high bilirubin levels a blood transfusion may be needed.

The decision to treat a newborn infant with jaundice depends on many factors, including the baby's weight, maturity, and health. Decisions to use phototherapy at home or in the hospital are always individualized, with many pediatricians relying on guidelines from the American Academy of Pediatrics. You can get the latest guidelines and information from http://aappolicy.aappublications.org. Helpful information is also available at http://bilitool.org. Table 7 shows a range of levels that pediatricians may use when they consider starting phototherapy.

Table 7: Guidelines for Considering Treatment of Bilirubin with Phototherapy	
Infant's Age	**Total Bilirubin Level (mg/dl)**
12 hours	5–10
24 hours	7–12
48 hours	10–15
72 hours	13–19
96 hours	14–20
5–7 days	More than 20

Eye Problems

Eye Redness, Burning, Itching, and Discharge

These symptoms usually signal **conjunctivitis**, or "pinkeye," an inflammation of the membrane that lines the eye and the inner surface of the eyelids. The inflammation may be due to an irritant in the air, an allergy to something in the air, or an infection (virus, bacteria, or chlamydia).

Irritants

Environmental pollutants in smog can produce burning and itching. These symptoms represent **chemical conjunctivitis** and affect anyone exposed to too much of a particular chemical. A smoke-filled room, chlorinated swimming pool, desert sandstorm, or sun glare on snow can cause similar irritation.

In contrast, **allergic conjunctivitis** affects only those people who are allergic. Almost always the allergen is in the air, and grass pollens are probably the most frequent offenders. Depending on the season for the offending pollen, this problem may occur in spring, summer, or fall and usually lasts for two to three weeks.

Infections

A minor conjunctivitis frequently accompanies a viral cold. Epidemics of conjunctivitis are most often caused by a virus. The eye discharge is not as thick as in more severe bacterial infections. Often a small swollen lymph gland will be found in front of the ear in **epidemic conjunctivitis**.

Conjunctivitis is also common in the first day or so of measles (page 422). Some viruses, such as herpes, may cause deep, painful ulcers in the cornea and may interfere with vision.

Bacterial infections cause pus to form, and a thick, plentiful discharge may run from the eyes. Often the eyelids are crusted over and "glued" shut upon awakening.

Chlamydia infections occur in the first few months of life. These infections require antibiotic treatment.

Some diseases affect the deeper layers of the eye—those that control the operation of the lens and the size of the pupillary opening. This condition is termed **iritis**, or "uveitis," and may cause irregularity of the pupil or pain when the pupil reacts to light. It is unusual in children. Medical attention is required.

Home Treatment

If allergic exposure is the cause of the symptoms, avoiding exposure will help. Special glasses that keep out pollen are available for severe cases. An antihistamine for the eyes is available—dopatadine (Patinol)—but should not be used for more than a few days. Murine, Visine, and other eyedrops seldom afford more than very temporary relief. Oral antihistamines obtained either over the counter (chlorpheniramine, brompheniramine, diphenhydramine, loratadine) may help, but don't expect total relief, and drowsiness may occur.

A viral infection related to a cold or flu will run its course in a few days, and it is best to be patient.

Although it is no longer considered medically necessary to keep children with conjunctivitis out of day care, this is still a common practice.

For very red eyes or a moderate discharge, a call to your physician is advisable. If the problem doesn't clear up, if the discharge is thick, or if there is eye pain or a problem with vision, see your doctor. Fever may be absent with a bacterial infection of the eye. Because the infection is superficial, washing the eye gently will help remove some of the bacteria, but you should still see the doctor.

What to Expect

The doctor will check vision, eye motion, the eyelids, and the reaction of the pupil to light. He or she may suggest an antihistamine (page 224) for an allergy. If a bacterial infection is likely, the doctor may prescribe antibiotic eyedrops or ointments. Steroid-containing eye ointments should be prescribed very infrequently. Certain infections (herpes) will get worse with these medicines. If herpes is diagnosed, usually by an ophthalmologist, special eyedrops and other medicines will be needed.

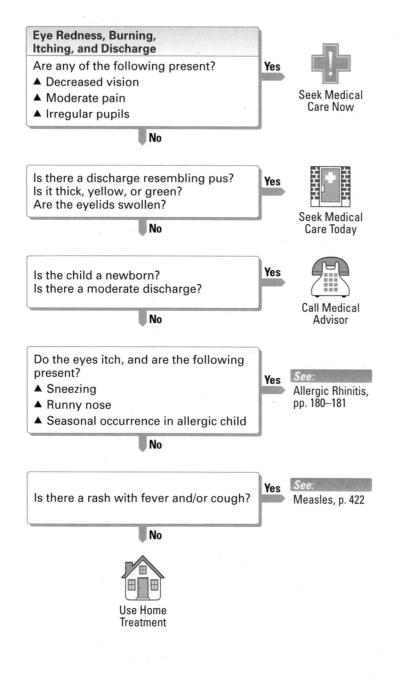

Eye Redness, Burning, Itching, and Discharge

Are any of the following present?
▲ Decreased vision
▲ Moderate pain
▲ Irregular pupils

Yes → Seek Medical Care Now

No

Is there a discharge resembling pus?
Is it thick, yellow, or green?
Are the eyelids swollen?

Yes → Seek Medical Care Today

No

Is the child a newborn?
Is there a moderate discharge?

Yes → Call Medical Advisor

No

Do the eyes itch, and are the following present?
▲ Sneezing
▲ Runny nose
▲ Seasonal occurrence in allergic child

Yes → *See:* Allergic Rhinitis, pp. 180–181

No

Is there a rash with fever and/or cough?

Yes → *See:* Measles, p. 422

No

Use Home Treatment

Swollen Eyes

It is easy and quite common for eyelids to become swollen. Not surprisingly, the most common reasons for swelling are linked to everyday events.

Irritants
Insect bites and stings (page 282) near the eye are notorious for causing eyelid swelling. Search carefully for a telltale bite near the affected eye. Usually, only one eyelid is swollen unless there has been a mosquito onslaught on your child's face.

Young children manage to rub a variety of irritating substances in their eyes, which can simultaneously cause redness of the eyes and lid swelling. Irritants can range from dirt to household cleansers to spices.

Allergies also contribute to swollen eyelids. Hay fever and allergic conjunctivitis usually include eye itching and redness along with eyelid swelling. Allergic problems tend to occur repeatedly, and parents can learn to treat them at home. If eyelid swelling accompanies swelling elsewhere in the body (for example, in the mouth, hands, or feet), this suggests a more widespread allergic reaction or an accumulation of fluid characteristic of certain kidney disorders. Obviously, both of these should receive immediate medical attention.

Infections
Certain infections such as **sinusitis** (in older children) and **conjunctivitis** (see page 321) characteristically produce eyelid swelling. Other, more serious infections also may be responsible for swollen eyes. **Periorbital cellulitis** is a serious bacterial infection carried by the blood that generally produces swelling of an area around the eyes. It is now rarely seen because of hemophilus immunizations. Usually, more than the eyelids are involved, the skin surrounding the eye may have a red or purple color, and fever is present. Even more unusual is infection of the eye cavity (orbit), which will, in addition to the above features, produce a bulging (sometimes painful) eye. This condition, which often follows trauma or sinusitis, merits immediate medical attention.

Home Treatment
For insect bites and other minor irritations, washing the area around the eye will be both cleansing and soothing. Allergic eye reactions can be helped with a variety of antihistamines (page 224), such as chlorpheniramine (Chlor-Trimeton), diphenhydramine (Benadryl), or loratadine (Claritin). Wraparound sunglasses may offer some protection in heavy pollen seasons.

What to Expect
The doctor will take a careful history and perform a physical examination, focusing on the eyes and face. He or she may order blood tests to check for indicators of serious infection or for bacteria in the blood. If sinusitis is suspected, the doctor may call for X rays. He or she will perform more extensive radiological evaluations for suspected orbital cellulitis or order a urinalysis if a kidney problem is suspected.

Antibiotics are commonly prescribed for milder infections. Daily injections or hospitalization for intravenous antibiotics is appropriate for serious infections.

Swollen Eyes

Are any of the following present?
- ▲ Protruding eye
- ▲ Fever
- ▲ Skin color change
- ▲ Eye pain
- ▲ Swelling after injury

Yes →

Seek Medical
Care Now

No ↓

Is there redness and discharge that is not clear, or are eyelids stuck together? (*See: Eye Redness, Burning, Itching, and Discharge, p. 321*)

Yes →

Seek Medical
Care Today

No ↓

Is swelling increasing, or are both eyelids swollen?

Yes →

Call Medical
Advisor

No ↓

Use Home
Treatment

Object in Eye/Eye Pain

All eye injuries should be taken seriously. If there is any question, visit the doctor; the stakes are too high.

A foreign body in the eye must be removed, or the threat of infection and loss of sight in that eye are present. Be particularly careful if the foreign body was caused by the striking of metal on metal. This can cause a small metal particle to enter the eye with great force and penetrate the eyeball.

Under a few circumstances, you can treat the injury at home. If the foreign body is minor, such as sand, and did not strike the eye with great velocity, it may feel as though it is still in the eye even when it is not. Small, round particles such as sand rarely stick behind the upper lid for long.

If it feels as though a foreign body is present but it is not, the covering of the eye (cornea) has been scraped or cut. A minor corneal injury will usually heal quickly without problems. A major one requires medical attention.

Even if you think the injury is minor, run through the questions on the decision chart daily. The eye repairs injury quickly, and most minor injuries will heal within 24–48 hours. If any symptoms at all are present after 48 hours and are not clearly resolving, see the doctor.

Eye pain is an unusual symptom that may signify a serious inflammation of the eye (iritis) or a serious infection with the herpes virus. Consult the doctor.

Home Treatment

Be gentle. Wash the eye out with water. Inspect the eye and have someone else check it as well. Use a good light and shine it from both the front and the side. Pay particular attention to the cornea—this is a clear membrane that covers the colored portion of the eye. Do not let your child rub the eye. If a foreign body is present, this will abrade or scratch the cornea.

Some doctors will recommend an eye patch to relieve pain. Usually, it is needed for 24 hours or less. Make the patch with several layers of gauze and tape it firmly in place. Check the child's vision each day and compare the two eyes. If you are not sure that all is going well, see the doctor.

What to Expect

The doctor will perform a vision check, inspect the eye, and inspect under the upper lid. This is not painful. Usually, the doctor will drop a fluorescent stain into the eye and then examine it under ultraviolet light. This too is not painful or hazardous.

If the physician finds a foreign body, he or she will remove it with a cotton swab, an eyewash solution, a small needle, or other appropriate eye instrument. Strong magnets are sometimes used to remove metallic objects. If these measures do not suffice, you may be referred to an ophthalmologist (a physician specializing in diseases of the eye). The doctor may apply an antibiotic ointment and provide the child with an eye patch.

If a foreign body is possibly inside the globe of the eye, the doctor may order ultrasound. If an iritis is present, he or she may use steroid drops, as well as special drops to dilate the pupil.

Object in Eye/Eye Pain

Are any of the
following present?

▲ The object can be
seen, and it remains
after gentle washing.

▲ The injury could
have penetrated the
globe of the eye.

▲ Blood can be seen
in the eye.

▲ It feels as though a
foreign body might
be trapped behind
the upper lid.

Yes

Seek Medical
Care Now

No

Is there any problem
with vision?

Yes

Seek Medical
Care Now

No

Is there eye pain?

Yes

Call Medical
Advisor

No

Use Home
Treatment

Styes and Blocked Tear Ducts

We might have called this problem "bumps around the eyes," because that is how they appear. Styes are infections (usually caused by staphylococcal bacteria) of the tiny glands in the eyelids. They are really small abscesses, and the bumps are red and tender. They grow to full size over a day or so.

Another type of bump in the eyelid, called a **chalazion**, appears more slowly over many days or even weeks and is not red or tender. A chalazion often requires drainage by a doctor, whereas most styes will respond to home treatment alone. There is no urgency to treat a chalazion, and home treatment will not cause any harm.

Tear Ducts

Tears are the lubricating system of the eye. The tear glands continually produce them, and they drain into the nose by the tear ducts. These ducts are often incompletely developed at birth, so the drainage of tears is blocked. When this happens, the tears may collect in the ducts and cause them to swell, appearing as bumps along the sides of the nose just below the inner corners of the eyes. These bumps are not red or tender unless they become infected. Most blocked tear ducts will open by themselves in the first month of life, and most of the remainder will respond to home treatment. Tears running down the cheek are seldom noted in the first month of life because the infant produces only a small volume of tears.

The eyeball itself is *not* involved in a stye or a blocked tear duct. Problems with the eyeball, and especially with vision, should not be attributed to these two relatively minor problems.

Home Treatment

Stye

Apply warm, moist compresses for 10 to 15 minutes at least three times a day. The compresses help the abscess to "point." This means that the tissue over the abscess becomes quite thin, and the pus in the abscess is very close to the surface. After an abscess points, it will often drain spontaneously. If this does not happen, it must be lanced by the doctor. Sometimes the stye goes away without coming to a point and draining.

Chalazions usually do not respond to warm compresses, but neither will they be harmed by compresses. If no improvement is noted with home treatment after 48 hours, see the doctor.

Blockage of Tear Ducts

Simply massage each bump downward with warm, moist compresses several times a day. If the bump is not red and tender (indicating infection), you may continue this treatment for up to several months. If the problem persists, discuss it with your doctor. If the bump becomes red and swollen, antibiotic drops will be needed.

What to Expect

If the stye is pointing and ready to be drained, the doctor will open it with a small needle. If it is not pointing, the doctor will usually recommend compresses and sometimes antibiotic eyedrops. Attempting to drain a stye that is not pointing is usually not very satisfactory.

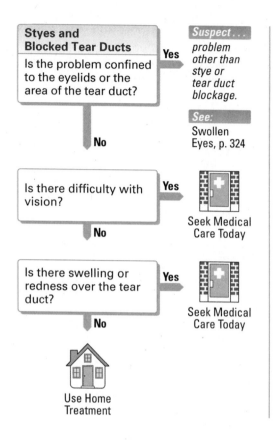

Styes and Blocked Tear Ducts

Is the problem confined to the eyelids or the area of the tear duct?

Yes → *Suspect...* *problem other than stye or tear duct blockage.*

See: Swollen Eyes, p. 324

No ↓

Is there difficulty with vision?

Yes → Seek Medical Care Today

No ↓

Is there swelling or redness over the tear duct?

Yes → Seek Medical Care Today

No ↓

Use Home Treatment

If the doctor feels that the problem is a chalazion, he or she may suggest that it be removed with minor surgery. You will have to decide whether your child should have the surgery. Chalazions are not dangerous, and the operation may be disturbing to the child.

If the child is older than six months and is still having problems with blocked tear ducts, they can usually be opened with a very fine probe. This procedure is successful on the first try in about 75% of cases and on subsequent attempts in the remainder. Only rarely is a surgical procedure necessary to establish an open tear duct. For red and swollen ducts, the doctor will usually recommend antibiotic drops and warm compresses.

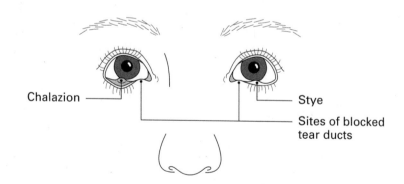

Chalazion — Stye

Sites of blocked tear ducts

Vision Problems

Although children can see at birth, the eye is not fully developed. The eye completes its development by about six months of age, and coordination between the two eyes is complete at about one year of age. It is difficult for most doctors to determine how clearly a child sees (visual acuity) before the age of three or four; however, ophthalmologists can test vision in younger children. Problems with vision may be suggested by the child's not reaching for objects or failing to follow a moving object with his or her eyes. Remember that the child's vision is still developing in the first months of life; do not be too quick in your judgment. Even in older children, significant problems with vision may not be detected without the use of eye tests. Eye tests are important for school-age children.

Crossed eyes may be striking in a newborn child. This occurs simply because muscle coordination between the eyes is not yet fully developed. The problem usually corrects itself by the sixth month of life. If crossed eyes persist beyond this age, discuss this with your doctor at a regular checkup.

Strabismus is a problem with the eye muscles that is also known as "lazy eye." One or both eyes may be involved. If the lazy eye is allowed to remain lazy, vision may be lost in that eye. Strabismus should be suspected in a child in which one or both eyes turn in or out after the age of four months. Ordinarily, a light shining from several feet in front of the child's eyes should reflect in the same location in both eyes.

Fortunately, sudden loss of vision is less frequent in children than in adults. When it does occur, an immediate trip to the doctor is warranted.

An optometrist and ophthalmologist are often involved in the care of these problems. Before referral, however, you should have the opportunity to discuss the problem with your doctor. This may help sort out the problem and will result in a referral if necessary.

Home Treatment

Home treatment is reserved for children under the age of six months who have crossed eyes. This problem is usually present at birth and gets better as the child gets older. Full correction may take as long as a year. Home treatment consists merely of observation to make sure the problem corrects itself. You should discuss crossed eyes that occur at any other age with your doctor.

What to Expect

The doctor will examine visual acuity, eye movement, and pupils. Eye charts with pictures are used for children too young to read. The doctor will alternately cover each eye while asking the child to look at a distant object. Charts may be used to check for simultaneous use of both eyes. Eye movement in a suddenly uncovered eye (cover-uncover test) is a sign of strabismus.

The doctor will examine the inside of the eye with a handheld instrument called an ophthalmoscope. He or she may use a special kind of microscope, called a slit lamp, to examine the front portion of the eye.

Most often, strabismus will be treated with an eye patch. The younger the age

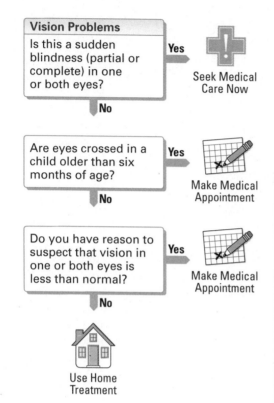

Vision Problems

Is this a sudden blindness (partial or complete) in one or both eyes?

Yes → Seek Medical Care Now

No ↓

Are eyes crossed in a child older than six months of age?

Yes → Make Medical Appointment

No ↓

Do you have reason to suspect that vision in one or both eyes is less than normal?

Yes → Make Medical Appointment

No ↓

Use Home Treatment

at which this condition is detected, the better the chances for saving the vision in the eye. Make sure your doctor always checks for visual acuity when your child is young.

If necessary, the doctor will prescribe corrective lenses, even for very small children. Sometimes surgery is required to correct crossed eyes and occasionally is necessary in cases of decreased vision.

Ear, Nose, and Throat Problems

Is It a Virus, a Bacterium, or an Allergy?

The following sections discuss upper respiratory problems, including colds and flu, sore throat, earaches, runny nose, cough, hoarseness, swollen glands, and nosebleeds. A central question is important to each of these complaints: Is it caused by a virus, a bacterium, or an allergic reaction? In general, only for bacterial infections does the doctor have more effective treatment than is available at home. Remember that viral infections and allergies do not improve with treatment with penicillin or other antibiotics. To demand a "penicillin shot" for a cold or allergy is to ask for a drug reaction, to risk a more serious "superinfection," and to waste time and money. Among the common problems that can be treated at home are the following:

▲ The common cold—often termed "viral URI (upper respiratory infection)" by doctors
▲ The flu, when uncomplicated
▲ Hay fever
▲ Mononucleosis—infectious mononucleosis, or "mono"

Medical treatment is commonly required for these illnesses:

▲ Strep throat
▲ Ear infection

How can you tell these conditions apart? Table 8 and the charts for the following problems will usually suffice. Here are some brief descriptions.

Viral Syndromes

Viruses usually involve several portions of the body and cause many different symptoms. Three basic patterns (or syndromes) are common in viral illnesses. Overlap of these three syndromes is not unusual. Your child's illness may have features of each.

Viral URI. This is the "common cold." It includes some combination of the following: sore throat, runny nose, stuffy or congested ears, hoarseness, swollen glands, and fever. One symptom usually precedes the others, and another (usually hoarseness or cough) may remain after the others have disappeared.

The flu. This is a combination of fever, headache, muscle pains, and fatigue. Fever may be quite high. Headache can be severe. Muscle aches and pain (especially lower back, calf muscles, and eye muscles) are equally troublesome. New tests allow immediate diagnosis of the flu. During flu season parents may want to have a sick child tested. The doctor may recommend possible treatment (in the first 48 hours) for the child and preventive medicines for other family members.

Viral gastroenteritis. This is the "stomach flu," with nausea, vomiting, diarrhea, and crampy abdominal pain. It may be incapacitating and can mimic a variety of other, more serious conditions, including appendicitis.

Table 8: Is It a Virus, a Bacterium, or an Allergy?

	Virus	Bacterium	Allergy
Runny nose	Often	Rarely	Often
Aching muscles	Usually	Rarely	Never
Headache (nonsinus)	Often	Rarely	Never
Fever	Often	Often	Never
Cough	Often	Sometimes	Rarely
Croup	Usually	Rarely	Never
Recurs in a particular season	Never	Never	Often
Antibiotics help	Never	Yes	Never
The doctor helps	Seldom	Yes	Sometimes
Dizziness	Often	Rarely	Rarely
Dry cough	Often	Rarely	Sometimes
Raising sputum	Rarely	Often	Rarely
Hoarseness	Often	Rarely	Sometimes
A single complaint (sore throat, earache, sinus pain, or cough)	Rarely	Usual	Rarely

Strep Throat

Strep throat is a bacterial infection caused by streptococcal bacteria. The infection causes a sore throat, often accompanied by symptoms outside the respiratory tract, most commonly fever and swollen lymph glands in the neck (from draining of the infected material). Abdominal pain or headache may be associated with a strep throat. Scarlet fever is a strep infection, and the scarlet fever rash may help to distinguish a streptococcal from a viral infection. This disorder should be diagnosed and treated, because serious heart and kidney complications can follow if adequate antibiotic therapy is not provided. (See Sore Throat, page 336.)

Remember, viral infections and allergies do not improve with the use of antibiotics.

Hay Fever (Allergic Rhinitis)

The seasonal runny nose, sneezing, and itchy eyes are well-known. As with viruses, this disorder is treated simply to relieve symptoms. Given enough time, the condition will run its course without doing any permanent harm. An allergy tends to recur whenever the child encounters pollen or another allergic substance. (See the discussion of allergic rhinitis on pages 180–181.)

Colds and Flu

All children have "colds," and most parents become experts in the treatment of their children's common viral upper respiratory infections rather quickly. Colds are almost invariably caused by viruses and do not require or respond to antibiotic treatment. An uncomplicated cold can hardly be considered an illness. In fact, a great many viral infections in children are so mild that you'll notice no symptoms at all. Viruses can cause headache (page 294), runny nose (page 346), sore throat (page 336), muscle aches (page 434), cough (page 349), vomiting (page 456), diarrhea (page 459), and eye discharges (page 321), among other symptoms. Consult these individual sections for further discussion.

Parents are frequently concerned that their children may have too many colds. Most healthy children have between six and nine viral infections each year. Some of these colds will be very short and mild, whereas others may last a week or longer. Children with frequent colds seldom have anything seriously wrong with them. These children do *not* need gamma globulin shots. Children who have real problems with their immune defense system most often have extremely serious illnesses rather than frequent mild illnesses. A child's immune system becomes stronger with each cold, so even a case of the sniffles has its positive side.

Complications

Most parents are worried about complications of colds. These do, of course, occur, but they are much less common than the uncomplicated illness. The most frequent complication is a blockage in the tube (Eustachian tube) that drains the middle ear and results in an ear infection. Other parents worry about colds progressing to pneumonia. The observant parent is often able to tell when a child is developing a complication of a cold.

- ▲ Children with a developing complication are often fussy and may be taking their food poorly.
- ▲ Younger children may tug at their ears or cry frequently if an ear infection is starting. Older children may complain of pain in their ears.
- ▲ A rapid breathing rate is an indication that a cold may be becoming complicated by pneumonia. See "How fast is your child breathing?" on page 241.

Home Treatment

A tired child needs **rest**, but most children will restrict themselves adequately. We see no reason for a child to be kept in bed if he or she feels well enough to be up and about. If a child feels well enough to go to school, he or she should be allowed to do so. Of course, if the child is coughing or having other problems that will interfere with schoolwork, it may be better to keep the child at home rather than to have the child sent home in the middle of the day. Colds are usually most contagious a day or two *before* symptoms appear, so keeping a child home until all the symptoms are gone is pointless; the other children have already been exposed.

The child should receive plenty of **fluids** during a cold. Don't worry about solid food if the child is not hungry. Treat fever appropriately (see Fever, page 288).

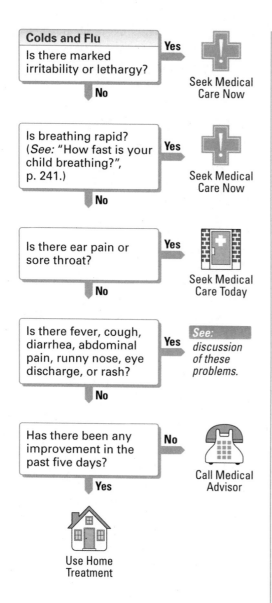

For the treatment of other symptoms, refer to the sections on those specific problems.

What to Expect

Simple colds do not require a visit to the doctor. If you are suspicious that your child may be developing a complication such as an earache or pneumonia, the doctor will perform a thorough examination.

Sore Throat

Sore throat is one of the most common complaints of childhood. Very often a sore throat is accompanied by fever, headache, or even abdominal pain. Infants seldom have sore throats, but as children approach school age, sore throats become more frequent.

Sore throats can be caused by viruses, bacteria, or special types of organisms such as mycoplasma and chlamydia. Most sore throats are caused by viruses. Often, especially in the winter, sleeping with an open mouth or mouth breathing can cause drying and irritation of the throat. This type of irritation subsides quickly after the pharynx becomes moist again. Post nasal drip can cause a sore throat that is worse in the morning.

Mono

Older children and adolescents frequently develop a viral sore throat known as infectious **mononucleosis**, or "mono." Despite the formidable-sounding name, complications seldom occur. The sore throat is often more severe than sore throats from other causes and often lasts longer than a week. The child also may feel particularly weak and have swollen lymph glands. Occasionally, the spleen, one of the internal organs in the abdomen, may enlarge during mononucleosis, and rest is important. A viral sore throat that does not resolve within a week might be caused by the virus responsible for mononucleosis.

Strep Throat

Although most sore throats are caused by viruses, virtually all bacterial sore throats are caused by streptococcal bacteria. These sore throats are commonly referred to as strep throat. A strep throat should be treated with an antibiotic because of possible complications.

An **abscess** in the throat is an extremely rare complication of strep throat, but it should be suspected if the child has extreme difficulty swallowing, has an excess of salivation, or has difficulty opening his or her mouth.

The more significant complications of strep throat occur from one to four weeks after the pain in the throat disappears.

Acute glomerulonephritis is an inflammation of the kidneys. Although antibiotics will not prevent this complication, they will prevent the strep from spreading to other family members or friends.

Rheumatic fever is rare today but still a problem in some parts of the country. Rheumatic fever is a complicated disease that causes painful swollen joints, unusual skin rashes, and heart damage in half of its victims. It can be prevented by antibiotic treatment of a strep throat.

Unfortunately, it is not possible to definitely distinguish a viral sore throat from strep throat on the basis of symptoms. Neither the height of the fever, the appearance of the throat, nor the amount of pain present clearly indicates whether a sore throat is due to a virus or strep. The only method of distinguishing a virus from strep is through a **throat test (rapid strep) or throat culture**.

In some offices, you can obtain a throat culture without paying for a doctor visit. If you have no other concerns about your child and merely need to know whether the child has strep throat, inquire about obtaining a throat culture without a full office visit.

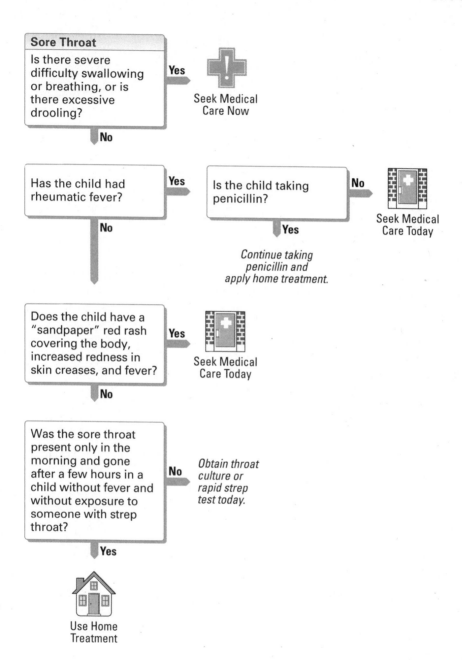

Sore Throat

Is there severe difficulty swallowing or breathing, or is there excessive drooling?

Yes → Seek Medical Care Now

No

Has the child had rheumatic fever?

Yes → Is the child taking penicillin?

No → Seek Medical Care Today

Yes

Continue taking penicillin and apply home treatment.

No

Does the child have a "sandpaper" red rash covering the body, increased redness in skin creases, and fever?

Yes → Seek Medical Care Today

No

Was the sore throat present only in the morning and gone after a few hours in a child without fever and without exposure to someone with strep throat?

No → *Obtain throat culture or rapid strep test today.*

Yes

Use Home Treatment

Home Treatment

Cold liquids and acetaminophen or ibuprofen are effective for the pain and fever of a sore throat. Home remedies include a saltwater gargle and honey or lemon in tea. Time is the most important healer for pain. A vaporizer may provide relief for some children.

What to Expect

The doctor will usually take a throat culture. Tests are also available to detect the streptococcal bacteria in just a few minutes. However, these tests are not quite as accurate as a throat culture. Your doctor may use either the rapid method or the culture technique; some will use both.

Most doctors will delay treating a sore throat until the test results are back. Delaying treatment by a day or two will not increase the risk of developing rheumatic fever. Furthermore, acetaminophen or ibuprofen (page 218) is as effective as an antibiotic in reducing the discomfort of a sore throat. Since the majority of sore throats are due to viruses, treating all sore throats with antibiotics would expose children needlessly to the risks of allergic reactions to antibiotics. Doctors often begin antibiotics immediately if there is a family history of rheumatic fever, the child has scarlet fever (a rash accompanying the sore throat), rheumatic fever is commonly occurring in the community at the time, or there are other compelling factors.

If one child has strep throat, chances are very good that other family members will also have strep throat, and it is common for doctors to take cultures from brothers and sisters.

Children diagnosed with strep throat should take penicillin or another effective antibiotic and should complete the entire prescribed course even if symptoms improve quickly.

Tonsils: In or Out?

Frequent and recurrent sore throats are common, especially in children between the ages of 5 and 10. There is no evidence that removing the tonsils decreases this frequency.

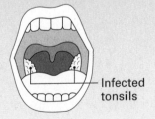
Infected tonsils

Earaches

Most children will have at least one earache while growing up, and many will have frequent earaches. Ear pain is caused by changes in pressure or a buildup of fluid in the child's middle ear. Under normal circumstances, the middle ear is drained by a short, narrow tube (the eustachian tube) into the nasal passages. Often during a cold, the eustachian tube will become swollen shut. This occurs most often in young children, in whom the tube is smaller.

Many infants are given bottles of milk while lying in bed. Drinking milk while lying down may, in some instances, cause the eustachian tube to become irritated and closed. When the tube closes, the fluid from the middle ear cannot drain normally, and it begins to accumulate. Bacteria grow rapidly in this stagnant fluid, and a bacterial infection often results.

Symptoms of an ear infection (otitis media) may include the following:

▲ Fever
▲ Ear pain
▲ Fussiness
▲ Increased crying
▲ Irritability
▲ Pulling at the ears

Because infants cannot tell you that their ears hurt, increased irritability, ear pulling, and frequent waking during sleep should make a parent suspicious of an ear infection.

Ear pain and ear stuffiness can also result from changes in altitude, as when descending in an airplane. Here again, the mechanism for the stuffiness or pain is obstruction of the eustachian tube. Swallowing frequently relieves this pressure. Closing the mouth and holding the nose closed while pretending to blow your nose is another method of opening the eustachian tube.

Parents are often concerned about hearing impairment after ear infections. Most children will have a temporary and minor hearing loss during and immediately following an ear infection, but there is seldom any permanent hearing loss with adequate medical management.

Home Treatment

Immunizations against hemophilus influenza B and pneumococcus have decreased the number of serious consequences from ear infections. Many ear infections are now caused by viruses or bacteria that seldom cause serious problems. Consequently there is a new approach to treating ear infections. For children over two years, if the child appears only minimally ill and has a temperature less than 102.2°F (39°C) observation without antibiotics is an option. In children from six months to two years it is often unclear whether they actually have an ear infection. If the diagnosis is uncertain in this group and the child does not appear ill or have a temperature elevation, observation without antibiotics may be recommended. Parents can begin pain and fever treatment with acetaminophen or ibuprofen. If the pain and fever persist more than two days you should consult a doctor to consider antibiotics.

Parents can begin pain and fever treatment with acetaminophen (page 218) immediately on suspecting an ear infection.

You can avoid some ear infections by not giving your baby a bottle at bedtime and by avoiding exposure to cigarette smoke.

What to Expect
The doctor will perform an examination of the ear, nose, and throat, as well as the bony portion of the skull behind the ears, known as the mastoid. Pain, tenderness, or redness of the mastoid signifies a serious infection (mastoiditis).

Because of immunizations, most serious bacterial cases of otitis media are a thing of the past. Most often antibiotics will not be prescribed unless the child is an infant, has had fever for more than 48 hours, or is experiencing modest pain. Decongestants (page 224) do not appear to be of value. Antihistamines (page 224) are seldom useful except in children known to be allergic. Antibiotic therapy generally is prescribed for ten days in younger infants and toddlers and five to seven days in older children. Be sure to give the child all of the antibiotic prescribed, and on schedule.

If your child still has a fever after two days of treatment, he or she may need a different antibiotic. Be sure to call your doctor. Children who have frequent ear infections may benefit from taking antibiotics daily for several months to prevent new infections. On occasion, surgical placement of tubes in the ear(s) may be recommended.

Occasionally, fluid in the middle ear will persist for a long time without infection. In this event, there may be a slight decrease in hearing. This condition is known as **serous otitis media** and is usually not treated with antibiotics but may require a procedure to open the eustachian tube and allow drainage. If this condition persists, the doctor may resort to the placement of ear tubes to establish proper functioning of the middle ear. Placing ear tubes sounds frightening, but it is actually a simple and very effective surgical procedure.

Some doctors will wish to reexamine your child's ears to make sure the infection has completely cleared and the child's hearing has returned to normal, but studies have shown that parents are excellent at knowing whether an infection is gone.

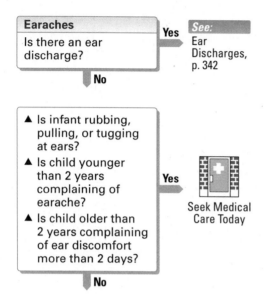

Earaches

Is there an ear discharge? — **Yes** → *See:* Ear Discharges, p. 342

No ↓

- ▲ Is infant rubbing, pulling, or tugging at ears?
- ▲ Is child younger than 2 years complaining of earache?
- ▲ Is child older than 2 years complaining of ear discomfort more than 2 days?

— **Yes** → **Seek Medical Care Today**

No ↓

Rethink your problem; consult table of contents for other symptoms.

Ear Discharges

Earwax is almost never a problem unless attempts are made to "clean" the child's ear canals. Earwax functions as a protective lining for the ear canal. Taking warm showers or washing the external ears with a washcloth dipped in warm water provides enough vapor to prevent the buildup of wax that is thick and caked. Children often like to push things into their ear canals. They may pack the wax tightly enough to prevent vibration of the eardrum and hence interfere with hearing. Well-meaning parents armed with cotton swabs often accomplish the same unfortunate result.

Ruptured Eardrum

In a young child or in an older child who has been complaining of ear pain, a white or yellow discharge is often the sign of a ruptured eardrum. Sometimes you will find a dry crusted material on the child's pillow. Here again, a ruptured eardrum may be the cause. Take your child to the doctor for antibiotic therapy. Do not be unduly alarmed; a ruptured eardrum is actually the first stage of a natural healing process, which the antibiotic will help. Children have remarkable healing powers, and most eardrums will heal completely within weeks.

Swimmer's Ear

In the summertime, ear discharges are commonly caused by swimmer's ear, an irritation of the ear canal and not a problem of the middle ear or eardrum. Children may complain that their ears are itchy. In addition, tugging on the ear will often cause pain. This can be a helpful clue to an inflammation of the outer ear and canal, such as swimmer's ear. Encourage the child not to scratch inside the ear, and caution the child against using hairpins or other such instruments to scratch because injury to the eardrum can result.

Home Treatment

Packed earwax can be removed by using a syringe, available at the drugstore, to flush the ears gently with warm water. A water jet, *set at the lowest setting,* can also be useful, but it can be frightening to young children and is dangerous at higher settings. We do not advise that parents attempt to remove impacted earwax unless they are dealing with an older child and can see the blackened wax.

Wax softeners such as Cerumenex and olive oil are useful. All commercial products can be irritating, however, if not used properly. Cerumenex, for example, must be flushed out of the ear within 30 minutes.

Two warnings:

▲ Water used to flush the ear must be close to body temperature. The use of cold water may result in dizziness and vomiting.

▲ You should never attempt to flush the ear if you have any question about the condition of the eardrum.

Although swimmer's ear (or other causes of similar *otitis externa*) is often caused by a bacterial infection, this infection does not usually require antibiotic treatment because the infection is very shallow. Instead, place a cotton wick soaked in Burow's solution in the ear canal overnight. In the morning, irrigate the ear briefly with warm water. For partic-

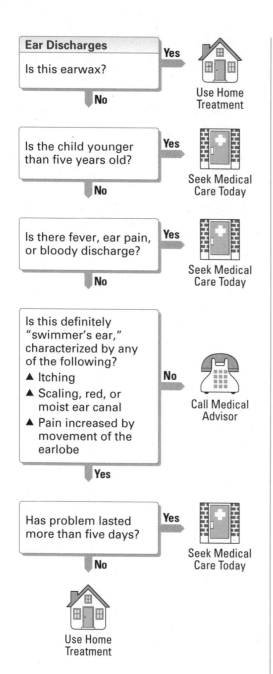

ularly severe, itchy, or persistent (more than five days) cases, a doctor's visit is advisable.

What to Expect

The doctor will examine the ear thoroughly. In severe cases, he or she may take a culture for bacteria. The doctor may prescribe corticosteroid and antibiotic preparations to be placed in the ear canal or recommend one of the regimens described under "Home Treatment." Physicians usually prescribe oral antibiotics if a perforated eardrum is causing the discharge.

Hearing Loss

Problems with hearing can be divided into two broad categories: sudden onset and slow onset. When a child five years old or older complains of difficulty hearing developing over a short time, the problem is usually a blockage in the ear. On the *outside* of the eardrum, such a blockage may be due to the accumulation of wax, a foreign object that the child has put in the ear canal, or an infection of the ear canal. On the *inside* of the eardrum, fluid may accumulate in the middle ear.

The other category includes hearing problems that develop slowly or are present from birth and become evident over a long period. Many parents become concerned when they suspect that an infant or small child is not hearing normally. Hearing can now be tested in a child of any age through the use of computers, which can analyze changes in brain waves in response to sounds or otoacoustic emissions.

More simply, a child with normal hearing will react in a characteristic manner to a noise. A hand clap, horn, or whistle can be used to produce the sound. From birth up to three months, the infant will blink or open the eyes, move the arms or legs, turn the head, or begin sucking in response to a sound. If a child is moving or vocalizing before the sound is made, these activities may stop. At three months, children begin to attempt to find a sound by moving the head and looking for it. The ability to find the sound no matter where it is (below, behind, or above the child) may not be fully developed until the age of two.

Normal speech development relies on hearing. A child whose speech is developing slowly or not at all may have difficulty hearing. A child who babbles continually without forming words for more than a year should also be suspected of hearing difficulties.

Most hospitals now screen all newborns shortly after birth for hearing loss.

Home Treatment

The need for an accurate ear examination usually requires a trip to the doctor. However, if you are certain that the problem is due to wax accumulation, you can treat it effectively at home. Simply flush the ear gently with warm water to wash out the wax.

Ear syringes or other devices for squirting water into the ear canal are available in drugstores. A water jet *set at the lowest setting* can be used with considerable success, but we do not recommend it for young children because of the frightening noise. Wax softeners such as Cerumenex may be needed when the wax is hard and impacted; follow the instructions on the label. (One softener, Debrox, has gained a reputation for irritating ear canals, perhaps unjustly.)

A few words of warning:

▲ Water used to flush the ear must be as close to body temperature as possible. The use of cold water may result in dizziness and vomiting.

▲ Never flush the ear if you have any doubt about the eardrum being intact and undamaged.

Always use caution when removing foreign objects. Unless the object is easily accessible and removing it clearly poses no threat of damage to the ear, do *not*

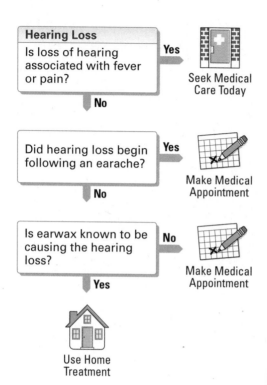

Hearing Loss

Is loss of hearing associated with fever or pain?

Yes → Seek Medical Care Today

No ↓

Did hearing loss begin following an earache?

Yes → Make Medical Appointment

No ↓

Is earwax known to be causing the hearing loss?

No → Make Medical Appointment

Yes ↓

Use Home Treatment

try to remove it. Never use sharp instruments to remove foreign objects. Many times efforts to remove an object at home lead to pushing the object farther into the ear or to damage of the eardrum.

What to Expect

A thorough examination of both ears often reveals the cause of a hearing loss. If it does not, the doctor may test the child's hearing in the manner described above or, if the child is older, recommend audiometry (an electronic hearing test).

Runny Nose

A runny nose is one of the most frequent childhood problems. Many infants will have a runny nose and sneeze during the first two weeks of life. The cause is unknown; it is certainly a natural phenomenon. Children also will have runny noses during crying episodes and sometimes after exercising. Runny noses in these instances are temporary and of no concern.

Infection

The hallmark of the common cold is the runny nose. It is intended by nature to help the body fight the viral infection. Nasal secretions contain antibodies that act against the virus. The profuse outpouring of fluid carries the virus outside the body.

Allergy

Allergy is another common cause of runny noses. Children whose runny noses are due to an allergy are deemed to have *allergic rhinitis*. Hay fever is one kind of allergic rhinitis, caused by ragweed pollen. The nasal secretions in this instance are often clear and very thin. Children with allergic rhinitis will often have other symptoms simultaneously, including sneezing and itchy, watery eyes. They will rub their noses so often that a crease in the nose may appear. A runny nose due to an allergy lasts longer than one due to a viral infection, often continuing for weeks or months, and it occurs most commonly during the season when pollen particles or other allergens are in the air. A great many other substances may aggravate allergic rhinitis, including dust, mold, and animal dander.

Other Causes

A runny nose may be due to a small object that a young child has pushed into the nose. Usually, this will produce a discharge from only one nostril. Often the discharge will be foul-smelling and yellow or green.

Another common cause of runny noses, as well as stuffy noses, is the prolonged use of medicated nose drops. This problem of excess medication is known as **rhinitis medicamentosum**. Medicated nose drops (page 226) should never be used for longer than three days.

Postnasal Drip

Complications from a runny nose are caused by excess mucus. The mucus may lead to postnasal drip and a cough that is most prominent at night. The mucus drip may plug the eustachian tube between the nasal passages and the ear, resulting in an ear infection and ear pain. It may plug the sinus passages, resulting in a secondary sinus infection and sinus pain.

Home Treatment

We do not recommend cold preparations. Antihistamines may cause drowsiness and interfere with sleep. A runny nose should be treated only when it is impairing the child's comfort. Often a tissue is the best approach. It has no side effects, is cheap, and helps get the virus outside the body.

Should you choose to treat a runny nose, saline nose drops are fine. Nose drops should never be used for longer than three consecutive days.

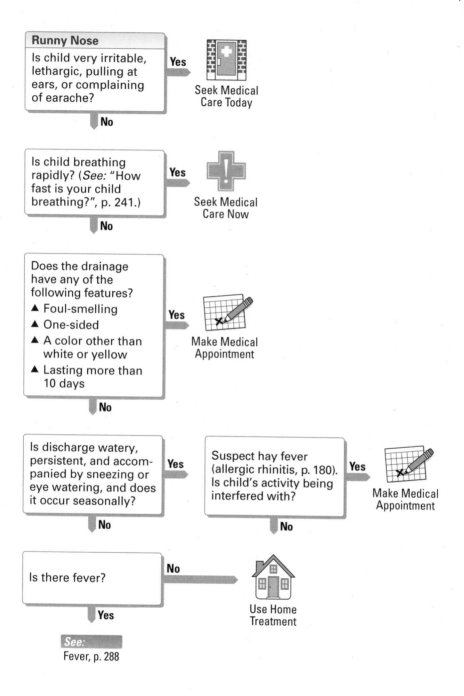

Runny Nose

Is child very irritable, lethargic, pulling at ears, or complaining of earache? **Yes** → Seek Medical Care Today

No

Is child breathing rapidly? (*See:* "How fast is your child breathing?", p. 241.) **Yes** → Seek Medical Care Now

No

Does the drainage have any of the following features?
▲ Foul-smelling
▲ One-sided
▲ A color other than white or yellow
▲ Lasting more than 10 days
Yes → Make Medical Appointment

No

Is discharge watery, persistent, and accompanied by sneezing or eye watering, and does it occur seasonally? **Yes** → Suspect hay fever (allergic rhinitis, p. 180). Is child's activity being interfered with? **Yes** → Make Medical Appointment

No → **No**

Is there fever? **No** → Use Home Treatment

Yes

See: Fever, p. 288

Keeping mucus thin may prevent plugging of the nasal passages. Using a vaporizer or humidifier to increase humidity in the air will help liquefy mucus. Inside a house, heated air is often very dry; cooler air contains more moisture and is preferable. Drinking a great deal of liquid also helps liquefy the secretions.

If symptoms persist beyond three weeks, contact your doctor.

What to Expect

The doctor will perform a thorough examination of the ears, nose, and throat and check for tenderness over the sinuses. He or she may take a swab of the nasal secretions to examine under a microscope. The presence of certain types of cells, known as eosinophils, will indicate the presence of allergic rhinitis. If the doctor finds allergic rhinitis, he or she may prescribe an antihistamine or nasal steroid, and explain a plan of dust, mold, dander, and pollen avoidance. (See the discussion of allergies on pages 174–183.)

Sneezing

Sneezing is healthy, for it removes germs, allergens, and dust from the child's nose. The only danger is that of infecting others with the same germ or virus. Teach children to cover their mouths with tissues or handkerchiefs before sneezing. And teach them to wash their hands afterward.

Cough

Coughing has several causes. In very young infants (less than 3 months), coughing is unusual and may indicate a serious lung problem. In older infants who are prone to swallowing foreign objects, an object may become lodged in the windpipe and cause coughing. Young children also tend to inhale bits of peanuts and popcorn, which can produce coughing and serious problems in the lungs. In some children, a chronic cough may be the first sign of asthma or sinusitis. Most coughs are produced by infections, usually viral.

Pneumonia

Is it pneumonia? This question worries parents more than any other. Pneumonia is a serious infection of the lungs that often requires antibiotics and hence a visit to the doctor. Fortunately, it is rare when the only symptom is a cough. Rapid breathing is often the best indicator of pneumonia. Difficulty breathing is also of concern. This problem may follow an ordinary upper respiratory infection (such as a cold) by a few days. If the fever from a simple cold doesn't go down after a few days, see the doctor.

Cough Reflex

The cough reflex is one of the body's best defense mechanisms. An irritation of the breathing tubes will trigger this reflex, and a violent rush of air will help clear material from the breathing tubes. Thus material that should not be present in the lungs is removed by coughing.

Often a minor irritation in the breathing tubes will trigger a cough reflex, even when there is no material to be expelled. At other times, mucus from the nasal passages will drip into the breathing tubes at night (postnasal drip) and start the cough reflex. Coughing that is interfering with a child's sleep can be counterproductive. This is the only type of cough that should be stopped.

Home Treatment

The goal of home treatment is to liquefy the secretions in the breathing tubes to enhance clearing of unwanted materials from the lungs. The mucus in the breathing tubes may be made thinner by several means. Increased humidity in the air may help; a cool-mist vaporizer can often provide this. Humidity may help in the severe "croupy" cough of small children (see Croup, page 352). Drinking large quantities of fluid may be helpful for a cough, particularly if a fever is present to dry out and dehydrate the body.

Oral cough medications (see page 225) do not help very much in liquefying secretions.

Children are often given cough suppressants containing dextromethorphan or codeine to allow them to get some rest. Studies have not proved the effectiveness of these preparations for children. However, buckwheat honey has been shown to be effective in one study.

What to Expect

The doctor will examine the ears, nose, throat, and chest. If the child is suspected of having inhaled a foreign body, or if pneumonia is suspected, the doctor will order a chest X ray. He or she will prescribe an antibiotic only if a bacterial infection (such as pneumonia or sinusitis) is suspected. The physician may recommend other evaluations and therapies if asthma is suspected.

Home Cure for Hiccups

Hiccups, which are caused by an irregularity in contractions of the diaphragm, may occasionally prove troublesome. Home remedies include drinking a large amount of water or drinking water in rhythmic sips. For older children, research indicates that the most effective treatment is as follows.

Insert a teaspoon containing a half teaspoon amount of granulated sugar into the child's mouth. When the spoon is above the rear third of the tongue, invert the spoon to dump the sugar. Placing the sugar on the front two-thirds of the tongue has not been shown to work.

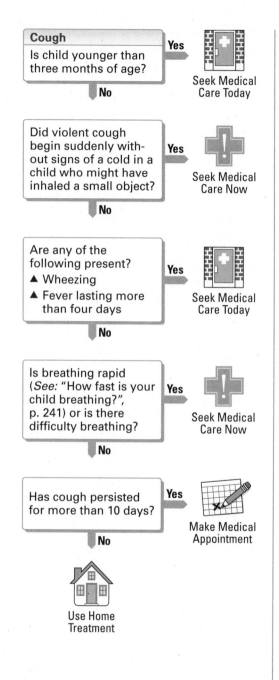

Cough
Is child younger than three months of age?

Yes → Seek Medical Care Today

No ↓

Did violent cough begin suddenly without signs of a cold in a child who might have inhaled a small object?

Yes → Seek Medical Care Now

No ↓

Are any of the following present?
▲ Wheezing
▲ Fever lasting more than four days

Yes → Seek Medical Care Today

No ↓

Is breathing rapid (*See:* "How fast is your child breathing?", p. 241) or is there difficulty breathing?

Yes → Seek Medical Care Now

No ↓

Has cough persisted for more than 10 days?

Yes → Make Medical Appointment

No ↓

Use Home Treatment

Croup

Croup can be one of the most frightening illnesses that parents will ever encounter. It generally occurs in children under the age of three or four. In the middle of the night, a child may sit up in bed gasping for air. Often there will be an accompanying cough that sounds like the barking of a seal. The child's symptoms are so frightening that panic is often the response. However, the most severe problems with croup usually can be relieved safely, simply, and efficiently at home.

Croup is usually caused by one of several viruses. The viral infection causes a swelling and outpouring of secretions in the larynx (voice box), trachea (windpipe), and larger airways going to the lungs. The swelling narrows the air passages of the young child, and this is further aggravated by the secretions, which may become dried out. This combination of swelling and thickened, dried secretions makes breathing extremely difficult. There may also be spasm of the airway passages, further complicating the problem. Treatment is designed to dissolve the dried secretions.

In some children, croup is a recurring problem. These children may have three or four bouts of croup. Seldom does this represent a serious underlying problem, but you should seek a doctor's advice. Children outgrow croup as the airway passages get larger. It is unusual after age seven.

Epiglottitis and Bacterial Tracheitis
Occasionally, a more serious obstruction caused by a bacterial infection and known as **epiglottitis** can be confused with croup. Epiglottitis is more common in children older than three. Epiglottitis is caused by the *Hemophilus influenzae* bacterium and is now preventable with immunization. It has become a rare disease in recent years. Children with epiglottitis often have more serious difficulty breathing. They may have an extremely hard time swallowing and will drool. Often they will assume a characteristic position, with the head tilted forward and the jaw pointed out, and will gasp for air. Bacterial tracheitis resembles croup but usually has a higher fever and is more severe.

Epiglottitis and bacterial tracheitis will not be relieved by the simple measures that bring the prompt relief of croup. They require medical attention immediately.

Home Treatment
Mist is the backbone of therapy for croup and is supplied efficiently by a cold-mist vaporizer. We prefer cold-mist to hot-steam vaporizers because of the possibility of scalding from the hot water.

If the breathing is very hard, you can get faster results by taking the child to the bathroom and running a hot shower to make thick clouds of steam. (*Do not put the child in the hot shower!*) Steam can be created more efficiently if there is some cold air in the room. Remember that

Night Air Can Help

In the case of croup, a trip to the doctor often cures a problem that was resistant to steam at home. Keep the car windows open a bit to let in the cool night air.

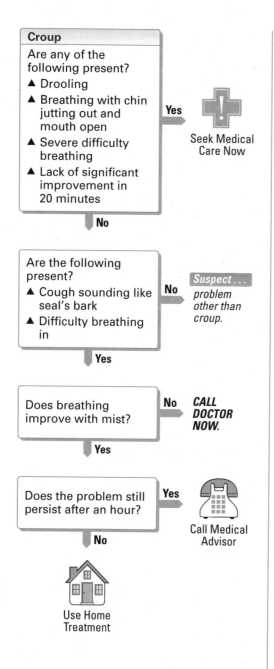

Croup

Are any of the following present?
- ▲ Drooling
- ▲ Breathing with chin jutting out and mouth open
- ▲ Severe difficulty breathing
- ▲ Lack of significant improvement in 20 minutes

Yes → Seek Medical Care Now

No

Are the following present?
- ▲ Cough sounding like seal's bark
- ▲ Difficulty breathing in

No → *Suspect…* *problem other than croup.*

Yes

Does breathing improve with mist?

No → *CALL DOCTOR NOW.*

Yes

Does the problem still persist after an hour?

Yes → Call Medical Advisor

No

Use Home Treatment

steam rises, so the child will not benefit from sitting on the floor.

Relief usually occurs promptly and should be noticeable within the first 10 minutes. Not becoming alarmed and keeping the child calm is also important. Holding the child may comfort him or her and may help relieve some of the airway spasm. If the child does not show significant improvement within 20 minutes, you should contact your doctor or the local emergency room immediately.

What to Expect

For moderate croup, the doctor may give the child a steroid injection. On occasion, children with severe croup may need hospitalization and inhalation treatments, including epinephrine, steroids, and oxygen.

X rays of the neck are a reliable way of differentiating croup from a rare case of epiglottitis. If epiglottitis is found, the child will be admitted to the hospital, an airway will be placed in the child's trachea to enable the child to breathe, and intravenous antibiotics directed at curing the bacterial infection will be started.

Wheezing

Wheezing is the high-pitched whistling sound produced by air flowing through narrowed breathing tubes (bronchi and bronchioles). It is most obvious when the child breathes out but may be present when he or she breathes both in and out. Wheezing comes from the breathing tubes deep in the chest, in contrast to the croupy, crowing, or whooping sounds that come from the area of the voice box in the neck (see Croup, page 352).

Most often, a narrowing of the breathing tubes in children is due to a viral infection or an allergic reaction, as in asthma (pages 176–180). In children younger than two years, bronchiolitis, or narrowing of the smallest air passages, can occur due to a viral infection. This is a very common problem in infants and toddlers caused by respiratory syncitial virus (RSV). Pneumonia can also produce wheezing.

Wheezing can follow an insect sting or the use of a medicine. If these allergic reactions occur, see the doctor. Any medication can cause the problem; some individuals even wheeze after taking aspirin.

Occasionally, a foreign body may be lodged in a breathing tube, causing a localized wheezing that is difficult to hear without a stethoscope.

The importance of wheezing lies in its being an indicator of difficult breathing. It should alert the parent to check carefully for shortness of breath. In a child with a respiratory infection, wheezing may occur before shortness of breath is marked. Therefore, when wheezing appears in the presence of a fever, early consultation with the doctor is advisable, even though the illness seldom turns out to be serious.

Treatment of wheezing addresses symptoms; there are no drugs that cure viral illnesses or asthma. Home treatment is an important part of this approach. However, the doctor's help is needed so that drugs that widen the breathing passages can be used. Intravenous fluids may be required on some occasions.

Home Treatment

Hydration with oral fluids is very important. The use of a vaporizer, preferably one that produces a cold mist, may help. If a vaporizer is not available, run a hot shower to produce steam. (*Do not put the child in the hot shower!*) Unfortunately, it is hard to get much vapor down to the small breathing tubes.

Encourage the child to take as much fluid as possible by mouth. Water is best, but fruit juices or soft drinks may be used if this will increase the amount taken. These measures will be part of the therapy the doctor will recommend and may be begun immediately, even though a visit to the doctor will be necessary.

What to Expect

Physical examination will focus on the chest and neck. The physician will ask questions not only about the current illness but also about a past history of allergies or asthma in the child or in the family. Measurement of oxygen in the blood may be done by a probe on the finger. The doctor also may investigate the possibility that the child has swallowed a foreign object.

Drugs to open up the breathing tubes may be given by injection, by mouth, or by

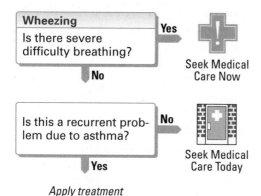

Wheezing

Is there severe difficulty breathing? — **Yes** → Seek Medical Care Now

↓ **No**

Is this a recurrent problem due to asthma? — **No** → Seek Medical Care Today

↓ **Yes**

Apply treatment recommended by doctor.

inhalation. (See the discussion of asthma on pages 176–180.) Occasionally, hospitalization will be necessary so that medications may be given intravenously or by inhalation, and oxygen may be required. Most important, hospital personnel can watch the child closely. Hospitalization is used as a precautionary measure against things getting worse before they get better.

Hoarseness

Hoarseness is usually caused by a problem in the vocal cords. In infants younger than three months of age, this can be due to a serious problem such as a birth defect or thyroid disorder. In young children, hoarseness is more often due to prolonged or excessive crying, which puts a strain on the vocal cords. In older children, viral infections are the most common causes of hoarseness.

If the hoarseness is accompanied by either difficulty breathing or a cough that sounds like a barking seal, it is considered a symptom of croup (page 352). Croup occurs most often in children under the age of four, whereas hoarseness by itself is more common in older children.

If hoarseness is accompanied by difficulty breathing, difficulty swallowing, drooling, gasping for air, or breathing with the mouth wide open and the chin jutting forward, see the doctor immediately, because this is a medical emergency. This problem, known as **epiglottitis**, is a bacterial infection that involves the entrance to the airway. It is becoming quite rare as children are being immunized to prevent hemophilus influenza infections.

Bacterial tracheitis may also cause hoarseness and is accompanied by fever. Like epiglottitis, it requires immediate medical attention.

Some children with strep throat may develop a peritonsillar abscess, which has similar symptoms to epiglottitis and also requires immediate medical attention.

In older children who develop hoarseness or laryngitis without any other symptoms, a virus is most often responsible.

Home Treatment

Hoarseness unassociated with other symptoms is very resistant to medical therapy. Nature must heal the inflamed area. Humidifying the air with a vaporizer or making sure the child drinks lots of fluids can offer some relief. However, the child must wait for healing to occur, and this may take several days. Resting the vocal cords makes sense; crying or shouting makes the situation worse. For the treatment of hoarseness associated with coughs, see Cough, page 349.

What to Expect

If the child is having severe difficulty breathing, the first order of business is to ensure that he or she has an adequate air passage. This may require placement, in the emergency room, hospital, or doctor's office, of a breathing tube. If X rays of the neck are taken, a doctor should accompany the child at all times. If a peritonsillar abscess is found, antibiotics will be given and the abscess drained.

In uncomplicated hoarseness that has persisted for a long period, the doctor will look at the vocal cords with the aid of a small mirror. Occasionally, a more extensive physical examination will help the doctor detect hormonal disorders caused by the thyroid or adrenal gland. These disorders must be confirmed by blood tests.

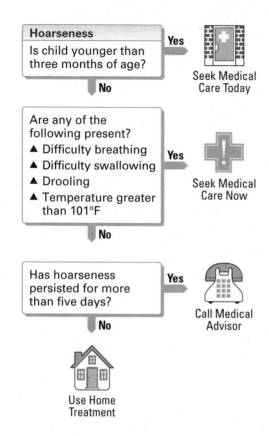

Hoarseness

Is child younger than three months of age? — **Yes** → Seek Medical Care Today

↓ **No**

Are any of the following present?
▲ Difficulty breathing
▲ Difficulty swallowing
▲ Drooling
▲ Temperature greater than 101°F
— **Yes** → Seek Medical Care Now

↓ **No**

Has hoarseness persisted for more than five days? — **Yes** → Call Medical Advisor

↓ **No**

Use Home Treatment

Swollen Glands

The most common types of swollen glands are lymph and salivary glands. The biggest salivary glands are located below and in front of the ears. When they swell, the characteristic swollen jaw appearance of mumps (page 424) is the result.

Lymph glands are part of the body's defense against infection. Swelling means a gland is taking part in the fight against infection. Glands may swell even if the infection is trivial or not apparent, although you can usually identify the infection that is causing the swelling. Occasionally, glands swell in response to a medicine (Dilantin) or because of a tumor.

▲ Swollen glands in the **neck** frequently accompany a sore throat or an ear infection.

▲ Glands in the **groin** enlarge when there is an infection in the feet, legs, or genital region. Sometimes the basic problem may be so minor as to be overlooked (see Athlete's Foot, page 394).

▲ Glands that swell in the **elbow** or **armpit** are usually due to an infection in the hand or chest.

▲ Swollen glands **behind the ears** are often the result of a scalp infection. Infectious mononucleosis (mono) and roseola can also cause swelling of the glands behind the ears. Immunizations have made rubella a rare cause.

Bacterial infection of either lymph or salivary glands themselves may also occur. If a swollen gland is red and tender, there may be a bacterial infection within the gland that requires antibiotic treatment.

Swollen glands otherwise require no treatment because they are merely fighting infections elsewhere. If there is an accompanying sore throat or earache, these should be treated as described under Sore Throat, page 336, or Earaches, page 339.

A bacterial infection is responsible for swollen red nodes that are part of cat scratch disease. Swollen glands located above the clavicle (collarbone) may represent a serious infection (tuberculosis) or other serious problem (cancer) and should prompt a doctor visit. Swollen glands and persistent fever accompanied by cracked lips with red or peeling palms may indicate a rare but treatable illness known as **Kawasaki disease**.

If you have noticed one or several glands progressively enlarging over a period of three weeks, consult the doctor.

Home Treatment

Merely observe the glands over several weeks to see whether they continue to enlarge or whether other glands become swollen. The vast majority of swollen glands that persist beyond three weeks are not serious, but see the doctor if the glands show no tendency to become smaller. Soreness in the glands will usually disappear in a couple of days; getting smaller takes longer.

What to Expect

The doctor will examine the glands and search for infections or other causes of the swelling. He or she will ask about fever, weight loss, or other associated symptoms. The doctor may decide to observe the glands for a time or order blood tests. Eventually, it might be necessary to remove or biopsy the glands.

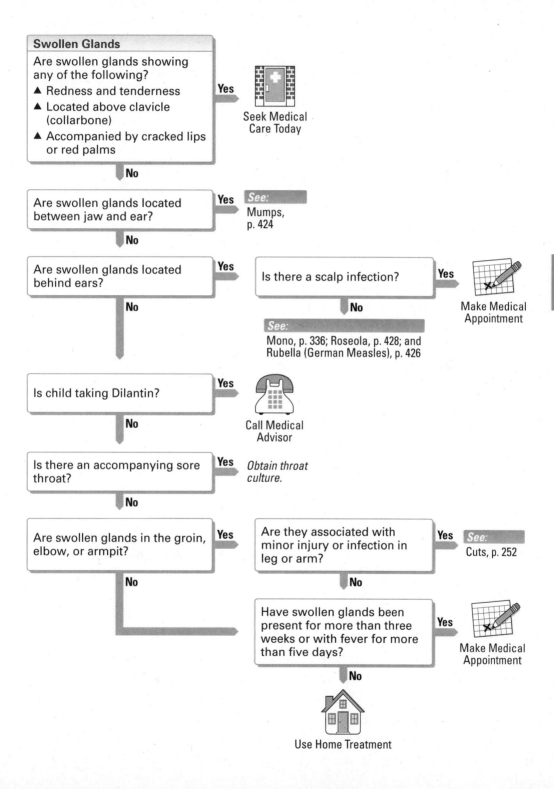

Swollen Glands

Are swollen glands showing any of the following?

▲ Redness and tenderness
▲ Located above clavicle (collarbone)
▲ Accompanied by cracked lips or red palms

Yes → Seek Medical Care Today

No

Are swollen glands located between jaw and ear?

Yes → *See:* Mumps, p. 424

No

Are swollen glands located behind ears?

Yes → Is there a scalp infection?

Yes → Make Medical Appointment

No → *See:* Mono, p. 336; Roseola, p. 428; and Rubella (German Measles), p. 426

No

Is child taking Dilantin?

Yes → Call Medical Advisor

No

Is there an accompanying sore throat?

Yes → *Obtain throat culture.*

No

Are swollen glands in the groin, elbow, or armpit?

Yes → Are they associated with minor injury or infection in leg or arm?

Yes → *See:* Cuts, p. 252

No → Have swollen glands been present for more than three weeks or with fever for more than five days?

Yes → Make Medical Appointment

No → Use Home Treatment

Nosebleeds

The blood vessels within the nose lie very near the surface, and bleeding may occur with the slightest injury. In children, picking the nose is a common cause. Keeping fingernails cut and discouraging the habit is good preventive medicine. Occasionally, a foreign body in the nose may be the cause of bleeding. Accidents and fights produce their share of nosebleeds, but more often than not, the onset is spontaneous.

Nosebleeds are frequently due to irritation by a virus or to vigorous nose blowing. The main problem in this case is a cold, and treatment of cold symptoms will reduce the probability of a nosebleed. If the mucous membrane of the nose is dry, cracking and bleeding are more likely.

Remember these key points.

▲ You can almost always stop the child's nosebleed yourself.
▲ The great majority of nosebleeds are associated with colds or minor injuries to the nose.
▲ Treatment such as packing the nose with gauze has significant drawbacks and should be avoided if possible.
▲ Investigation into the cause of recurrent nosebleeds is not urgent and is best accomplished when the nose is *not* bleeding.

Home Treatment

The nose consists of a bony part and a cartilaginous part: a "hard" portion and a "soft" portion. The area of the nose that usually bleeds lies within the "soft" portion, and compression will control the nosebleed. Simply squeeze the nose between your thumb and forefinger just below the hard portion of the nose. Apply pressure for at least five minutes. The child should be seated. Holding the head back is not necessary; it merely directs the blood flow backward rather than forward. Cold compresses or ice applied across the bridge of the nose may help. Almost all nosebleeds can be controlled in this manner if *sufficient time* is allowed for the bleeding to stop.

Nosebleeds are more common in the winter, when both viruses and dry, heated indoor air are common. A cooler house and a vaporizer to return humidity to the air help many children.

If nosebleeds are a recurrent problem, are becoming more frequent, and are not associated with a cold or another minor irritation, consult the doctor on a nonurgent basis. You need not see the doctor immediately after the nosebleed, because examination at that time may simply restart the bleeding.

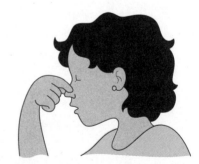

To stop a nosebleed. Have the child sit down while you or the child squeezes with thumb and forefinger just below the hard portion of the nose. Hold for five minutes. The child need not tilt his or her head back.

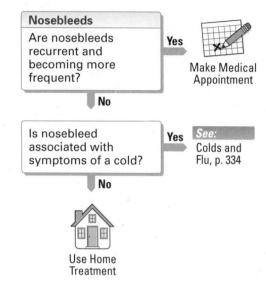

Nosebleeds

Are nosebleeds recurrent and becoming more frequent?

Yes → Make Medical Appointment

No

Is nosebleed associated with symptoms of a cold?

Yes → *See:* Colds and Flu, p. 334

No

Use Home Treatment

What to Expect

The child will be seated, with his or her head back and nostrils compressed. This will be done even if the child has been doing it at home, and it will usually work. Packing the nose or attempting to cauterize a bleeding point is less desirable. If the nosebleed cannot be stopped, the doctor will examine the nose to see if he or she can identify a bleeding point. If the physician finds a bleeding point, he or she may attempt coagulation by either electrical or chemical cauterization. If this is not successful, packing the nose may be unavoidable. Such packing is uncomfortable and may lead to infection. The child must be observed carefully for a possible infection. Some physicians recommend Vaseline or antibiotic ointments in the nostrils if the nose is packed.

If you see the doctor because of recurrent nosebleeds, you can expect questions about events preceding the bleeds and a careful examination of the nose itself. Depending on the child's history and the physical examination, the doctor may, on rare occasions, order blood-clotting tests.

Bad Breath

Children seldom have the problem with bad breath in the morning that is so common among adults, and regular toothbrushing should eliminate bad breath in children. Other causes may be more important to identify.

Infections of the mouth and sore throats may cause bad breath. Because of the possibility of bacterial infection, consult the doctor.

A common cause of prolonged bad breath is a foreign body in the child's nose. This is especially common in toddlers who have inserted some small object. Often, but not always, there is a white, yellowish, or bloody discharge from one or both nostrils.

A sinus infection or even tonsillitis also can be responsible for bad breath. A severely decaying tooth may cause bad breath. Finally, unusual problems such as abscesses of the lungs or heavy worm infestations have been reported to cause bad breath, although we have not seen these in our practices.

Home Treatment

Proper dental hygiene will prevent most cases of bad breath. If this does not eliminate the odor, a foreign body in a young child's nose is possible, and a trip to the doctor will be necessary. Although some foreign bodies may be seen very close to the child's nostril, most are located deep within the nasal cavity, where they are extremely difficult to remove.

Do not use mouthwashes to perfume the breath. These cover up, but do not treat, the underlying problem.

What to Expect

The doctor will perform a thorough examination of the mouth and nose. If the child has a sore throat or mouth sores, the doctor may take a culture and prescribe an antibiotic. If there is an object in the nose, the doctor will use a special forceps to remove it. Older children should be evaluated for sinusitis and pharyngitis.

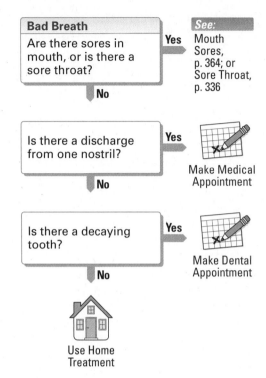

Bad Breath

Are there sores in mouth, or is there a sore throat?

Yes → *See:* Mouth Sores, p. 364; or Sore Throat, p. 336

No ↓

Is there a discharge from one nostril?

Yes → Make Medical Appointment

No ↓

Is there a decaying tooth?

Yes → Make Dental Appointment

No ↓

Use Home Treatment

Mouth Sores

Problems in the mouth are very common in children. Doctors frequently use the term *lesion* to describe anything that may be wrong, be it a sore, a patch, or a pimple. In infants, large white spots may appear on the roof or sides of the mouth or the tongue due to a monilial yeast infection commonly referred to as **thrush**. Thrush can be treated effectively by medication, but it often disappears by itself.

Bacteria and viruses can also be responsible for mouth lesions. A bacterial infection more common in older children and adults is commonly known as **trench mouth**. Lesions in trench mouth often occur on the gums.

Lesions of the gum are more likely to be caused by a **herpes** virus. Herpes lesions often start as blisters and then change to small spots with ulcerous white centers surrounded by redness. In the first infection, they may be found on the gums, inner parts of the lips, cheeks, and even tongue. In repeat infections, it is more usual for the virus to involve only the lips. Because these herpes infections are almost always accompanied by a fever, they are known as fever blisters. The blisters have usually ruptured, and generally parents observe only the remaining underlying sore.

A **canker sore** often follows an injury, such as accidentally biting the inside of the lip or the tongue, or it may appear without obvious cause. These problems are minor and disappear in a short time.

Another virus that can cause mouth lesions is the **Coxsackie virus**. Lesions from this virus are often accompanied by spots on the hands and feet, hence the name "hand-foot-mouth syndrome." Again, this problem will go away by itself.

Allergic reactions to drugs may cause mouth ulcers. In such cases, a skin rash may be present on other parts of the body as well. Consult the doctor if you suspect an allergic reaction.

Home Treatment

Mouth sores caused by viruses heal by themselves. The goal of treatment is to reduce fever, relieve pain, and maintain adequate fluid intake.

Children will seldom want to eat when they have painful mouth lesions. Although children can go several days without taking in solid foods, it is imperative that they maintain an adequate liquid diet. Cold liquids are the most soothing, and Popsicles or frozen juices often are helpful.

For sores inside the lips and on the gums, a preparation called Orabase, available over the counter, may be applied for protection. For cold sores and fever blisters on the outside of the lips, one of the phenol and camphor preparations (Blistex, Camphophenique) may provide relief, especially if applied early. If one of these preparations appears to cause further irritation, discontinue its use. If the external sores have crusted over, apply cool compresses to remove the crusts.

Mouth sores usually resolve in one to two weeks. Any sore that persists beyond three weeks requires a doctor visit.

What to Expect

The doctor will perform a thorough examination of the mouth. He or she will usually prescribe a drug called nystatin for thrush. If the doctor suspects a bacterial cause of trench mouth, he or she may

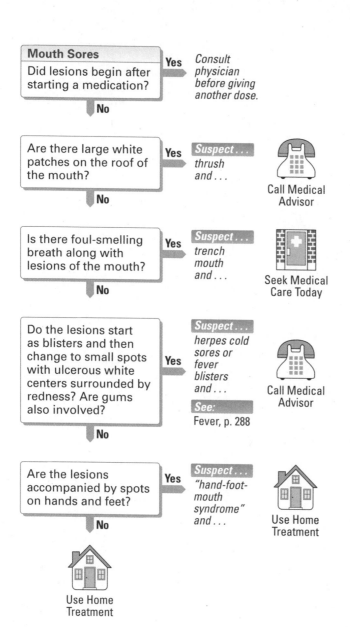

Mouth Sores

Did lesions begin after starting a medication? — **Yes** → *Consult physician before giving another dose.*

No ↓

Are there large white patches on the roof of the mouth? — **Yes** → *Suspect...* thrush and... → Call Medical Advisor

No ↓

Is there foul-smelling breath along with lesions of the mouth? — **Yes** → *Suspect...* trench mouth and... → Seek Medical Care Today

No ↓

Do the lesions start as blisters and then change to small spots with ulcerous white centers surrounded by redness? Are gums also involved? — **Yes** → *Suspect...* herpes cold sores or fever blisters and... *See:* Fever, p. 288 → Call Medical Advisor

No ↓

Are the lesions accompanied by spots on hands and feet? — **Yes** → *Suspect...* "hand-foot-mouth syndrome" and... → Use Home Treatment

No ↓

Use Home Treatment

Thrush. Suspect thrush if there are large white patches on the roof of the mouth or on the tongue.

prescribe an antibiotic. For most viral infections, doctors have no more to offer than home remedies. Under certain circumstances, doctors may use acyclovir to treat herpes infections. .

We caution against the use of oral anesthetics such as viscous Xylocaine. This anesthetic can interfere with proper swallowing and can lead to inhalation of food into the lungs.

Toothaches

A toothache is the sad result of a poor program of dental hygiene. Although resistance to tooth decay is partly inherited, the majority of dental problems are preventable. (See the discussion of dental care on pages 183–187.)

Dental Problems

If you can see a decayed tooth or an area of redness surrounding a tooth, a toothache is most likely. Tapping on the teeth with a wooden Popsicle stick will often accentuate the pain in an affected tooth, even though it appears normal.

If your child appears ill, has a fever, and has swelling of the face or jaw or redness surrounding the tooth, an abscess is likely, and antibiotics will be necessary in addition to proper dental care. In such circumstances, a visit to the doctor may be in order before seeing the dentist. Alternatively, see the dentist.

Other Causes

Occasionally, it is difficult to distinguish a toothache from other sources of pain. Earaches (page 339), sore throats (page 336), mumps (page 424), sinusitis, and injury to the joint that attaches the jaw to the skull may all be confused with a toothache. If a pain occurs every time your child opens his or her mouth wide, it is likely that the joint of the jaw has been injured. This can occur from a blow or just by trying to eat too big a sandwich.

Home Treatment

Acetaminophen or ibuprofen (page 218) can be used for pain when a toothache is suspected and while a dental appointment is being arranged. Acetaminophen is also helpful for problems in the joint of the jaw.

What to Expect at the Dentist's Office

The dentist will fill or extract the tooth. He or she will usually extract a baby tooth. A root canal, as opposed to an extraction, is more likely for a permanent tooth if the problem is severe. If there is fever or swelling of the jaw, the dentist usually will prescribe an antibiotic.

Toothaches

Are any of the following present?

▲ Fever

▲ Earache

▲ Facial swelling

Yes →

Call Medical
Advisor

No ↓

*SEE DENTIST
TODAY.*

Skin Problems

Identifying Skin Problems

Skin problems must be approached somewhat differently from other medical problems. Decision charts that proceed from complaints such as "red bumps" can be developed, but the charts are complicated and somewhat unsatisfactory. This is because most people, including doctors, identify skin diseases by recognizing a particular pattern. This pattern is composed of not only what the skin problem looks like at a particular time but also how it began, where it spread, and whether it is associated with other symptoms such as itching or fever. Also important are elements of the medical history that may suggest an illness to which the child has been exposed. Fortunately, many times you already have a good idea of the source of a problem, and it is possible to proceed immediately with the question of whether this problem is indeed present—say, poison ivy or ringworm. If you are confused about what skin problem is present, we provide help in the accompanying decision chart and Table 9 (pages 370–371).

Each decision chart in this chapter begins with the question of whether the problem is compatible with the essentials of the pattern for that skin disease. (Note that a more complete description of the pattern is given in the text that accompanies the chart.) If it is not, you are directed to reconsider the problem and to consult Table 9.

Most cases of a particular skin disease do not look exactly as a textbook says they should, so in general we have not provided you with pictures. We have tried to allow for a reasonable amount of variation in the descriptions, and you will have to use your common sense a good deal. Don't be afraid to ask for other opinions. Your mother, grandmother, and friends have probably seen a lot of skin problems over the years and know what the problems we describe in print look like in the flesh. Google Images is also an excellent resource. For each problem we discuss you will be able to see a broad range of how the condition will appear on the skin. Be aware that many of the images represent worst case scenarios.

We have listed some of the more common problems, but this is by no means a comprehensive list. If your child's problem doesn't seem to fit any of the descriptions, common sense—about whether the problem is serious and whether to call the doctor—will take you a long way.

Finally, because every case is at least a little different, even the best doctors will not be able to identify all skin problems immediately. Simple office laboratory methods can help distinguish different conditions. Fortunately, the vast majority of skin problems are minor, last only a short time, and pose no major threat to the child's health.

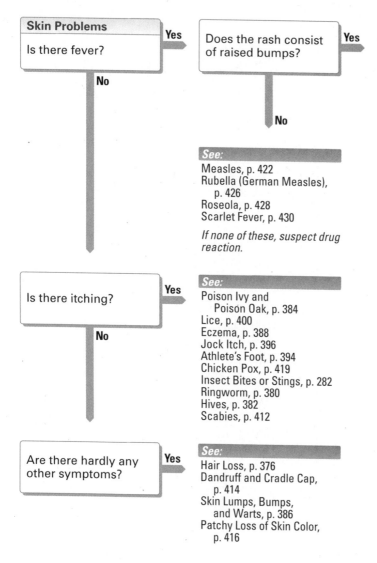

Skin Problems

Is there fever?

Yes

Does the rash consist of raised bumps?

Yes

See:
Chicken Pox, p. 419
Mouth Sores, p. 364
Impetigo, p. 378
Boils, p. 390
Insect Bites or Stings, p. 282

If none of these, suspect drug reaction.

No

No

See:
Measles, p. 422
Rubella (German Measles),
    p. 426
Roseola, p. 428
Scarlet Fever, p. 430

If none of these, suspect drug reaction.

Is there itching?

Yes

See:
Poison Ivy and
    Poison Oak, p. 384
Lice, p. 400
Eczema, p. 388
Jock Itch, p. 396
Athlete's Foot, p. 394
Chicken Pox, p. 419
Insect Bites or Stings, p. 282
Ringworm, p. 380
Hives, p. 382
Scabies, p. 412

No

Are there hardly any other symptoms?

Yes

See:
Hair Loss, p. 376
Dandruff and Cradle Cap,
    p. 414
Skin Lumps, Bumps,
    and Warts, p. 386
Patchy Loss of Skin Color,
    p. 416

Table 9: Skin Problems

	Fever	Itching	Elevation
Baby Rashes (p. 372)	No	Sometimes	Slightly raised dots
Diaper Rash (p. 374)	No	No	Only if infected
Impetigo (p. 378)	Sometimes	Occasionally	Crusts on sores
Ringworm (p. 380)	No	Occasionally	Slightly raised rings
Hives (p. 382)	No	Intense	Raised with flat tops
Poison Ivy and Poison Oak (p. 384)	No	Intense	Blisters are elevated
Eczema (p. 388)	No	Moderate to intense	Occasional blisters when infected
Acne (p. 392)	No	No	Pimples, cysts
Athlete's Foot (p. 394)	No	Mild to intense	No
Scabies (p. 412)	No	Intense	Slight
Dandruff and Cradle Cap (p. 414)	No	Occasionally	Some crusting
Chicken Pox (p. 419)	Yes	Intense during pustular stage	Flat, then raised, then blisters, then crusts
Measles (p. 422)	Yes	None to mild	Flat
Rubella (German Measles) (p. 426)	Yes	No	Flat or slightly raised
Roseola (p. 428)	Yes	No	Flat, occasionally with a few bumps
Scarlet Fever (p. 430)	Yes	No	Flat, feels like sandpaper
Fifth Disease (p. 432)	No	No	Flat, lacy appearance

Color	Location	Duration of Problem	Other Symptoms
White or red dots; surrounding skin may be red	Trunk, neck, skin folds on arms and legs	Until controlled	
Red	Under diaper	Until controlled	
Golden crusts on red sores	Arms, legs, face first, then most of body	Until controlled	
Red	Anywhere, including scalp and nails	Until controlled	Flaking or scaling
Pale raised lesions surrounded by red	Anywhere	Minutes to days	
Red	Exposed areas	7 to 14 days	Oozing; some swelling
Red	Elbows, wrists, knees, cheeks	Until controlled	Moist; oozing
Red	Face, back, chest	Until controlled	Blackheads
Colorless to red	Between toes	Until controlled	Cracks; scaling; oozing blisters
Red crust	Arms, legs, trunks; Infant: head, neck, hands, feet	Until controlled	
White to yellow to red	Scalp, eyebrows, behind ears, groin	Until controlled	Fine, oily scales
Red	May start anywhere; most prominent on trunk and face	4 to 10 days	Lesions progress from flat to tiny blisters, then become crusted
Pink, then red	First face, then chest and abdomen, then arms and legs	4 to 7 days	Preceded by fever, cough, red eyes
Red	First face, then trunk, then extremities	2 to 4 days	Swollen glands behind ears; occasional joint pains in older children and adults
Pink	First trunk, then arms and neck; very little on face and legs	1 to 2 days	High fever for 3 days that disappears with rash
Red	First face, then elbows; spreads rapidly to entire body in 24 hours	5 to 7 days	Sore throat; skin peeling afterward, especially palms
Red	First face, then arms and legs, then rest of body	3 to 7 days	"Slapped-cheek" appearance, rash comes and goes

Baby Rashes

The skin of a newborn child may exhibit a wide variety of bumps and blotches. Fortunately, almost all of these are harmless and clear up by themselves. If the baby was delivered in a hospital, many of these conditions may occur before discharge, so advice will be readily available from nurses or doctors.

Heat Rash

Heat rash is caused by blockage of the pores that lead to the sweat glands. It can occur at any age but is most common in very young children, in whom the sweat glands are still developing. When heat and humidity rise, these glands attempt to provide sweat as they normally would. Because of the blockage, however, this sweat is held within the skin and forms little red bumps. Heat rash is also known as "prickly heat" or "miliaria."

Milia

The "little white bumps of milia" are composed of normal skin cells that have over-accumulated in some spots. As many as 40% of children have these bumps at birth. Eventually, the bumps break open, the trapped material escapes, and the bumps disappear without requiring any treatment.

Erythema Toxicum

Erythema toxicum is an unnecessarily long and frightening term for the flat, red splotches that appear in up to 50% of all babies. These splotches seldom appear after five days of age and have usually disappeared by seven days. They require no treatment. The children affected are perfectly normal, and whether any real toxin is involved is not clear.

Baby "Pseudo" Acne

Because the baby is exposed to the mother's adult hormones, a mild case of acne may develop, just as may occur when a child begins to produce adult hormones during adolescence. (The little white dots often seen on a newborn's nose represent an excess amount of normal skin oil, *sebaceous gland hyperplasia,* that has been produced by the hormones.) Acne usually becomes evident at between two and four weeks of age and clears up spontaneously within six months to a year. Recent studies suggest some cases may be caused by a mild fungal infection (cephalic pustulosis).

Home Treatment

For treatment of these rashes, less is best.

You can treat heat rash simply by providing a cooler and less humid environment. Powders carefully applied do no harm but are unlikely to help. Ointments and creams should be avoided because they tend to keep the skin warmer and block the pores.

Acne should *not* be treated with the medicines used by adolescents and adults. Usually, normal washing is all that is required.

Fever should not be associated with any of these problems. With the exception of minor discomfort from heat rash, these problems should be painless. If you have any questions about these conditions, call the doctor.

Baby Rashes

Are there small white bumps scattered over forehead, nose, and cheeks?

Yes → **Suspect...** *milia and...*

Use Home Treatment

No ↓

Are there small red bumps in skin folds, especially on the neck and upper chest?

Yes → **Suspect...** *heat rash and...*

Use Home Treatment

No ↓

Are there red splotches on chest, back, face, and extremities appearing before five days of age?

Yes → **Suspect...** *erythema toxicum and...*

Use Home Treatment

No ↓

Does this appear to be acne on forehead, cheeks, and chin appearing at two to four weeks of age?

Yes → **Suspect...** *baby acne and...*

Use Home Treatment

No ↓

Suspect... *problem other than those listed and...*

Call Medical Advisor

What to Expect

Discussion of these problems can usually wait until the next scheduled well-baby visit. The doctor can confirm your diagnosis at that time. If cephalic pustulosis is suspected, an antifungal cream may be recommended.

Diaper Rash

The only children who never have diaper rash are those who never wear diapers. An infant's skin is particularly sensitive and likely to develop an irritation caused by dampness and the interaction of urine and skin. An additional irritant is thought to be the ammonia in urine.

Two factors that tend to keep the baby's skin wet and exposed to the irritant promote diaper rash:

▲ Continuously wet diapers
▲ The use of plastic pants

Treatment consists of reversing these two factors.

The irritation of simple diaper rash may become complicated by an infection due to **yeast** (candida) or bacteria. When yeast is the culprit, small red spots may be seen. Also, small patches of the rash may appear outside the area covered by the diaper, as far away as the chest. Infection with bacteria leads to development of large fluid-filled blisters. If the rash is worse in the skin creases (intertrigo), a mild underlying skin problem known as **seborrhea** may be present. Yeast (candida) may also flourish in the skin creases. Seborrhea is also responsible for cradle cap and dandruff (page 414).

Occasionally, parents will notice blood or what appear to be blood spots when boys have diaper rash. This is due to an irritating rash at the urinary opening at the end of the penis.

Home Treatment

Treatment of diaper rash is aimed at keeping the skin dry. The first things to do are to change the baby's diapers more frequently and to discontinue the use of plastic pants. Leaving a diaper off altogether for as long as possible will also help. Cloth diapers should be washed in a mild soap and rinsed thoroughly. Occasionally, the soap residue left in diapers will act as an irritant. Adding ½ cup (120 ml) of vinegar to the last rinse cycle may help counter the irritating ammonia in urine. Cloth and paper diapers are equivalent insofar as causing diaper rash. Moisture and not material is the culprit.

Complete clearing of the rash will take several days, but definite improvement should be noted within the first 48 to 72 hours. If this is not the case or if the rash is severe, consult the doctor.

To prevent diaper rash, some parents use zinc oxide cream (Desitin) or A & D ointment. Others use baby powder. (**Caution:** Talc dust can injure the lungs.) Caldesene powder is helpful in preventing seborrhea and monilial rashes. Always place powder in your hand first, then pat it on the baby's bottom. We do not feel that all babies need powders and creams.

Sometimes a rash will not heal until a precipitating problem, such as diarrhea, has resolved. Dealing with the diarrhea is the initial approach to healing the diaper rash.

Many skin preparations are now available without a prescription. If candida is the culprit, nystatin (Mycolog, Mycostatin, Mytrex, Nilstat, Nystatin) is effective and inexpensive, as is clotrimazole (Lotrimin).

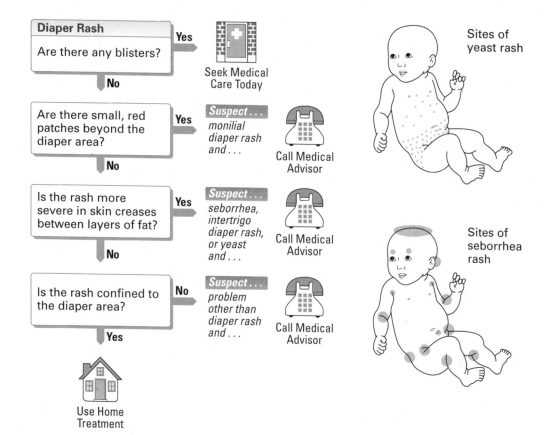

Diaper Rash

Are there any blisters? — **Yes** → Seek Medical Care Today

No ↓

Are there small, red patches beyond the diaper area? — **Yes** → *Suspect...* monilial diaper rash and... → Call Medical Advisor

No ↓

Is the rash more severe in skin creases between layers of fat? — **Yes** → *Suspect...* seborrhea, intertrigo diaper rash, or yeast and... → Call Medical Advisor

No ↓

Is the rash confined to the diaper area? — **No** → *Suspect...* problem other than diaper rash and... → Call Medical Advisor

Yes ↓

Use Home Treatment

Sites of yeast rash

Sites of seborrhea rash

What to Expect

The doctor will inspect all of the baby's skin. Occasionally, he or she may look at a scraping from the involved skin under the microscope. If a yeast (monilial) infection has complicated the diaper rash, the doctor will prescribe a medication to kill the yeast (nystatin cream and occasionally oral nystatin, clotrimazole cream, or miconazole cream). If a bacterial infection has occurred, the doctor will recommend an antibiotic. If the rash is very severe or seborrhea is suspected, he or she may advise using a steroid cream. In any case, you may begin home therapy before seeing the doctor.

Hair Loss

Hair loss may cause concern in childhood. Hair loss is common in infants. Many lose their hair by three months; others develop bald spots in the back of their heads due to sleeping appropriately on their backs.

Hair pulling by a child, or occasionally by a friend, often is responsible for hair loss. Tight braids or ponytails also may cause some hair loss. If your child constantly pulls out his or her hair, you should consider this unusual behavior and discuss it with the doctor.

Types of hair loss that may need treatment by a doctor are characterized by abnormalities in the scalp or the hairs themselves. The most frequent problem in this category is **ringworm** (page 380). Ringworm may be red and scaly, or there may be oozing pustules. The ringworm fungus infects the hairs so that they become thickened and break easily. Whenever the scalp or the hairs themselves appear abnormal, the doctor may be able to help.

Often all the hair in one small area will be completely lost, but the scalp underneath will be normal. This problem is called **alopecia areata**, and its cause is unknown. Usually, the hair will grow back completely within 12 months, although about 40% of children will have a similar loss within the next four to five years. This problem resolves itself. Cortisone creams may make the hair grow back faster, but the new hair will fall out again when the treatment is stopped, so these creams are of little use.

Home Treatment

In this instance, home treatment is reserved for presumed alopecia areata and consists of watchful waiting. The skin in the involved area must be completely normal to make a diagnosis of alopecia areata. Should the appearance of the scalp or hairs become abnormal, consult the doctor.

What to Expect

An examination of the hair and scalp is usually sufficient to determine the nature of the problem. Occasionally, the doctor may examine the hairs under the microscope. Certain types of ringworm can be identified because they fluoresce (glow) when viewed under a special ultraviolet light called a Wood's lamp. Ringworm of the scalp will require the use of an oral drug, griseofulvin, because creams and lotions applied to the affected area will not penetrate into the hair follicles to kill the fungus. Griseofulvin should be taken with fatty foods and will need to be taken for at least six weeks. Don't expect to see any results sooner. Simultaneously, topical therapy may be given to prevent the fungus from spreading to other parts of the scalp or to other family members.

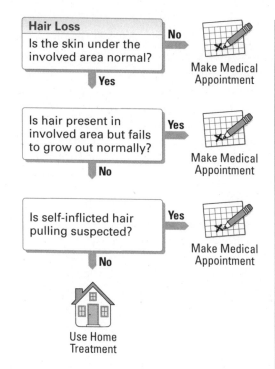

Hair Loss

Is the skin under the involved area normal?

No → Make Medical Appointment

Yes ↓

Is hair present in involved area but fails to grow out normally?

Yes → Make Medical Appointment

No ↓

Is self-inflicted hair pulling suspected?

Yes → Make Medical Appointment

No ↓

Use Home Treatment

Impetigo

Impetigo is particularly troublesome in the summer and especially in warm, moist climates. It can be recognized by the characteristic appearance of the lesions. These lesions begin as small red spots and progress to tiny blisters that eventually rupture, producing an oozing, sticky, honey-colored crust. The lesions are usually spread very quickly by scratching fingers. Another characteristic of impetigo is that it is extremely contagious, and children pass it on to brothers, sisters, and playmates very easily.

Impetigo is a skin infection usually caused by streptococcal bacteria and sometimes by staphylococcal bacteria. If impetigo spreads, it can be a very uncomfortable problem. There is usually a great deal of itching, and scratching hastens the spread of the lesions. After the sores heal, there may be a slight decrease in skin color at the site. Skin color usually returns to normal, so this need not concern you.

Complication in the Kidneys
Of greatest concern is a rare, complicating kidney problem known as **glomerulonephritis**, which occasionally occurs in epidemics. Glomerulonephritis will cause the urine to turn a dark brown (cola) color and is often accompanied by a headache and elevated blood pressure. Although this problem has a formidable name, the kidney problem is short-lived and heals completely in most children.

Unfortunately, antibiotics will not prevent glomerulonephritis, but they can prevent the impetigo from spreading to other children, thus protecting them from both impetigo and glomerulonephritis. Antibiotics are effective in healing impetigo.

Although there is some debate on this matter, many doctors believe that if only one or two lesions are present and they are not progressing, home treatment may be used for impetigo. The exception to this rule is if an epidemic of glomerulonephritis is occurring within your community.

Home Treatment
Bacitracin, an antibiotic ointment, may prevent the spread of impetigo to others. If lesions do not show prompt improvement, or if they seem to be spreading, see the doctor without delay.

What to Expect
After examining the sores and taking an appropriate medical history, the doctor usually will prescribe either an effective topical agent (mupirocin) or an antibiotic to be taken orally. Cephalexin (Keflex), sulfamethoxazole/trimethoprim (Septra, Bactrim), or clindamycin (Cleocin) may be prescribed. Some doctors may check the blood pressure or urine to examine for early signs of glomerulonephritis.

Impetigo

Does the child have small, crusted, yellow sores with or without a tiny surrounding area of redness?

No → *problem other than impetigo. Check Skin Problems Table on pp. 370–371.*

Yes ↓

Has anyone in your family or neighborhood had glomerulonephritis (blood in the urine) recently?

Yes → Seek Medical Care Today

No ↓

Is there fever?

Yes → Seek Medical Care Today

No ↓

Are there only one or two lesions?

No → Make Medical Appointment

Yes ↓

Are the lesions healing and not spreading to other family members?

No → Make Medical Appointment

Yes ↓

Use Home Treatment

Ringworm (Tinea corporis— body; Tinea capitis—scalp)

Ringworm is a shallow fungal infection of the skin. Worms have nothing whatsoever to do with this condition. The designation "ringworm" is derived from the characteristic red ring that appears on the skin.

Ringworm can generally be recognized by its pattern of development. The lesions begin as small, round, red spots and get progressively larger. When they are about the size of a pea, the center begins to clear. When the lesions are about the size of a dime, they have the appearance of a ring. The border of the ring is red, elevated, and scaly. Often there are groups of infections so close together that it is difficult to recognize them as individual rings.

Ringworm may also affect the scalp or the nails. These infections are more difficult to treat but are not seen as often. Epidemics of ringworm of the scalp were common many years ago.

Home Treatment

Tolnaftate (Tinactin) applied to the skin is an effective treatment for ringworm. Clotrimazole (Desenex, Lotrimin, Mycelex) and miconazole (Fungoid, Micatin) are also highly effective. Apply either the cream or the solution of these products two or three times a day. Only a small amount is required for each application. Resolution of the problem may require several weeks of therapy, but you should note improvement within a week. Ringworm that shows no improvement after a week of therapy or that continues to spread should be checked by a doctor.

What to Expect

The diagnosis of ringworm can be confirmed by scraping the scales, soaking them in a potassium hydroxide solution, and viewing them under the microscope. Some doctors may culture the scrapings. Results of the cultures may take several weeks to come back. Treatment is usually begun before the cultures are ready. Occasionally, a prescription oral medicine (griseofulvin) may be needed.

In infections involving the scalp, an ultraviolet light (called a Wood's lamp) will cause affected hairs to become fluorescent (glowing). The Wood's lamp may be used to make the diagnosis; it does not treat the ringworm. More than 90% of ringworm does not fluoresce, so your doctor need not perform this test. Ringworm of the scalp must be treated by griseofulvin, taken orally, usually for at least a month. This medication is also effective for fungal infections of the nails but must be taken for 6 to 18 months.

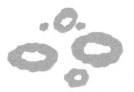

Ringworm. Lesions begin as small, round, red spots. When they are about the size of a dime, they will have the appearance of a ring.

Ringworm

Are all of the following conditions present?

▲ Rash begins as a small, red, colorless, or depigmented circle that becomes progressively larger.

▲ The circular border is elevated and perhaps scaly.

▲ The center of the circle begins healing as the circle becomes larger.

No →

Suspect...
problem other than ringworm. Check Skin Problems Table on pp. 370–371. For foot infections, see p. 394.

Yes ↓

Is the scalp infected?　**Yes** →

Make Medical Appointment

No ↓

Use Home Treatment

Hives

Hives are an allergic reaction. Unfortunately, the reaction can be to almost anything, including cold or heat and even emotional tension. Unless you already have a good idea what is causing the hives or your child has just taken a new drug, the doctor is unlikely to be able to determine the cause. Most often a search for a cause is fruitless.

Here is a list of some frequently mentioned causes of hives.

▲ Drugs
▲ Eggs
▲ Milk
▲ Wheat
▲ Chocolate
▲ Pork
▲ Shellfish
▲ Freshwater fish
▲ Berries
▲ Cheese
▲ Nuts
▲ Pollens
▲ Insect bites or stings

The only sure way to know whether one of these is the culprit is to expose the child to it on purpose. The problem with this approach is that if an allergy does exist, the allergic response may include not only hives but also dangerous reactions that cause difficulty breathing or circulation problems.

As indicated by the decision chart, a **systemic reaction** (trouble breathing, swallowing, dizziness) along with hives is a potentially dangerous situation, and you should consult the doctor immediately. Avoid exposure to a suspected cause to see if attacks cease. Such "tests" are difficult to interpret because attacks of hives are often separated by long periods. Actually, most people have only one attack, lasting from a few hours to weeks.

Home Treatment

Determine whether there has been any pattern to the appearance of hives. Do they appear after meals? After exposure to the cold? During a particular season of the year? If you can identify possible causes, eliminate them and see what happens.

Antihistamines such as oral diphenhydramine are often helpful.

If the reactions seem to be related to foods, an alternative is available. Lamb and rice virtually never cause allergic reactions. The child may be placed on a diet consisting only of lamb and rice until completely free of hives. Add foods back to the diet one at a time, and observe the child for the development of hives.

Itching may be relieved by cold compresses, oatmeal baths (Aveeno), calamine lotion (page 227), or antihistamines (page 224) such as diphenhydramine (Benadryl).

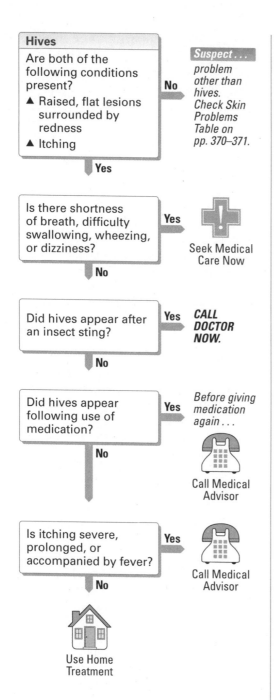

Hives

Are both of the following conditions present?
▲ Raised, flat lesions surrounded by redness
▲ Itching

No → *Suspect...* problem other than hives. Check Skin Problems Table on pp. 370–371.

Yes ↓

Is there shortness of breath, difficulty swallowing, wheezing, or dizziness?

Yes → Seek Medical Care Now

No ↓

Did hives appear after an insect sting?

Yes → *CALL DOCTOR NOW.*

No ↓

Did hives appear following use of medication?

Yes → Before giving medication again... Call Medical Advisor

No ↓

Is itching severe, prolonged, or accompanied by fever?

Yes → Call Medical Advisor

No ↓

Use Home Treatment

What to Expect

If the child is suffering a systemic reaction with difficulty breathing or dizziness, the doctor may give him or her injections of adrenaline and other drugs. If such a reaction follows an insect sting, several approaches are available, including the following:

▲ Desensitization to the insect through injections
▲ Instructions in the use of an emergency epinephrine injection kit

In the more usual case of hives alone, the doctor can do two things for your child. First, he or she can prescribe an antihistamine or use adrenaline injections to relieve swelling and itching. Second, the doctor can review the history of the reaction to try to find an offending agent and advise you of treatments such as those under "Home Treatment." Remember that most often the cause of hives goes undetected.

Poison Ivy and Poison Oak

Poison ivy and poison oak need little introduction. The itching skin lesions that follow contact with these and other plants of the genus *Rhus* are the most common example of a larger category of skin problems known as **contact dermatitis**. Contact dermatitis simply means that something that has been applied to the skin has caused the skin to react to it. An initial exposure is necessary to "sensitize" the patient. A subsequent exposure will result in an allergic reaction if the plant oil remains in contact with the skin for several hours. The resulting rash begins after 12 to 48 hours and persists for about 2 weeks.

Contact may be indirect, from pets, contaminated clothing, or the smoke from burning plants. It can occur during any season.

Home Treatment

The best approach is to teach your children to recognize and avoid the plants, which are hazardous even in the winter, when they have dropped their leaves.

Next best is to remove the plant oil from the skin as soon as possible. If the oil has been on the skin for less than six hours, thorough cleansing with ordinary soap, repeated three times, will often prevent a reaction. Alcohol-based cleansing tissues, available in prepackaged form (Alco-wipe) are very effective in removing the oil. If a large area has been exposed, use rubbing alcohol on a washcloth. Wash the child's clothes thoroughly because oils can remain on fabric and shoe leather.

To relieve itching, many doctors recommend cool compresses of Burow's solution (Domeboro, BurVeen, Bluboro) or baths with Aveeno or oatmeal (1 cup, or 230 g, in a tubful of water). Acetaminophen (Tylenol) and ibuprofen (Motrin, Advil) are also useful (page 218). The old standby, calamine lotion (page 227), is sometimes helpful in treating early lesions, but it may spread the plant oil. (**Caution**: Do not use Caladryl or Zyradryl. They cause allergic reactions in some people. Use only calamine lotion.) Be sure to cleanse the skin, as above, even if you are too late to prevent the rash entirely. The cleanser Tecnu is quite effective for both prevention and the itch. Some children may be relieved by 1% hydrocortisone cream.

Another useful method of obtaining symptomatic relief for older children is the use of a hot bath or shower. Heat releases histamine, the substance in the skin cells that causes the intense itching. A hot shower or bath will cause intense itching as the histamine is released. The heat

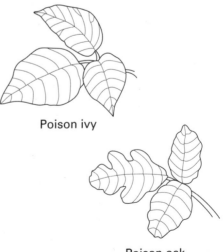

Poison ivy

Poison oak

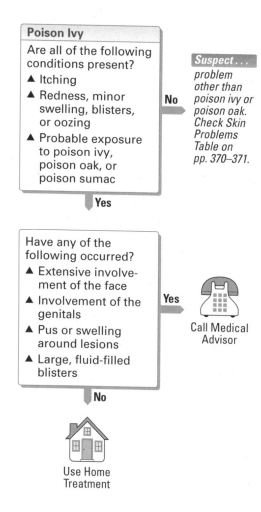

Poison Ivy

Are all of the following conditions present?

▲ Itching

▲ Redness, minor swelling, blisters, or oozing

▲ Probable exposure to poison ivy, poison oak, or poison sumac

No → *Suspect...* problem other than poison ivy or poison oak. Check Skin Problems Table on pp. 370–371.

Yes ↓

Have any of the following occurred?

▲ Extensive involvement of the face

▲ Involvement of the genitals

▲ Pus or swelling around lesions

▲ Large, fluid-filled blisters

Yes → Call Medical Advisor

No ↓

Use Home Treatment

should be gradually increased to the maximum level tolerable and continued until the itching has subsided. This process will deplete the cells of histamine, and the child will obtain up to eight hours of relief from the itching. This method has the advantage of not requiring frequent applications of ointments to the lesions and is a good way for the child to get some sleep at night.

Whether or not any medication is used, poison ivy or poison oak will persist for the same length of time. If a secondary bacterial infection occurs, healing will be delayed; hence scratching is not helpful. Cut the child's nails to avoid damage to the skin through scratching.

Poison ivy is not contagious. It cannot be spread once the oil has been absorbed by the skin or removed.

If the lesions are too extensive to be treated easily, if home treatment is ineffective, or if the itching is so severe that the child can't tolerate it, a visit to the doctor may be necessary.

What to Expect

After taking a history and performing a physical examination, the doctor may prescribe a steroid cream to be applied to the lesions four to six times a day. This is often of moderate help.

An alternative is to give the child a steroid (such as prednisone) by mouth for a short time. A rather large dose is given the first day, and the dose is then gradually reduced. We are reluctant to recommend oral steroids except in children with previous severe reactions to poison ivy or poison oak or with extensive exposure.

The itching may be treated symptomatically with an antihistamine such as diphenhydramine (Benadryl) or hydroxyzine (Atarax, Vistaril), an anti-inflammatory agent such as ibuprofen, or a cleanser such as Tecnu. Antihistamines may cause drowsiness and interfere with sleep.

Skin Lumps, Bumps, and Warts

Lumps and bumps are common at all ages. The lump may be:

▲ Above the skin, as with warts, moles, and insect bites

▲ Within the skin, as with boils and certain kinds of moles

▲ Under the skin, as in the case of swollen lymph glands or small collections of fat called lipomas

If there is only one lump and it is red, hot, tender, and swollen (inflamed), it should be considered a boil until proven otherwise. (See Boils, page 390.)

A dark mole that appears to be enlarging or changing color might be a melanoma, a kind of skin cancer, although melanomas are extremely unusual in children.

The most commonly found lumps in children are swollen lymph glands. These are discussed in more detail under Swollen Glands, page 358.

Warts are caused by viral infections and often resolve by themselves but may take several years. However, warts can occasionally be troublesome, especially if they are on the fingers, where they may interfere with writing, or on the face, where they are cosmetically disturbing. Warts on the soles of the feet (plantar warts) can be painful.

Home Treatment

Treatment of many lumps and bumps is discussed under Insect Bites or Stings, page 282; Boils, page 390; Swollen Glands, page 358; and Arm and Leg Lumps, page 444.

Warts can be treated with over-the-counter medicines used consistently and carefully. Available preparations include salicylic acid plasters, Compound W, Vergo, TransVerSal, and preparations with salicylic acid and lactic acid (DuoFilm). Covering warts with duct tape also works. On your child's next visit to the doctor, ask about any skin lumps or warts that are of concern to you. These are seldom worth a special trip.

What to Expect

The doctor may be able to make the diagnosis simply by inspecting the lump or wart and asking you a few questions. A wart may be removed by freezing it with liquid nitrogen, by using an electric needle, or by chemical cauterization. It is seldom treated surgically because warts are caused by viruses; cutting them out may leave the virus to cause a later recurrence of the wart. A recurrence of warts is common, and repeated treatments may be necessary.

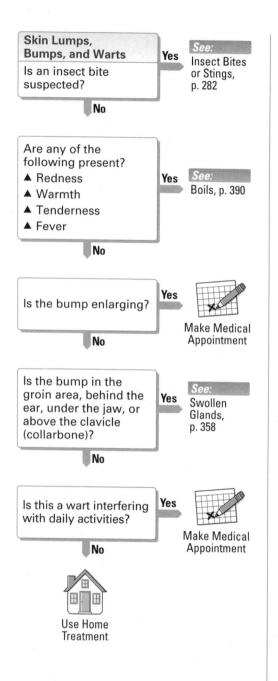

Skin Lumps, Bumps, and Warts

Is an insect bite suspected?

Yes → *See:* Insect Bites or Stings, p. 282

No ↓

Are any of the following present?
▲ Redness
▲ Warmth
▲ Tenderness
▲ Fever

Yes → *See:* Boils, p. 390

No ↓

Is the bump enlarging?

Yes → Make Medical Appointment

No ↓

Is the bump in the groin area, behind the ear, under the jaw, or above the clavicle (collarbone)?

Yes → *See:* Swollen Glands, p. 358

No ↓

Is this a wart interfering with daily activities?

Yes → Make Medical Appointment

No ↓

Use Home Treatment

Eczema

Eczema, also known as **atopic dermatitis**, is commonly found in children with a family history of either eczema, hay fever, or asthma. The underlying problem is the inability of the skin to retain adequate amounts of water. The skin of children with eczema is consequently very dry, which causes the skin to itch.

Children with atopic dermatitis have skin that responds to changes in the environment, allergic substances in food, and emotional stress with intense itching. Most of the manifestations of eczema are a consequence of scratching. Atopic skin also has an increased tendency to swell and ooze when scratched.

In young infants who are unable to scratch, the most common manifestation is red, dry, mildly scaling cheeks. Although the infant cannot scratch his or her cheeks, the cheeks can be rubbed by moving against the sheets and thus become red. In infants, eczema may also be found in the area where plastic pants meet the skin. The tightness of the elastic produces the characteristic red scaling lesion. In older children, it is very common for eczema to involve the area behind the knees and in front of the elbows.

If there is a fair amount of weeping or crusting, the eczema has become infected with bacteria, and a visit to the doctor will most likely be required.

The course of eczema is quite variable. Some children have only a brief mild problem; others have manifestations throughout their lives.

Home Treatment

Attempts must be made to prevent the skin from becoming too dry. Frequent baths dry out the skin. Although a child with eczema will feel comfortable in the bath, itching will become more intense after the bath because of the drying effect. Lubricating substances help keep the skin moist. The products should be unscented and hypoallergenic. They include Keri and Lubriderm lotions, Aquaphor, Keri and Nivea creams, and Eucerin paste.

Sweating aggravates eczema. Consequently, children should not be overdressed so that they perspire. Light night clothing is important. Contact with wool or silk seems to aggravate eczema in some children and should be avoided.

When inflammation is prominent—the skin is red, swollen, oozing, and itching—wet dressings of Burow's solution and oatmeal baths (Aveeno) can be applied. A 1% hydrocortisone cream is also effective on troublesome areas. For itching, oral diphenhydramine is often effective. Nails should be kept trimmed short to minimize the effects of scratching. In older children who help with household chores, rubber gloves can help prevent drying of the hands after washing dishes or the car.

Washing is best accomplished with a cleansing and moisturizing agent such as Cetaphil lotion. Many soaps aggravate eczema. Dove soap is milder and less drying than most.

Freshwater or pool swimming can aggravate eczema by causing loss of skin moisture, but ocean swimming does not do so and can be undertaken freely. (Also see the discussion of allergies on pages 174–183.)

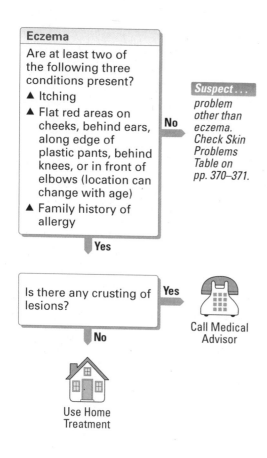

Eczema

Are at least two of the following three conditions present?

▲ Itching

▲ Flat red areas on cheeks, behind ears, along edge of plastic pants, behind knees, or in front of elbows (location can change with age)

▲ Family history of allergy

No → *Suspect...* problem other than eczema. Check Skin Problems Table on pp. 370–371.

Yes ↓

Is there any crusting of lesions? **Yes** → Call Medical Advisor

No ↓

Use Home Treatment

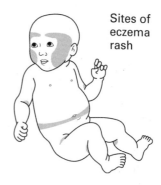

Sites of eczema rash

What to Expect

By history and examination of the lesions, the doctor can determine whether the problem is eczema. If home treatment has not improved the problem, the doctor may prescribe steroid creams and ointments. Although these are effective, they are not curative; eczema is characterized by repeated occurrences. If crusted or weeping lesions are present, a bacterial infection is likely, and the doctor will prescribe an oral antibiotic. Hydroxyzine (Atarax, Vistaril) is an antihistamine that is often used to reduce itching. Cetirizine (Zyrtec) makes fewer children drowsy and can be used in school-age children.

Boils

A boil is a localized infection due to staphylococcus. Usually, a strain of the bacteria that is resistant to many antibiotics (MRSA or methicillin-resistant staphylococcus aureus) is responsible. When this particular bacteria inhabits the child's skin, recurrent problems with boils may persist for months or years. Often several family members will be affected at about the same time.

Boils may be single or multiple, and they may occur anywhere on the body. They range from the size of a pea to the size of a walnut or larger. The surrounding red, thickened, and tender tissue increases the problem even further. The infection begins in the tissue beneath the skin and develops into an abscess pocket filled with pus. Eventually, the pus pocket "points" toward the skin surface and finally ruptures and drains. Then it heals.

Boils often begin as infections around hair follicles, hence the term **folliculitis** for minor infections. Often areas under pressure (such as the buttocks) are likely spots for boils to begin. A boil that extends into the deeper layers of the skin is called a **carbuncle**.

Special consideration should be given to boils on the face because they are more likely to lead to severe complicating infections.

Home Treatment

Boils are handled gently because rough treatment can force the infection deeper inside the body. Warm, moist soaks are applied gently several times a day to speed the development of the pocket of pus and to soften the skin for the eventual rupture and drainage. Once drainage begins, the soaks will help keep the opening in the skin clear. The more drainage, the better. Frequent, thorough soaping of the entire skin helps prevent reinfection. *Ignore all temptation to squeeze the boil.*

What to Expect

If there is fever or if the boil is on the face, in multiple places, or large, the doctor will usually prescribe an antibiotic.

If the boil feels as if fluid is contained in a pocket but it has not yet drained, the doctor may lance the boil. In this procedure, a small incision is made to allow the pus to drain. After drainage, the pain is reduced, and drainage alone can be the cure. Although "incision and drainage" is not a complicated procedure, it is tricky enough that you should not attempt it yourself. The doctor may take a culture of the fluid to make sure the antibiotic works. If the boil does not heal your doctor may prescribe antibiotics such as cephalexin (Keflex), trimetoprim/sulfamethoxazole (Bactrim, Septra), or clindamycin (Cleocin) and may even consider intravenous antibiotics in a sick child.

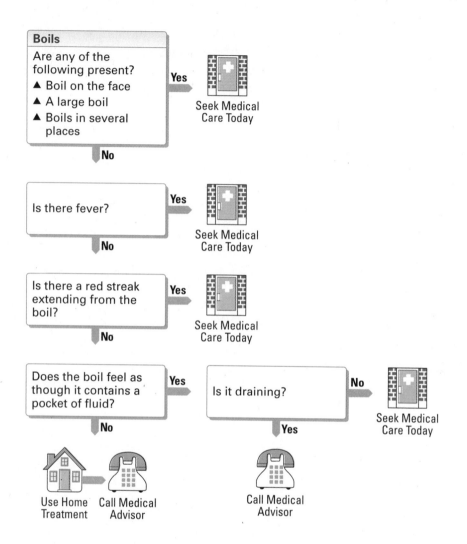

Boils

Are any of the following present?
▲ Boil on the face
▲ A large boil
▲ Boils in several places

Yes → Seek Medical Care Today

No ↓

Is there fever?

Yes → Seek Medical Care Today

No ↓

Is there a red streak extending from the boil?

Yes → Seek Medical Care Today

No ↓

Does the boil feel as though it contains a pocket of fluid?

Yes → Is it draining?

No → Seek Medical Care Today

No ↓ (from "Does the boil feel...")

Use Home Treatment   Call Medical Advisor

Yes ↓ (from "Is it draining?")

Call Medical Advisor

Acne

Acne is a skin eruption caused by a combination of factors. It is triggered by the hormonal changes of puberty and is common in children with oily skin. The increased skin oils (sebum) accumulate below plugs in the openings of the hair follicles and oil glands. In this area below the plug, secretions accumulate, and bacteria grow. These normal bacteria cause changes in the secretions that make them irritating to the surrounding skin. The result is usually a **pimple**, but sometimes it may develop into a larger pocket of secretions, or **cyst**.

Blackheads are formed when a pigment known as melanin is deposited on keratin plugs. Skin irritation is minimal.

Home Treatment

Although excessive dirt will aggravate acne, scrupulous cleaning will not prevent it. With acne, the face should be washed several times daily with a warm washcloth and a mild soap (Dove) to remove skin oils and keratin plugs. The rubbing and heat of the washcloth help dislodge the plugs. Diet is no longer considered a cause of acne.

Acne Medicines

Benzoyl peroxide is the most effective preparation currently available. Benzoyl peroxide acts by causing a mild peeling of the skin and assists in promoting unplugging of the sebaceous glands. It also has some activity against bacteria and is able to interfere with some of the chemical processes involved in the formation of papules and pustules. It can be irritating,

especially if used with abrasive soaps, which is why we do not recommend coarse and gritty soaps. As many as 2% of children may be allergic to this product, so it is not for everyone.

It takes a number of weeks for benzoyl peroxide to produce any results. This is important to bear in mind, for the first few weeks can be discouraging. The goal is to produce a mild dryness of the skin. The best way to achieve this is to begin applications every other day. Begin with the 5% lotion. If there is no skin irritation and the acne persists, use every day. The most potent forms are available in gels.

Some cosmetics can aggravate acne. It is best to avoid them as much as possible, especially when treating the skin with benzoyl peroxide or tretinoin. Look for products labeled non-comodogenic.

Sun Lamps

Acne appears to get better in the summer. Although this is most likely due to increased exposure to sunlight, other factors may be involved. We do *not* recommend the routine use of sun lamps, the primary effect of which is to induce peeling of the skin. This can be done much more safely with peeling agents such as benzoyl peroxide and tretinoin. Sun lamps can produce severe burns.

Acne and Diet

Diet is not an important factor in most cases of acne, but if certain foods tend to aggravate the problem, avoid them. There is scant evidence that chocolate aggravates acne.

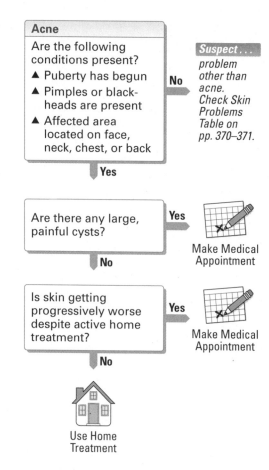

Acne

Are the following conditions present?
▲ Puberty has begun
▲ Pimples or black-heads are present
▲ Affected area located on face, neck, chest, or back

No →

Suspect . . .
problem other than acne. Check Skin Problems Table on pp. 370–371.

Yes ↓

Are there any large, painful cysts?

Yes → Make Medical Appointment

No ↓

Is skin getting progressively worse despite active home treatment?

Yes → Make Medical Appointment

No ↓

Use Home Treatment

What to Expect

If acne continues as a problem after home treatment, your doctor may prescribe tretinoin (Retin-A) to apply to the skin. Its actions are similar to those of benzoyl peroxide, but it is slightly more irritating. In resistant cases, an oral antibiotic (tetracycline, erythromycin, minocycline, or doxycycline) may be prescribed; they are used for more extensive involvement, especially for the back, where other products are hard to apply. Some doctors call for antibiotics to be applied to the skin; erythromycin and clindamycin are often used. In the most severe and resistant cases, isotretinoin (Accutane) may be used.

"Acne surgery" is a term generally applied to the doctor's removal of blackheads with a suction device and an eyedropper. Large cysts are sometimes arrested with the injection of steroids. Such procedures should be required only in severe cases and are more usually performed on the back than on the face.

Athlete's Foot (Tinea pedis)

Athlete's foot is very common during adolescence and relatively uncommon before. It is the most common of the fungal infections and is often persistent. The fungi responsible for ringworm (page 380) and jock itch (page 396) also cause athlete's foot. When athlete's foot involves toenails, it can be difficult to treat.

Friction and moisture are important in aggravating the problem. In fact, there is evidence that bacteria and moisture are most responsible for this problem. The fungus is responsible only for getting things started.

When many people share locker-room and shower facilities, exposure to the fungus is impossible to prevent, and infection is the rule rather than the exception. But you don't have to participate in sports to contact this fungus; it's all around.

Home Treatment

Scrupulous hygiene, without resorting to drugs, is often effective. *Twice a day*, have the child wash the space between the toes with soap, water, and a cloth. Have him or her dry the entire area carefully with a towel, particularly between the toes (despite the pain), and put on clean socks.

The child should wear shoes that allow evaporation of moisture. Plastic linings must be avoided. Sandals or canvas sneakers are best. Changing shoes every other day to allow them to dry out completely is a good idea.

Over-the-counter products such as Desenex powder or cream may be effective. The powder has the virtue of helping keep the toes dry. If Desenex is not effective, a more expensive over-the-counter medication, tolnaftate (Tinactin), is available in either cream or lotion. Tinactin powder is better as a preventive than as a curative preparation. Clotrimazole and miconazole are also effective treatments. Burow's solution is helpful if applied to blistering areas.

Keeping the feet dry with the use of a powder is helpful in preventing reinfection.

What to Expect

Through history and physical examination, and possibly laboratory examination of a skin scraping, the doctor will establish the diagnosis. Several other problems, notably a condition called **dyshidrosis**, may mimic athlete's foot. If home treatment has failed, the doctor may prescribe a skin cream such as ciclopirox. For severe cases, the doctor may prescribe oral griseofulvin, which works well against fungal infections of the nails.

Athlete's Foot

Are both of the following conditions present?

▲ Redness and scaling between toes (may have cracks and small blisters)

▲ Itching

No →

Suspect . . .
problem other than athlete's foot.
Check Skin Problems Table on pp. 370–371.

↓ **Yes**

Have any of the following occurred?

▲ Blisters or pus oozing from toes

▲ Difficulty walking

▲ Progression despite home treatment

Yes →

Call Medical Advisor

↓ **No**

Use Home Treatment

Jock Itch
(Tinea cruris)

We might wish for a less picturesque name for this condition, but the medical term, *tinea cruris*, is understood by relatively few. Jock itch is a fungal infection of the pubic region. It is aggravated by friction and moisture. For the most part, this is a male disease. It usually does not involve the scrotum or penis, nor does it spread beyond the groin area. Frequently, the fungus grows in an athletic supporter turned old and moldy in a locker room far from a washing machine. The preventive measure for such a problem is obvious.

Home Treatment
The problem should be treated by removing the contributing factors, friction and moisture. This is done by wearing boxer-type shorts rather than briefs, by applying a powder to dry the area after bathing, and by frequently changing soiled or sweaty underclothes. It may take up to two weeks to clear up the problem, and it may recur. The powder-and-clean-shorts treatment will usually be successful without any medication. Tolnaftate (Tinactin) will eliminate the fungus if the problem persists.

What to Expect
Occasionally, a yeast infection will mimic jock itch. By examination and history, the doctor will attempt to establish the diagnosis and may make a scraping to identify a yeast. Medicines used for this problem are virtually always applied to the affected skin. Clotrimazole (Lotrimin) is an effective over-the-counter product.

Oral drugs or injections are rarely used. The prescription creams and lotions haloprogin (Halotex), miconazole (Micatin, Monistat-Derm), and ciclopirox (Loprox) are effective against both fungi and certain yeast infections.

Jock Itch

Are all of the following conditions present?

▲ Involves only groin and thighs

▲ Redness, oozing, or some peripheral scaling

▲ Itching

No →

Suspect...
problem other than jock itch. Check Skin Problems Table on pp. 370–371.

↓ **Yes**

Are there signs of infection?

▲ Pus

▲ Crusting

Yes →

Call Medical Advisor

↓ **No**

Use Home Treatment

Sunburn

Sunburn is common, painful, and *avoidable*. Rarely, people with sunburn have eye swelling and difficulty with vision. If so, they should call the doctor. Otherwise, a visit to the doctor is unnecessary unless the pain is extraordinarily severe or unless extensive blistering (not peeling) has occurred. Blistering indicates a **second-degree burn** and rarely follows sun exposure (see Burns, page 278).

The pain of sunburn is worst between 6 and 48 hours after sun exposure. Peeling of injured layers of skin occurs later, between 3 and 10 days after the burn. The real danger is malignant melanoma; the most dangerous risk factor is three blistering sunburns before the age of 18. This is a particularly dangerous form of cancer.

Prevention

Sunburn is better prevented than treated. Infants in particular should be shielded because they can burn rapidly. We recommend keeping babies younger than six months out of direct sunlight and covered with clothing and hats. It is unclear whether sunscreen should be used in infants younger than six months. Protective clothing and sunscreen offer the best protection for young children. For teens insisting on a summer tan, gradual exposure is permissible. Start with only 15 minutes daily, and increase exposure time gradually. Remember that water, snow, and high altitude intensify sun exposure. Cloud covering offers only a modest decrease in sun exposure. Sunscreen should *always* be used. Although babies with darker skin do not burn as easily and are less likely to develop melanoma later in life, they can still have problems.

Sunscreen products are classified by a number known as the sun protection factor (SPF), with 2 being minimal and over 30 being maximal; the latter does not permit tanning. For children, we recommend a sunscreen with an SPF of at least 30. Some sunscreens contain para-aminobenzoic acid (PABA). Effective preparations contain at least 5% PABA. Because of allergic reactions to PABA, new products now dominate the shelves. Benzophenone is another sunscreen that

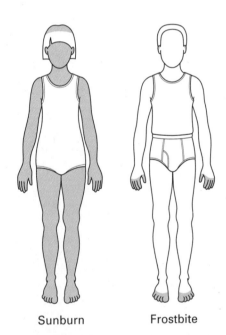

Sunburn   Frostbite

Sites of sunburn and frostbite. Sunburn (left) can occur on any unprotected part of the body, including the scalp in children with a part in the hair or in babies with little or no hair. Frostbite (right) most often affects the fingers and toes. The top of the ears is another vulnerable spot.

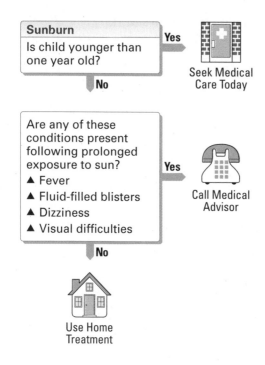

Sunburn

Is child younger than one year old? — **Yes** → Seek Medical Care Today

No ↓

Are any of these conditions present following prolonged exposure to sun?
▲ Fever
▲ Fluid-filled blisters
▲ Dizziness
▲ Visual difficulties
— **Yes** → Call Medical Advisor

No ↓

Use Home Treatment

shields a wider spectrum of light rays, although it is less effective against damaging ultraviolet light than PABA. Opaque white sunscreens that contain zinc oxide are quite effective but not very attractive.

Home Treatment

Cool compresses or cool baths with Aveeno (1 cup, or 230 g, in a tubful of water) may be useful. Ordinary baking soda (½ cup, or 115 g, in a tubful of water) is nearly as effective. Lubricants such as petroleum jelly feel good to some children but retain heat and should not be used the first day. Avoid products that contain benzocaine. These can cause irritation of the skin and may actually prolong healing. Acetaminophen or ibuprofen may ease pain and thus help sleep.

Frostbite

Frostbite is rare in children and easy to prevent. Have your children wear warm clothing, including mittens and windproof garments, in cold weather. Don't forget face masks on especially bitter days. When one's torso is warm, blood flows better to the fingers and toes, where frostbite usually occurs. Teach your children to come in from the cold whenever their fingers, noses, or toes start to hurt.

If your child's extremities begin to numb, they are starting to get frostbite. In the extreme case, the affected tissues turn black; see the doctor immediately. Otherwise, warm up the frostbitten area as quickly as possible with warm water, 100–104°F (38–40°C). Do not rub the affected area. As the blood flow resumes, the frostbitten part will begin to hurt, sometimes a lot. This is a good sign, since the tissues are obviously still alive. Your child may have leftover numbness for months after minor frostbite, but this does not require medical attention.

What to Expect

The doctor will determine the extent of the burn and the possibility of other heat-related injuries, such as sunstroke. If the doctor finds only first-degree burns, he or she may prescribe steroid lotion. This is not of particular benefit. The rare second-degree burns may be treated with antibiotics in addition to analgesics or sedation. There is no evidence that steroid lotions or antibiotic creams help in the *usual* case of sunburn. Most doctors prescribe therapy that is available at home.

Lice

Lice are found in the best of families. Lack of prejudice with respect to social class is as close as lice come to having a virtue. At best, they are a nuisance; at worst, they can cause real disability.

Lice themselves are very small and are seldom seen without the aid of a magnifying glass. There are three types of lice that infect children's hair, bodies, or pubic areas.

Head lice are quite common in day care centers and schools. Lice are very small and difficult to see. Usually, it is easier to find the "nits," which are clusters of **louse eggs**. Without magnification, nits will appear as tiny white lumps on hair strands. Sometimes other skin particles on the hair shaft can be confused with nits. These particles usually slide off the hair easily, but nits do not. During epidemics of head lice, children should be cautioned about sharing hats. Clothing should not be hung in closely crowded areas.

Pubic lice are not a "venereal disease," although they may be spread from person to person during sexual contact. Unlike syphilis and gonorrhea, lice can be spread by toilet seats, infected bedding, and other sources. Pubic lice bear some resemblance to crabs, hence the use of the name "crabs" to indicate a lice infestation of the pubic hair. Lice like to be close to a warm body all the time and will not live for long periods in clothing not being worn, unused bedding, and so on.

Body lice are uncommon in children but cause severe itching that may lead to skin infection.

Home Treatment

Permethrin (1%) is the most effective product and is available over the counter as a cream rinse (Nix). Apply it to the child's scalp for 10 minutes. Because it lasts for 2 weeks, one treatment is usually all that is needed.

Other over-the-counter preparations containing pyrethrins are also effective against lice. These include A-200, RID, and R & C shampoo. RID has the advantage of supplying a fine-tooth comb, a rare item these days. Repeat treatment 7 to 10 days later is needed with these products.

Bedding and clothing must be changed simultaneously and should be washed in water hotter than 130°F (54°C) or stored in plastic bags for 10 days. Sexual partners should be treated at the same time.

Most failures of home treatment are not due to using the wrong shampoo but failure to remove the eggs with a fine-tooth comb and reinfection through unwashed clothes and linens.

What to Expect

If lice are the suspected problem, the doctor will make a careful inspection to see if he or she can find nits or the lice themselves.

Lice

Is either of the following conditions present?
▲ Lice seen on skin or in clothing
▲ Nits seen on hair shafts

Yes →

Use Home Treatment

↓ **No**

Suspect...

problem other than lice. Check Skin Problems Table on pp. 370–371.

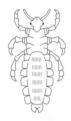

Head louse (approx. 10x)

Head louse (approx. size)

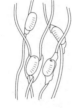

Louse eggs on hair

Pubic louse (approx. 10x)

Pubic louse (approx. size)

Bedbugs

Bedbug bites cause itchy red bumps. The adult bedbug is flat, wingless, oval in shape, reddish in color, and about ¼ inch (6 mm) in length. Like lice, bedbugs stay alive by sucking blood. Unlike lice, they feed for only 10 to 15 minutes at a time and spend the rest of the time hiding in crevices and crannies.

Bedbugs feed almost entirely at night because that is when bodies are in bed and because they have a real aversion to light. They have such a keen sense of the nearness of a warm body that the U.S. Army has used them to detect the approach of an enemy at ranges of several hundred feet! Catching these pests out in the open is very difficult and may require some curious behavior. One technique is to dash into the bedroom at bedtime, flip on the lights, and pull back the bedcovers in an effort to catch them in anticipation of their next meal.

The bite of a bedbug leaves a firm bump. Usually, two or three bumps are clustered together. Occasionally, a child may develop a sensitivity to these bites, in which case itching may be severe and blisters may form.

Home Treatment
Because bedbugs don't hide on the body or in clothes, you should treat the bed and the bedroom. Contact your local health department for information. Some chemical sprays are dangerous, especially for children. Simply getting the exposed bedding outdoors and exposed to the sun and air for several days may work as well.

What to Expect
The doctor will be hard-pressed to make a certain diagnosis of bedbug bites without information from you that bedbugs have been seen in the house. However, the bumps may be suggestive, and you and the doctor may decide to assume that the problem is bedbugs. If this is the case, the doctor will recommend treatment with an insecticide (see "Home Treatment").

Bedbugs

Have bedbugs been seen on or near the bed?

Yes →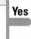
Use Home Treatment

No ↓

Suspect...
problem other than bedbugs. Check Skin Problems Table on pp. 370–371.

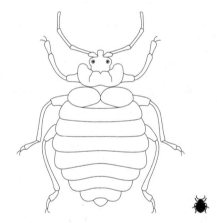

Bedbug
(approx. 10x)

Bedbug
(approx. size)

Ticks

Outdoor living has its dangers. Although you can usually avoid bears, mountain lions, and vertical cliffs, the shrubs and tall grasses that hide tiny insects eager for blood from a passing animal or person are hard to avoid. Ticks are among the most common of the small hazards. The tick achieved celebrity status with its appearance on the cover of *Newsweek* some years back. *Notoriety* is a more appropriate term for the tick's role in transmitting an organism causing Lyme disease (page 406).

Ticks are rather easily seen, and a tick bite usually has the obvious cause sticking out of it. Ticks are about ¼ inch (6 mm) long. The tick buries its head and crablike pincers beneath the skin, with the body and legs protruding. Ticks feed on passing animals such as dogs, deer, and people.

Practice tick prevention with your children. When they go out into the woods, they should wear protective clothing such as long-sleeved shirts, long slacks or trousers, and socks. If possible, tuck the trousers into the socks to prevent ticks from getting near the skin. In tick-infested areas, it is helpful to check your child's hair periodically. You may be able to catch the ticks before they become embedded by checking after hikes.

Tick-Borne Diseases

Besides Lyme disease, ticks can carry other diseases, such as **Rocky Mountain spotted fever**. If a fever, rash, or headache follows a tick bite by a few days or weeks, consult the doctor.

If a pregnant female tick is allowed to remain feeding for many days, under certain circumstances a peculiar condition called **tick paralysis** may result. The female tick secretes a toxin that can cause temporary paralysis. The condition will clear up shortly after the tick is removed. This complication is quite rare and can happen only if the tick stays in place for many days.

Home Treatment

For advice on preventing ticks, see Lyme Disease, page 406.

Ticks should be removed, although they will eventually "fester" out, and complications are unusual. The trick is to get the tick to "let go" with the pincers and not to kill the tick before getting it out. If the mouthparts and pincers remain under the skin, healing may take several weeks.

Make the tick uncomfortable with its new home. Alcohol, acetone, oil, or gentle heat from a heated paper clip are home remedies that have occasionally worked. We prefer to use tweezers to grasp the tick and remove it slowly with a straight pulling motion. If you inadvertently leave the head under the skin, have the child

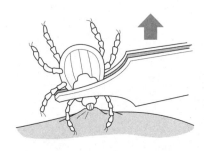

Removing a tick

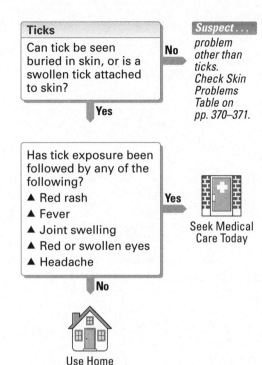

Ticks

Can tick be seen buried in skin, or is a swollen tick attached to skin?

No →

↓ **Yes**

Has tick exposure been followed by any of the following?
▲ Red rash
▲ Fever
▲ Joint swelling
▲ Red or swollen eyes
▲ Headache

Yes →

Seek Medical
Care Today

↓ **No**

Use Home
Treatment

soak the spot gently with warm water twice a day until healing is complete.

Call the doctor if your child gets a fever, rash, or headache within three weeks of the tick bite. (See Lyme Disease, page 406.)

What to Expect

The doctor can remove the tick but cannot prevent any illness that might have been transmitted. You can do as well with home treatment. We always seem to be removing ticks from unusual places, such as armpits and belly buttons, but the scalp is the most common location. The technique is exactly the same, no matter where the tick is.

If the doctor suspects Lyme disease or Rocky Mountain spotted fever, he or she will do blood tests and administer antibiotics, if required.

Lyme Disease (Ticks)

First discovered as a disease in 1975 and named for its town of origin in Connecticut, Lyme disease has become a distressingly common illness. Whereas only 11 states reported several hundred cases in 1982, Lyme disease was reported in more than 27,000 individuals in 47 states in 2007. The Northeast, from Massachusetts to Maryland, and parts of the upper Midwest (Minnesota and Wisconsin) have the biggest populations of infected ticks and highest rates of Lyme disease.

The disease is caused by the *Borrelia burgdorferi* bacteria and infects people by hitching a ride in a tick. When an infected tick bites an unfortunate person, the bacteria may be transferred to the blood of the host. Fortunately for the millions of people who give free rides to ticks every spring and summer, only a small number of ticks are infected, and it takes a prolonged feed (generally more than two days) to transfer the bacteria. Young, small ticks are most likely to transmit Lyme disease, in part because they are much smaller and therefore harder to find than adult ticks while they feed.

Home Treatment

As usual, prevention is preferred to treatment. In areas where there are many infected ticks, take the following steps.

▲ Dress children in clothing that covers the arms and legs. It's easier to spot ticks on light-colored clothing.

▲ You can spray permethrin on clothes to discourage ticks and use insect repellents containing DEET on uncovered skin.

▲ If you are hiking on a trail, stay in the center to avoid brush on the sides.

▲ Check children after every outdoor experience during tick season. The hair is a favorite hiding place.

▲ Ticks also enjoy dogs (which can also develop Lyme disease), so don't forget to check your pets.

▲ Removing dead leaves, tall grass, and brush from around your home may reduce your tick tenants (and will also reduce the fire risk).

Ticks can be removed with tweezers, using a strong steady pull (see Ticks, page 404).

If you suspect that your child may have been bitten by a tick, watch for symptoms. The most serious symptoms are a circular lesion wider than $1\frac{1}{2}$ inches (4 cm) in the area of the bite, numbness, stiff neck, and weak face muscles.

What to Expect

Lyme disease is difficult to diagnose. An early manifestation usually involves a large red rash around the tick bite, accompanied by fever, headache, joint pain, and swollen lymph glands. The early disease may occur a few days or a month after the bite of an infected tick. Late Lyme disease can occur weeks to years after infection and may include arthritis, nervous system problems, and even heartbeat difficulties.

If your child develops the characteristic bull's-eye rash and other symptoms of Lyme disease after a known or suspected tick encounter, your doctor can

Lyme Disease

Following a known or suspected tick bite, does your child show any of these symptoms?

▲ Circular lesion larger than 1½ inches (4 cm) in area of bite
▲ Numbness
▲ Stiff neck
▲ Weak face muscles

Yes → Seek Medical Care Today

No ↓

Following a known or suspected tick bite, does your child show any of these symptoms?

▲ Chills and fever
▲ Headache
▲ Muscle and joint pain
▲ Swollen lymph glands

Yes → Call Medical Advisor

No ↓

Use Home Treatment

Deer tick (approx. 10x)   approx. size

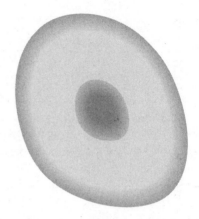

Lyme disease cause and effect. The deer tick (top) can carry the bacteria that cause Lyme disease. A "bull's-eye" rash (bottom) in the area of the tick bite is a characteristic symptom and indicates the need for a prompt visit to the doctor.

order a variety of tests to check for Lyme disease. If Lyme disease is confirmed, the doctor will prescribe one of several antibiotics. Doxycycline and amoxicillin are commonly used for localized or early disease. Other antibiotics are used for more complicated cases.

West Nile Virus (Mosquitoes)

Although previously just a nuisance of summer, mosquitoes are now responsible for one of the latest epidemics in the United States, West Nile Virus. This virus was first noted to cause disease in a woman in the West Nile District of Uganda in 1937. It did not arrive in the United States until 1999. In 2007 more than 3,600 cases were reported in the United States, with 124 deaths. Most serious cases occurred in persons over age 50. One third of the cases were in California while most New England states did not have any cases. Infections generally occur in the late summer and early fall.

The virus is carried by mosquitoes who have previously fed on infected birds. Fortunately, most people who acquire the virus after a mosquito bite will never have any symptoms. Only about 1 in 5 infected persons develop symptoms. About half will have fever alone or fever associated with swollen glands. The other half will have involvement of the nervous system with symptoms such as severe headache, neck stiffness, dizziness, and, potentially, seizures and coma.

Home Treatment

Prevention is the way to avoid this illness. A variety of approaches are effective to minimize mosquito bites.

▲ Dress children in clothes that cover arms and legs.
▲ Spray permethrin on clothes (not skin) to discourage mosquitoes.
▲ Use insect repellent on uncovered skin. Products containing DEET or Picaridin are very effective. Higher concentration products (more than 20% DEET) last longer (about 5 hours) than low concentration (5%) products, which last about 1½ hours. Oil of lemon eucalyptus is comparable to low concentration DEET.
▲ Be aware that peak mosquito biting times begin at dusk and continue till dawn. Be extra cautious during those times.
▲ Drain standing water. This is where mosquitoes breed and lay eggs.
▲ Install or repair window screens. Keep mosquitoes out of your home.
▲ Call local authorities if you find a dead bird. Birds die for many reasons (including encounters with household cats). But some may be infected with West Nile virus.

For regular mosquito bites, keeping the area clean is important. Calamine lotion may relieve some of the itching. If there is a growing area of redness around the bite it may have become infected and you should contact your physician. (See Impetigo, page 378.)

What to Expect

West Nile Virus is uncommon in children but does occur. If your child is having fever or swollen glands (common symptoms with the disease) it is unlikely that West Nile Virus is the culprit and equally unlikely your doctor will order the laboratory tests to identify the virus. However, in unexplained nervous system diseases such as meningitis that occur in the late summer, a blood test might be ordered. Treatment is directed at minimizing the symptoms and keeping the patient supported until the illness resolves. As is the case with most viruses, there is not a specific medicine available to fight West Nile virus.

West Nile Virus

In a child probably bitten by a mosquito, are any of the following present?
▲ High fever
▲ Severe headache
▲ Stiff neck
▲ Disorientation
▲ Coma
▲ Muscle weakness
▲ Muscle tremors
▲ Seizures

Yes

Seek Medical
Care Now

No

Is there redness around mosquito bite?

Yes

Call Medical
Advisor

No

Use Home
Treatment

Chiggers

Chiggers are small red mites, sometimes called "red bugs." Their bite contains a chemical that eats away at the skin, causing a tremendous itch. Usually, the small red sores are around the belt line or other openings in clothes. Careful inspection may reveal the tiny red larvae in the center of the itching sore. Chiggers live on grasses and shrubs.

Home Treatment

Chiggers are better avoided than treated. Using insect repellents, wearing clothing that covers the arms and legs, and bathing after exposure help cut down on the frequency of bites. Once you get chiggers, they itch, often for several weeks. Keep the sores clean and soak them with warm water twice a day. A-200 and RID applied during the first few days will help kill the larvae, but the itch will persist.

What to Expect

Doctors usually prescribe Kwell for chiggers, which is perhaps slightly more effective than A-200 or RID but does not stop the itching either. The doctor may prescribe an antihistamine (page 224) if intense itching persists despite home treatment with acetaminophen, ibuprofen, warm baths, oatmeal soaks, and calamine lotion (page 227).

Chiggers

Are any of the following present?

▲ Itchy red sores around belt line or other opening in clothes

▲ Itchy red sores following contact with grass or shrubs

▲ Small red mites seen on skin or red spot in center of sore

No → **Suspect . . .** *problem other than chiggers. Check Skin Problems Table on pp. 370–371.*

Yes

Use Home Treatment

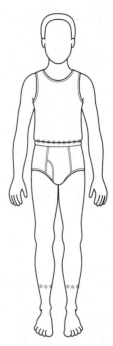

Sites of chigger bites

Scabies

Scabies is an irritation of the skin caused by a tiny mite related to the chigger. The itching is intense. No one knows why, but scabies seems to be on the rise in this country. As with lice, scabies is no longer related to hygiene. It occurs in the best of families and in the best of neighborhoods. The mite is easily spread from person to person or by contact with items such as clothing and bedding that may harbor the mite. Epidemics often spread through schools despite strict precautions against contact with known cases.

Scabies affects children differently depending on their age:

▲ Young children—head, neck, shoulders, palms, and soles of feet
▲ Older children—hands, wrists, and belly

The mite burrows into the skin to lay eggs. These burrows may be evident, especially at the beginning of the problem. However, the mite soon causes the skin to have a reaction to it, so that redness, swelling, and blisters follow within a short time. Intense itching causes scratching, and the scratch marks may become infected from bacteria on the skin. Thus the telltale burrows are often obscured by scratch marks, blisters, and a secondary infection.

If you can locate something that looks like a burrow, you might be able to see the mite with the aid of a magnifying lens. This is the only way to be absolutely sure that the problem is scabies. The diagnosis in most children is made on the basis of a problem that is consistent with scabies and the fact that scabies is known to be in the community.

Home Treatment
There is no effective home remedy to eliminate the scabies mite. However, symptoms can be minimized.

For itching, we recommend cool soaks and calamine lotion (page 227). Hydrocortisone cream is effective in relieving symptoms. Antihistamines (page 224) such as chlorpheniramine (Chlor-Trimeton) or diphenhydramine (Benadryl) are available without a prescription but often cause drowsiness. Follow the directions that come with the package. As in the case of poison ivy, warmth makes the itching worse by releasing histamine, but if all the histamine is released, then relief may be obtained for several hours. (See Poison Ivy and Poison Oak, page 384.)

What to Expect
The doctor should examine the entire skin surface for signs of the problem and may examine the area with a magnifying lens in an attempt to identify the mite. He or she may scrape the lesion to examine it under the microscope. Usually, the doctor will be forced to make a decision based on the probability of various kinds of diseases and then treat it much as you would at home. The proof of the pudding will be whether the treatment is successful.

The first-line drug against scabies is 5% permethrin (Elimite). Other effective drugs include crotamiton cream (Eurax) and gamma benzene hexachloride (Kwell). Kwell is prescribed with caution for infants because of its potential toxicity. Hydroxyzine (Atarax, Vistaril) may be prescribed for intense itching.

Scabies

Are the following conditions present?

▲ Intense itching

▲ Raised red skin in a line (represents a burrow) and possibly blisters or pustules

▲ Located on hands (especially between fingers); in elbow crease, armpit, or groin crease; or behind knees

▲ Exposure to scabies

No →

Suspect . . .
problem other than scabies. Check Skin Problems Table on pp. 370–371.

Yes

Make Medical Appointment

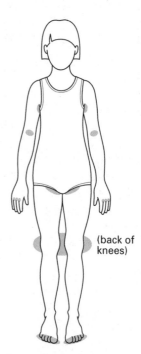

(back of knees)

Sites of scabies bites

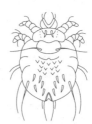

Scabies mite, greatly enlarged (approx. size: ·)

Dandruff and Cradle Cap

Although they look somewhat different, cradle cap and dandruff are really part of the same problem, called **seborrhea**. It occurs when the oil glands in the skin have been stimulated by adult hormones, leading to oiliness and flaking of the scalp. Children will frequently have redness and scaling of the eyebrows and behind the ears as well.

Seborrhea itself is a somewhat ugly but relatively harmless condition. However, it may make the skin more susceptible to infection with yeast or bacteria. Cradle cap occurs in infants because of exposure to the mother's hormones. Dandruff occurs in older children when they begin to make their own adult hormones. However, seborrhea does occur between these two ages. Once a child has the problem, it tends to recur.

Lookalike Problems

Occasionally, this condition is confused with **ringworm** of the scalp (page 380). Careful attention to the conditions listed in the decision chart will usually help you avoid this confusion. Remember also that ringworm is unusual in a newborn or a very young child.

Psoriasis often stops at the hairline. Furthermore, the scales of psoriasis are on top of raised lesions called "plaques," which is not the case with seborrhea. Psoriasis requires a doctor's help.

Home Treatment

Dandruff

One of the most effective ingredients for treating dandruff is selenium sulfide. Selsun (available by prescription only) and Selsun Blue are brand names of shampoos that contain selenium sulfide. Selsun Blue is available over the counter, and, though weaker than Selsun, it is just as good if you apply more of it more frequently. When using these shampoos, it is important to follow the directions carefully, because they can cause oiliness and a yellowish discoloration of the hair.

Sebutone and Pragmatar contain salicylic acid—sulfur combinations that are not quite as effective. Least effective are products that contain only tar.

The heavily advertised antidandruff shampoos such as Head & Shoulders contain zinc pyrithione and are helpful in mild to moderate cases of dandruff.

Cradle Cap

Cradle cap is best treated with a scrub brush. If the cradle cap is thick, rub in warm baby oil, cover with a warm towel, and let sit for 15 minutes. Use a fine-tooth comb or scrub brush to help remove the scale. Then shampoo with Sebulex or one of the preparations listed above. Be careful to avoid getting shampoo in the child's eyes.

No matter what you do, the problem will often return, and you may have to repeat the treatment. If the problem gets worse despite home treatment over several weeks, see the doctor.

What to Expect

Severe cases of seborrhea may require more than the medications listed above. A prescription cream such as ketoconazole (Nizoral) may be prescribed. Consult the doctor to clear up any confusion concerning the diagnosis. The doctor will usually make a diagnosis on the basis of the

**Dandruff
and Cradle Cap**

In an infant, are all
of the following
conditions present?

▲ Thick, adherent,
oily, yellowish,
scaling or crusting
patches

▲ Located on the scalp,
behind the ears, or
(less frequently) in
the skin creases of
the groin

▲ Only mild redness
in involved areas

Yes →

Suspect...
*problem
other than
cradle cap.
Check Skin
Problems
Table on
pp. 370–371.*

In an older child
(especially an adoles-
cent), are all of the
following conditions
present?

▲ Fine, white, oily
scales

▲ Confined to scalp
and/or eyebrows

▲ Only *mild* redness
in involved areas

No →

Suspect...
*problem
other than
dandruff.
Check Skin
Problems
Table on
pp. 370–371.*

↓ **No**

Use Home
Treatment

appearance of the rash. Occasionally, he or she will look at scrapings from the involved areas under the microscope. Drugs by mouth or by injection are not indicated for seborrhea unless a bacterial infection has complicated the problem.

Patchy Loss of Skin Color

Children are constantly getting minor cuts, and scrapes, insect bites, and other minor skin infections. During the healing process, it is common for the skin to lose some of its color. With time (months to years), the skin coloring generally returns.

In the summertime, many light-skinned children appear to develop small, round, colorless spots on the face. The white spots have probably been present for some time, but tanning reveals them. This condition is known as **pityriasis alba**. The cause is unknown, but it is believed to be a mild inflammation of cosmetic concern only. The condition may take many months to disappear and may recur, but there are virtually never any long-term effects.

If there are lightly scaled, tan, pink, or white patches on the neck or back, the problem is most likely due to a very minor and superficial fungal infection known as **pityriasis (tinea) versicolor**.

Occasionally, **ringworm**, a fungal infection, will begin as a small round area of scaling with associated loss of skin color. (See Ringworm, page 380.)

Vitiligo is an unusual problem characterized by complete loss of skin color with the skin appearing white.

Home Treatment

Waiting is the most effective home treatment for loss of skin color. Pityriasis (tinea) versicolor can be treated by applying Selsun Blue shampoo to the affected area once every day or so until the lesions are gone. Follow the directions for application on the shampoo bottle. Unfortunately, this condition almost always comes back. Pityriasis alba often gets better with 1% hydrocortisone cream.

What to Expect

The doctor will take a history and perform a careful examination of the skin. He or she may take scrapings of the lesions, because tinea versicolor can be identified from these scrapings. Pityriasis alba should be distinguished from more severe fungal infections that may occur on the face. Pityriasis versicolor may be treated with higher strength (2.5%) selenium sulfide or other topical antifungals. Again, scrapings will help identify the fungus. For vitiligo, steroids may be prescribed as well as ultraviolet therapy.

Patchy Loss of Skin Color

Are the following conditions present?

▲ Scaling edges

▲ Circular, enlarging areas

▲ Clearing of center

Yes → *See:* Ringworm, p. 380

No ↓

Are the following conditions present?

▲ Lightly scaled, tan, pink, or white patches

▲ Confined to the neck and upper back

Yes → *Suspect...* pityriasis (tinea) versicolor and...   Use Home Treatment

No ↓

Are the following conditions present?

▲ White scaly patches on face

▲ More noticeable with suntan

▲ No signs of infection (crusting, redness, oozing, or fever)

Yes → *Suspect...* pityriasis alba and...   Use Home Treatment   → *If no response...*   Make Medical Appointment

No ↓

Is there complete loss of skin color?

Yes → *Suspect...* vitiligo and...   Make Medical Appointment

No ↓

Did loss of skin color follow cut or infection?

Yes → Use Home Treatment

No ↓

Call Medical Advisor

"Classic" Childhood Diseases

Chicken Pox

Chicken pox is now preventable with an immunization. However, some children are not yet immunized.

It is valuable to know the signs of chicken pox because you can then avoid taking your child to the doctor for these symptoms. As soon as you recognize chicken pox, do *not* give your child aspirin during the course of the disease. Use acetaminophen or ibuprofen instead (page 218).

How to Recognize Chicken Pox

Before the Rash. Usually there are no symptoms before the rash appears, but occasionally there is fatigue and a mild fever 24 hours before the rash is noted.

The Rash. The typical rash goes through the following stages.

1. It may appear as flat red splotches.

2. The splotches become raised and may resemble small pimples.

3. They develop into small blisters, called vesicles, which are very fragile. They may look like drops of water on a red base. The tops are easily scratched off.

4. The vesicles tend to appear in crops, with 2 to 4 crops appearing within 2 to 6 days. All stages may be present in the same area. They often appear first on the scalp and the face and then spread to the rest of the body, but they may begin anywhere. They are most numerous over the shoulders, chest, and back. They are occasionally found on the palms of the hands or the soles of the feet. They may also be found in the mouth or in the vagina. There may be only a few sores, or there may be hundreds.

5. As the vesicles break, the sores become "pustular" and form a crust. (The crust is made of dried serum, not true pus.) This stage may be reached within several hours of the first appearance of the rash. Itching is often severe in the pustular stage. The crust falls away between the 9th and the 13th days.

Fever. After most of the sores have formed crusts, the fever usually subsides.

How Chicken Pox Spreads

Chicken pox spreads very easily in un-immunized children—more than 90% of brothers and sisters catch it! It may be transmitted from 24 hours before the rash appears up to about 6 days after. It is spread by droplets from the mouth or throat or by direct contact with contaminated articles of clothing. It is not spread by dry scabs. The time from exposure to signs of illness is 10 to 21 days. Chicken pox leads to lifelong immunity with rare exceptions.

The same virus that causes chicken pox also causes **shingles** (herpes zoster), and anyone with a history of chicken pox may develop shingles later in life.

Chicken pox can be a serious problem in children with cancer or those receiving drugs that affect the immune system. See page 170 for information about immunizations for chicken pox.

Most of the time, chicken pox should be treated at home. Complications are rare. The specific questions on the decision chart deal with complications that may require more than home treatment: encephalitis (viral infection of the brain), pneumonia, and severe bacterial infection of the lesions. Encephalitis and pneumonia are rare.

Home Treatment

The major problem in dealing with chicken pox is control of the intense itching. Warm baths containing Aveeno or baking soda (½ cup, or 115 g, in a tubful of water) frequently help. Calamine lotion (page 227) may be temporarily helpful. The use of antihistamines (page 224) is sometimes necessary and may require contact with your doctor. Check by phone before exposing other children in a doctor's office. **Caution:** *Do not give your child aspirin, because of the associated risk of Reye syndrome* (page 220). Use acetaminophen or ibuprofen (page 218) for fever.

Cut fingernails or use gloves to prevent scarring from scratching. When lesions occur in the mouth, gargling with salt water (½ teaspoon salt in 1 cup, or 240 ml, water) may help. Wash the child's hands three times a day, and keep the skin gently but scrupulously clean to prevent a complicating bacterial infection. A minor bacterial infection will respond to soap and time. If it becomes severe and results in the return of a fever, see the doctor.

What to Expect

Do not be surprised if the doctor is willing and even anxious to treat the case over the phone. Doctors are concerned about exposure to other children who have chronic medical problems. If it is necessary to bring the child to the doctor's office, try to keep him or her separate from other children. In healthy children, chicken pox has few lasting ill effects, but in children with other serious illnesses, it can be a devastating or even fatal disease. A visit to the doctor's office may not be necessary unless a complication seems possible.

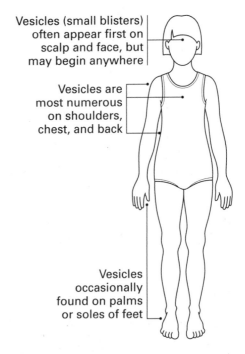

Vesicles (small blisters) often appear first on scalp and face, but may begin anywhere

Vesicles are most numerous on shoulders, chest, and back

Vesicles occasionally found on palms or soles of feet

Chicken pox. Usually there are no symptoms before the rash. Do not give aspirin during the course of the disease.

Chicken Pox

Are there convulsions, a stiff neck, severe lethargy, or severe headaches? **Yes** →
Seek Medical Care Now

No ↓

Is breathing rapid? (*See:* "How fast is your child breathing?", p. 241.) **Yes** →
Seek Medical Care Now

No ↓

Do any of the lesions appear seriously infected (surrounded by a large area of redness or draining pus)? **Yes** →
Seek Medical Care Today

No ↓

Has there been exposure to chicken pox in a child:
▲ With cancer?
▲ Taking steroids?
▲ With an immunity problem?
▲ Who is a newborn whose mother has chicken pox? **Yes** → *CALL DOCTOR NOW.*

No ↓

Has a pregnant woman been exposed? **Yes** → *Have her call doctor today.*

No ↓

Use Home Treatment

Measles

This type of measles is also called "red measles," "7-day measles," or "10-day measles," as opposed to German, or 3-day, measles (page 426). Unlike some of the other childhood illnesses, measles can be quite severe. It is a preventable disease. The results of more than three decades of immunizing children are remarkable, with the elimination of 99% of cases. Make sure your child is immunized against measles.

How to Recognize Measles
Early Signs. Measles is a viral illness that begins with a fever, weakness, a dry "brassy" cough, and inflamed eyes that are itchy, red, and sensitive to the light. These symptoms begin three to five days before the appearance of the rash.

Another early sign of measles is the appearance of fine white spots on a red base inside the mouth opposite the molars (Koplik's spots). These fade as the skin rash appears.

Rash. The rash begins on about the fifth day as a pink, blotchy, flat rash. The rash first appears around the hairline, on the face, on the neck, and behind the ears. The spots, which fade on pressure early in the illness, become somewhat darker and tend to merge into larger red patches as they mature.

The rash spreads from head to chest to abdomen and finally to arms and legs. It lasts four to seven days and may be accompanied by mild itching. There may be some light brown coloring to the skin lesions as the illness progresses.

How Measles Spreads
Measles is a highly contagious viral disease. It is spread by droplets from the mouth or throat and by direct contact with articles freshly soiled by nose and throat secretions. It may be spread during the period from 3 to 6 days before the appearance of the rash to several days after. Symptoms begin in an exposed susceptible person approximately 8 to 12 days after exposure to the virus.

There are many complications of measles. Sore throats, ear infections, and pneumonia are all common. Many of these complicating infections are due to bacteria and will require antibiotic treatment. The pneumonia can be life threatening. A very serious problem that can

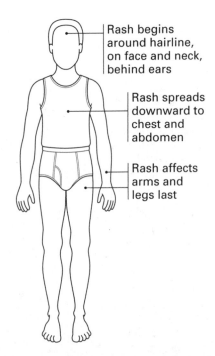

Rash begins around hairline, on face and neck, behind ears

Rash spreads downward to chest and abdomen

Rash affects arms and legs last

Measles. Early signs include red, itchy eyes; "brassy" cough; and Koplik's spots inside mouth.

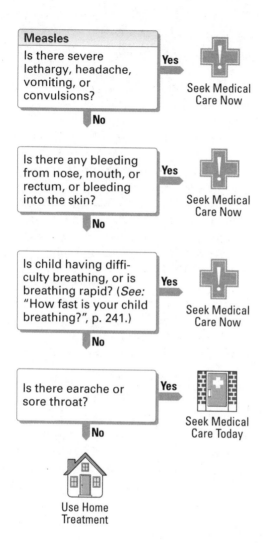

Measles

Is there severe lethargy, headache, vomiting, or convulsions? — **Yes** → Seek Medical Care Now

↓ **No**

Is there any bleeding from nose, mouth, or rectum, or bleeding into the skin? — **Yes** → Seek Medical Care Now

↓ **No**

Is child having difficulty breathing, or is breathing rapid? (*See:* "How fast is your child breathing?", p. 241.) — **Yes** → Seek Medical Care Now

↓ **No**

Is there earache or sore throat? — **Yes** → Seek Medical Care Today

↓ **No**

Use Home Treatment

lead to permanent damage is **measles encephalitis** (infection of the brain). Life-support measures and treatment of seizures are necessary when this rare complication occurs.

Home Treatment

Symptomatic measures are all that is needed for uncomplicated measles. Give the child acetaminophen or ibuprofen (page 218) to keep the fever down, and use a vaporizer (page 223) to relieve a cough. Dim lighting in the room often makes the child feel more comfortable because of the eyes' sensitivity to light. He or she should be isolated until the end of the contagious period. All unimmunized children who come in contact with the sick child should be brought to be immunized immediately after symptoms begin in the first child.

What to Expect

The doctor will direct the history and physical examination at determining the diagnosis of measles and the nature of any complications. Bacterial complications, such as ear infections and pneumonia, are usually treated with antibiotics. A child with symptoms suggestive of encephalitis (lethargy, stiff neck, convulsions) will be hospitalized, and a spinal tap will be performed. Very rarely, there may be a problem with blood clotting, so that bleeding occurs, usually first apparent as dark purple splotches on the skin. It is best to avoid these problems with measles immunization, which is discussed on page 166.

Mumps/ Swollen Salivary Glands

Mumps is a viral infection of the salivary glands. It can be prevented with an immunization, and few children today will be troubled with mumps. Only 100 children a year develop mumps. However, other infections may involve the salivary glands.

The major salivary glands are located directly below and in front of the ear. Before any swelling is noticeable, the child may have a low fever, complain of a headache or an earache, or experience weakness. Fever is variable; it may be only slightly above normal or as high as 104°F (40°C). After several days of these symptoms, one or both salivary glands (parotid glands) may swell.

It is sometimes difficult to distinguish mumps or other salivary gland infections from swollen lymph glands in the neck. In mumps, you will not be able to feel the edge of your child's jaw beneath the ear. Chewing and swallowing may produce pain behind the ear. Sour substances, such as lemons and pickles, may make the pain worse. When swelling occurs on both sides, children take on the appearance of chipmunks!

Mumps is quite contagious during the period from 2 days before the first symptoms to the complete disappearance of the parotid gland swelling (usually about a week after the swelling has begun). Mumps will develop in a susceptible exposed person approximately 16 to 18 days after exposure to the virus. In children, it is generally a mild illness.

The decision chart is directed toward detection of the rare complications of mumps, which include encephalitis (viral infection of the brain), pancreatitis (viral infection of the pancreas), kidney disease, deafness, and involvement of the testicles or ovaries. Complications are far more frequent in adults than in children.

Home Treatment

The pain may be reduced with acetaminophen or ibuprofen (page 218). The child may have difficulty eating, but adequate fluid intake is important. Avoid giving the child sour foods, including orange juice. Adults who have not had mumps should avoid exposure to the child until complete disappearance of the swelling. Many adults who do not recall having mumps as a child may have had an extremely mild case and consequently are not at risk of developing mumps.

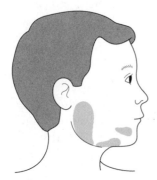

Sites of swelling in mumps

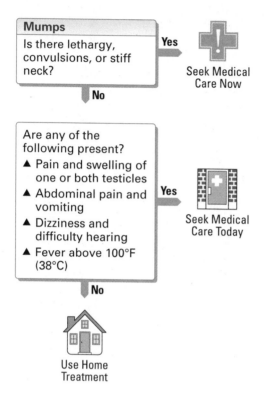

Mumps

Is there lethargy, convulsions, or stiff neck?

Yes → Seek Medical Care Now

No ↓

Are any of the following present?
▲ Pain and swelling of one or both testicles
▲ Abdominal pain and vomiting
▲ Dizziness and difficulty hearing
▲ Fever above 100°F (38°C)

Yes → Seek Medical Care Today

No ↓

Use Home Treatment

What to Expect

If you suspect a complication of mumps, see the doctor. He or she will direct the history and physical examination at confirming the diagnosis or the presence of a complication. The rare complication of a right ovarian infection may be confused with appendicitis, and blood tests may be required.

Because mumps is a viral disease, there is no medicine that will directly kill the virus. Supportive measures may be necessary for some of the complications. Fortunately, these occur rarely, and permanent damage to hearing or other functions is unusual. Mumps very rarely produces sterility in men or women, even with complicating involvement of the testes or ovaries. Mumps vaccination is discussed on page 168.

If salivary gland infection from bacteria is suspected, antibiotics will be given.

Rubella (German Measles)

Rubella is also known as "German measles" and "3-day measles." (See Measles, page 422.)

How to Recognize Rubella

Before the Rash. There may be a few days of mild fatigue. Lymph nodes at the back of the neck may be enlarged and tender.

Rash. The rash first appears on the face as flat or slightly raised red spots. It quickly spreads to the trunk and the extremities, and the discrete spots tend to merge into large patches. The rash of rubella is highly variable and is difficult for even the most experienced parents and doctors to recognize. Often there is no rash.

Fever. The fever rarely goes above 101°F (38.3°C) and usually lasts less than two days.

Pain. Joint pain occurs in about 10 to 15% of older children and adolescents. The pain usually begins on the third day of the illness.

How Rubella Spreads

German measles is a mild viral infection that is not as contagious as measles or chicken pox. It is usually spread by droplets from the mouth or throat. The incubation period is 12 to 21 days, with an average of 16 days.

The specific questions on the decision chart are addressed to possible complications, which are extremely rare. The main concern with German measles is an infection in an unborn child. If 3-day measles occurs during the first month of pregnancy, there is a 50% chance that the fetus will develop an abnormality such as cataracts, heart disease, deafness, or mental deficiency. By the third month of pregnancy, this risk decreases to less than 10%, and it continues to decrease throughout the pregnancy. Because of the problem of congenital defects, a vaccine for German measles was developed. Rubella immunization is discussed on page 167.

Home Treatment

Usually no therapy is required. Occasionally, fever will require the use of acetaminophen or ibuprofen (page 218). Isolation is usually not imposed.

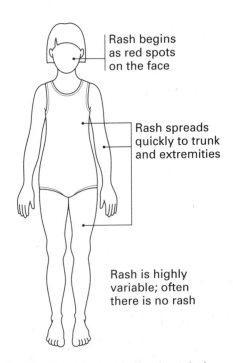

Rash begins as red spots on the face

Rash spreads quickly to trunk and extremities

Rash is highly variable; often there is no rash

Rubella. For a few days before the rash, the child may experience mild fatigue and have enlarged, tender lymph nodes at the back of the neck.

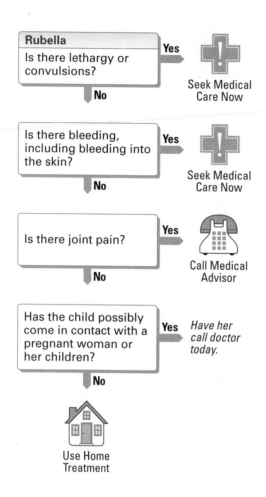

Rubella

Is there lethargy or convulsions? — **Yes** → Seek Medical Care Now

↓ **No**

Is there bleeding, including bleeding into the skin? — **Yes** → Seek Medical Care Now

↓ **No**

Is there joint pain? — **Yes** → Call Medical Advisor

↓ **No**

Has the child possibly come in contact with a pregnant woman or her children? — **Yes** → *Have her call doctor today.*

↓ **No**

Use Home Treatment

Avoid any exposure of the child to women who could be pregnant. If a question of such exposure arises, the pregnant woman should discuss the risk with her doctor. Blood tests are available that will indicate whether a pregnant woman has had rubella in the past and is immune, or whether problems with the pregnancy might be encountered.

What to Expect

Visits to the doctor's office are seldom required for uncomplicated German measles. Questions about possible infection of pregnant women can often be discussed over the telephone.

Roseola

Roseola is most common in children under the age of three but may occur at any age. Its main significance lies in the sudden high fever, which may cause a convulsion (page 312). Such a convulsion does not indicate that the child has epilepsy. Prompt treatment of the fever is essential. (See Fever, page 288.)

How to Recognize Roseola

Fever. There are usually several days of sustained high fever, and sometimes this fever can trigger a convulsion or seizure in a susceptible child. Otherwise, the child appears well.

Rash. The rash appears as the fever is decreasing or shortly after it is gone. It consists of pink, well-defined patches that turn white on pressure and first appear on the trunk. It may be slightly bumpy. It spreads to involve the arms and neck but is seldom prominent on the face or legs. The rash usually lasts less than 24 hours.

Other Symptoms. Occasionally, there is a slight runny nose, throat redness, or swollen glands at the back of the head, behind the ears, or in the neck. Most often there are no other symptoms.

This disease has been found to be caused by human herpes virus 6. Consequently, this condition, long known as **exanthem subitum**, has become sixth disease. It is contagious. Keep the child out of contact with other children until the fever has passed. The incubation period is 7 to 17 days.

Encephalitis (infection of the brain) is a very rare complication of roseola, which is basically a mild disease.

Home Treatment

Home treatment is based on two principles. The first is effective treatment of the fever. The second is careful watching and waiting. This approach assumes that the child appears reasonably well and has no other significant symptoms when the fever is controlled. Watch for an ear infection (a complaint of pain or tugging at the ear), a cough (see Cough, page 349), or lethargy (fatigue). If these occur, consult the appropriate sections of this book. If

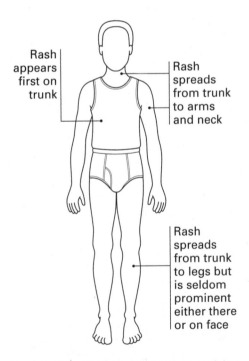

Rash appears first on trunk

Rash spreads from trunk to arms and neck

Rash spreads from trunk to legs but is seldom prominent either there or on face

Roseola. The child may experience several days of sustained high fever before the onset of the rash.

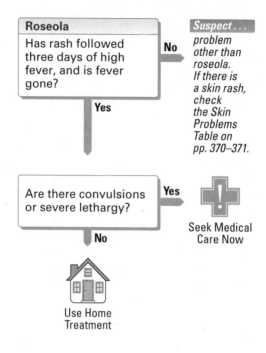

Roseola

Has rash followed three days of high fever, and is fever gone?

No → **Suspect...** *problem other than roseola. If there is a skin rash, check the Skin Problems Table on pp. 370–371.*

Yes ↓

Are there convulsions or severe lethargy?

Yes → **Seek Medical Care Now**

No ↓

Use Home Treatment

the problem still is not clear, a phone call to the doctor may be necessary.

Remember that roseola should not last more than four or five days. Consult your doctor about a persistent problem.

What to Expect

The doctor often sees the child soon after the onset of the high fever. As noted, at this stage there is little else to be found in roseola. Typically, the diagnosis of roseola cannot be made until after the fever has gone and the rash appears. The doctor should examine the ears, nose, throat, and chest. If the fever remains the only finding, the physician may order tests and will recommend home treatment (control of the fever with careful waiting and watching to see if the roseola rash appears). There is no medical treatment for roseola other than that available at home.

Scarlet Fever

Scarlet fever derived its name more than 300 years ago from its characteristic red rash. The illness is caused by a streptococcal infection, usually of the throat. Strep throats are discussed under Sore Throat, page 336.

How to Recognize Scarlet Fever

The Rash. The rash appears 12 to 48 hours after the illness begins. It starts on the face, trunk, and arms and generally covers the entire body by the end of 24 hours. It is red, very fine, and covers most of the skin surface. If you touch it with your eyes closed, it has the feeling of fine sandpaper. The area around the mouth is pale. Skin creases, such as in front of the elbow and the armpit, are more deeply red. Pressing on the rash will produce a white spot lasting several seconds. The intense redness of the rash lasts for about five days.

Peeling. Peeling of the skin can go on for weeks. It is not unusual for peeling, especially of the palms, to last for more than a month.

Other Symptoms. Fever and weakness are often accompanied by a headache, stomachache, and vomiting. A sore throat is usually but not always present. Examination often reveals a red throat, spots on the roof of the mouth (soft palate), and a fuzzy white tongue, later becoming swollen and red. There may be swollen glands in the neck.

Home Treatment

Because scarlet fever is due to a streptococcal infection, a medical visit is required for antibiotic treatment. Streptococcal infections are quite contagious, and other children within the home also should have throat cultures. Besides antibiotics, you will wish to reduce the fever with acetaminophen or ibuprofen (page 218), keep up with fluid requirements, and give the child plenty of cold liquids to help soothe the throat.

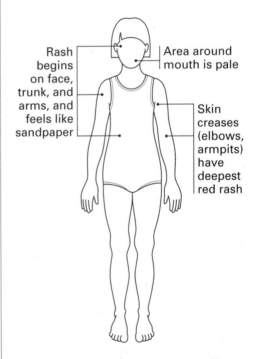

Rash begins on face, trunk, and arms, and feels like sandpaper

Area around mouth is pale

Skin creases (elbows, armpits) have deepest red rash

Scarlet fever. Fever and weakness are often accompanied by headache, stomachache, vomiting, and sore throat.

Scarlet Fever

Are both of the following present?

▲ Fever

▲ Fine red rash on trunk and extremities that feels like sandpaper

No →

Suspect...
problem other than scarlet fever. If there is a skin rash, check the Skin Problems Table on pp. 370–371.

Yes
↓

Seek Medical Care Today

What to Expect

Several rashes can be confused with scarlet fever, including those of measles and drug reactions. If the rash is sufficiently typical of scarlet fever, the doctor probably will prescribe an antibiotic, usually penicillin (or erythromycin if the child is allergic to penicillin), and may take throat cultures from the rest of the family. If the doctor is uncertain of the cause of the rash, he or she may take a throat culture before beginning treatment. Treatment that is delayed by a day or two while waiting for the culture results will still prevent the complication about which we are most concerned: rheumatic fever (see page 336).

Fifth Disease

Consider the strange case of fifth disease, whose only claim to fame is that it might be mistaken for another disease. It is so named because it was always listed last among the five very common contagious rashes of childhood. Its medical name, *erythema infectiosum*, is easily forgotten. The agent responsible for this illness is parvovirus B19.

Fifth disease comes very close to not being a disease at all. It has no symptoms other than a rash, has few complications, and needs no treatment. Rare complications include joint pain and nervous system involvement.

The disease causes a characteristic "slapped cheek" appearance in children. The rash often begins on the cheeks and is later found on the backs of the arms and legs. It often has a very fine, lacy, pink appearance. It tends to come and go and may be present one minute and absent the next. It is prone to recur for days or even weeks, especially as a response to heat (warm bath or shower) or irritation. In general, however, the rash around the face will fade within four days of its appearance, and the rash on the rest of the body within three to seven days.

Although the disease is a minor annoyance for children, it poses a slight risk to the fetus in pregnancy. Pregnant women who have come in contact with children with fifth disease can be tested to see if they have already had parvovirus.

This rash might worry you or cause you to make an avoidable trip to the doctor. It is very contagious; epidemics of fifth disease have resulted in unnecessary school closings. The incubation period is usually 4 to 14 days.

No Longer Last or Least

In previous editions of this book, we described fifth disease as "last and least" among childhood diseases. The discovery of the virus responsible for roseola has earned it the name "sixth disease," but there is another, more serious reason we do not use the "last and least" subhead for fifth disease anymore. Pregnant women exposed to parvovirus B19 can have serious problems. Call your physician immediately if you are exposed to this disease while pregnant.

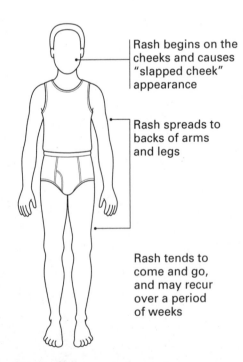

Rash begins on the cheeks and causes "slapped cheek" appearance

Rash spreads to backs of arms and legs

Rash tends to come and go, and may recur over a period of weeks

Fifth disease. Apart from rash, there are no symptoms.

Fifth Disease

Are all of the following conditions present?

▲ No fever.

▲ Rash is the first and only symptom.

▲ Palms and soles are not involved.

No → *Suspect...* *problem other than fifth disease. If there is a skin rash, check the Skin Problems Table on pp. 370–371.*

Yes ↓

Has a pregnant woman been exposed?

Yes → *Have her call doctor today.*

No ↓

Use Home Treatment

Home Treatment

There is none. Just watch and wait to make sure you are dealing with fifth disease. Check that there is no fever (fever is very unusual with fifth disease). No restrictions on activities are necessary.

What to Expect

The doctor may be able to distinguish fifth disease from other rashes. If the rash fits the description given in this section, the doctor is going to make the same diagnosis that you might have made. He or she will take the child's temperature and look at the rash. Because there are no tests for the known cause, laboratory tests are unlikely. Waiting and watching are the means of dealing with fifth disease.

Bones, Muscles, and Joints

Pain in the Limbs, Muscles, or Joints

Arm and leg pains are quite common in school-age children. Physical exertion can stress bones, joints, and muscles and result in muscle pains and muscle aches (myalgias). Some viruses cause muscle infections that also cause myalgia (myositis). Influenza often causes calf pain in young children. Severe pain of sudden onset often signifies a muscle cramp.

"Growing pains" are found in the mid-portion of the upper and lower legs, generally at night, in children from 6 to 12 years of age. Growing pains do not involve joints. The cause is unknown, but millions of children have them, and they are of absolutely no medical significance.

Joint Pains

In children, very seldom does pain in the joint mean arthritis. The word **arthritis** comes from *arthron*, meaning "joint," and *itis*, meaning "inflammation of" and denotes that a joint is red, warm, swollen, and painful to move.

The word **arthralgia** means pain in the joint without redness, warmth, or swelling.

Because injuries are so common in children, they are the most common causes of joint pain and are discussed under the specific injury (see, for example, Knee Injuries, page 270).

Most true arthritis in children is caused by infection. Occasionally, arthralgia may precede the arthritis by a day or two. This is often true in **gonococcal arthritis**, which may occur in adolescents.

Arthritis accompanied by a fever occurs in **rheumatic fever** (see page 336). Arthritis accompanied by abdominal pain and a blotchy, dark rash most prominent on the legs can be part of a rare illness in children, Henoch-Shönlein-purpura, that temporarily affects the small blood vessels. Arthritis may also occur in children with **sickle-cell disease**. In addition, arthritis somewhat similar to the rheumatoid arthritis of adults occurs occasionally in children.

Arthralgia (pain without swelling) is a common temporary complaint in many viral illnesses. It can occur with rubella (German measles, page 426) and may be accompanied by swollen lymph glands behind the ears as well as the rubella rash. If rubella is suspected, make sure the child is not exposed to any pregnant women.

A cause of knee pain in active adolescents is **Osgood-Schlatter disease**. This problem is caused by a strong set of thigh muscles pulling at their insertion on the tibial bone in the knee. Resting the leg is the treatment of choice. Some diseases of children and adolescents that cause pain in the knees actually may have their origins in the hips. For persistent arthralgia, see the doctor.

Home Treatment

Heat will often relax sore muscles caused by strenuous exercise. Stretching exercises may prevent cramps, especially in the calves. Acetaminophen or ibuprofen (page 218) is often effective in relieving the muscle pain of viral illness. Do not

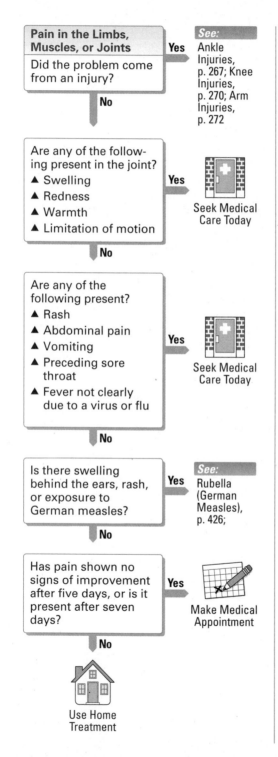

Pain in the Limbs, Muscles, or Joints

Did the problem come from an injury?

Yes → *See:* Ankle Injuries, p. 267; Knee Injuries, p. 270; Arm Injuries, p. 272

No ↓

Are any of the following present in the joint?
▲ Swelling
▲ Redness
▲ Warmth
▲ Limitation of motion

Yes → Seek Medical Care Today

No ↓

Are any of the following present?
▲ Rash
▲ Abdominal pain
▲ Vomiting
▲ Preceding sore throat
▲ Fever not clearly due to a virus or flu

Yes → Seek Medical Care Today

No ↓

Is there swelling behind the ears, rash, or exposure to German measles?

Yes → *See:* Rubella (German Measles), p. 426;

No ↓

Has pain shown no signs of improvement after five days, or is it present after seven days?

Yes → Make Medical Appointment

No ↓

Use Home Treatment

give children aspirin to relieve the muscle ache of influenza because of the risk of Reye syndrome.

A combination of the above remedies may provide relief of severe "growing pains." Home treatments for various injuries are discussed in those particular sections. All arthritis in children requires a visit to the doctor immediately, because of the potential serious consequences of the underlying infection. For the arthralgia that accompanies viral illnesses such as rubella or that follows rubella immunization, ibuprofen may afford some pain relief.

What to Expect

The doctor will take a history and perform a physical examination of the joints. He or she may make a more complete examination depending on the specific history. The doctor may order blood tests and X rays depending on the nature of the condition. If a joint contains fluid, the physician may remove and test the fluid. Treatment of serious infections will very often require administration of antibiotics in the hospital.

Limp

Many children will experience periods when they are not walking as well as usual.

When children are first learning to walk, there may be several setbacks. Most children will improve steadily, but on rare occasions, a child particularly favoring one leg may have a **developmental hip dysplasia** that was not detected during routine child health-supervision visits. In this condition, the head of the femur (leg bone) is not developing normally in the hip socket.

Although the initial glimpse of an offspring suddenly limping conjures up images of Charles Dickens's Tiny Tim, there is seldom reason to panic. Sometimes the cause is apparent or is offered by the child ("Megan bit me"). Usually, some investigating is warranted. Bare feet have a knack for acquiring splinters and becoming irritated from other sources. Warts or blisters may be the culprits.

Trauma is frequently involved (see Broken Bones, page 264). Often an evening of jumping off the couch may result in a morning limp without obvious evidence of trauma. Very active children who run distances on hard surfaces may develop shinsplints, which are actually very tiny fractures.

Another common source of a limp may be an injection into the thigh muscle. The muscle may develop a slight swollen reaction to the medication or immunizing agent. Rarely, an abscess may develop.

Infections may also develop in bones (osteomyelitis), joints (arthritis), or muscles (myositis), leading to a limp. In these situations, fever or redness will alert you to the possibility.

Home Treatment

Injuries involving the leg are discussed elsewhere (see Broken Bones, page 264; Ankle Injuries, page 267; and Knee Injuries, page 270). Rest, ice, compression, elevation, and protection are in order. Acetaminophen and ibuprofen (page 218) are useful for pain relief in injuries.

Splinters can usually be removed with tweezers or a needle sterilized with alcohol or heating. Distraction during this home surgery is generally the most effective anesthetic. Splinters left in usually work their way to the surface, but the limp may go on longer than is necessary.

What to Expect

A careful history and examination will provide probable diagnoses for most limps. The doctor will spend much of the visit inspecting, prodding, and rotating your child's feet, ankles, legs, knees, thighs, and hips. He or she may order X rays to detect possible fractures, dislocations, or developmental hip dysplasia.

Blood tests are possible if fever or redness accompanies the limp. In certain instances, the doctor may place a needle inside a joint or bone to remove fluid so that he or she can evaluate a potentially serious infection.

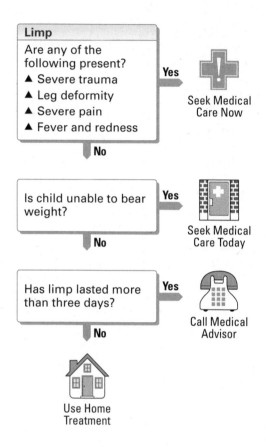

Limp

Are any of the
following present?
▲ Severe trauma
▲ Leg deformity
▲ Severe pain
▲ Fever and redness

Yes → Seek Medical
Care Now

No

Is child unable to bear
weight?

Yes → Seek Medical
Care Today

No

Has limp lasted more
than three days?

Yes → Call Medical
Advisor

No

Use Home
Treatment

Neck Pain

A variety of problems can be responsible for children having pain or difficulty moving their necks.

Newborn infants often have considerable pressure applied to their necks during delivery. A small amount of bleeding in one of the neck muscles can produce both swelling and difficulty moving the neck. This may not become apparent in a baby for several weeks.

Other types of muscle problems may affect older children, especially spasm that may follow an injury or occur spontaneously. These neck problems are known as **torticollis**, or wryneck.

Infection

Often children will complain of neck pain or refuse to move their necks because of an infection. Pneumonia or pharyngitis (sore throat) are two of the more common infections that produce this symptom. A swelling that feels like a lima bean represents a swollen lymph node and usually signals an infection. On occasion, inability to move the neck represents a very serious infection, meningitis; one form of meningitis (meningococcal) will often occur with a purple rash.

If your child experiences difficulty touching the chin to the chest or is irritable, drowsy, lethargic, or vomiting, an immediate doctor visit is necessary. Unwillingness to move the neck may be a protective reaction to **epiglottitis**, a rare infection causing swelling of the opening of the trachea. (Epiglottitis is discussed under Croup, page 352.) Difficulty breathing in and drooling are other symptoms of this problem.

Home Treatment

For minor aches and muscle spasm, heat can be soothing, and pain relievers such as acetaminophen and ibuprofen (page 218) are quite helpful. If your infant has developed torticollis, you will probably receive instructions from your doctor on how to perform gentle stretching exercises.

What to Expect

After your doctor carefully examines the neck muscles and movement of the head, his or her course of action will depend on whether muscle spasm, trauma, or infection seems most likely. If the doctor suspects trauma, he or she may order X rays of the neck, collarbones, and shoulders. Depending on the location of the suspected infection, the physician may call for a throat culture, chest X ray, CT scan, or evaluation of swollen lymph glands (see Swollen Glands, page 358).

An abscess may also occur in or around the tonsils or the back of the throat. Either location will require antibiotics and possible surgery.

If the doctor suspects meningitis, he or she will need to do a lumbar puncture (spinal tap) immediately. Although this is a terrifying procedure to contemplate, it is extraordinary how low the risks are. More important, it is a crucial procedure that must be done without delay if meningitis is suspected.

Neck Pain

Are any of the following present?
- ▲ Vomiting
- ▲ Irritability
- ▲ Drowsiness or lethargy
- ▲ Inability to touch chin to chest
- ▲ Drooling
- ▲ Difficulty breathing
- ▲ Neck injury
- ▲ Onset with purple rash

Yes → Seek Medical Care Now

No ↓

Has there been a recent non-neck injury?

Yes → *CALL DOCTOR NOW.*

No ↓

Is there a swollen gland, cough, or fever over 101°F (38°C) without other aching muscles?

Yes → Seek Medical Care Today

No ↓

Has pain lasted more than two days?

Yes → Call Medical Advisor

No ↓

Use Home Treatment

Bowlegs and Knock-Knees

These problems are quite common and almost never need treatment. Practically all normal infants and toddlers have some bowing of the legs. The bowing is worst at about one year of age and usually disappears by age two. The strengthening of the leg muscles that occurs in the first year of walking appears to be responsible for correcting bowing. Bowed legs are often more apparent than real and may disappear merely by placing the ankles together.

Knock-knees usually develops a year or so later. It appears the worst at about age three and is often accompanied by pigeon toes (page 442), which are actually a compensating balancing response. Knock-knees tends to correct itself without any treatment by age six.

Many years ago, a vitamin D deficiency (**rickets**) sometimes caused bowlegs, but this is unusual in an adequately nourished child in the United States today. In some parts of the eastern United States, a hereditary form of rickets still occurs. Because nursing is becoming more common and breast milk does not contain vitamin D, cases of rickets are again being seen. Vitamin D also comes from sunshine. Dark skin hampers the absorption of sunlight, so breast-fed infants, especially those with dark skin, need vitamin D supplements.

Bowlegs rarely requires medical treatment, but in cases that do, the bowing is severe and tends to get worse as time goes by. Knock-knees also rarely requires medical treatment. A proper decision to treat is made after careful measurements indicate that the problem is getting worse and the deformity is more than mild. You can usually discuss this problem during a regular doctor visit, and it seldom requires a separate appointment.

Home Treatment
Watching is usually all that is required. Remember that bowlegs tends to be most apparent during the first year of life and tends to resolve thereafter. Adequate walking and other exercises that will strengthen the leg muscles are important for the overall health of your child, as well as for proper leg development.

What to Expect
The doctor will carefully examine the back, hips, and legs, taking the appropriate measurements. He or she also will observe the child's gait. If there is excess bowing, the doctor may order an X ray or refer the child to an orthopedic surgeon. Only very rarely treatment may consist of having the child use a nighttime brace (Denis Browne splint). Most cases require no treatment. Surgery is rarely needed. Surgical intervention in a severe case of knock-knees may be recommended before age eight or nine.

Bowlegs

With the ankles touching, is the distance between the knees more than 1½ inches (4 cm)?

Yes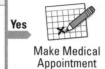

Make Medical Appointment

No

Use Home Treatment

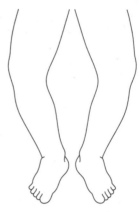

Bowlegs. This condition usually corrects itself after the child begins walking. It rarely requires medical treatment.

Knock-Knees

With the knees touching, is the distance between the ankles more than 2 inches (5 cm)?

Yes

Make Medical Appointment

No

Use Home Treatment

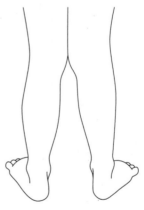

Knock-Knees. Like bowlegs, this rarely requires medical treatment. Knock-knees usually corrects itself by age six.

Pigeon Toes and Flat Feet

As a nation, we have a fascination with feet. Most concerns about feet can be allayed by understanding normal development.

Infants

When children are born, their feet often turn in because of the cramped uterine environment. You should be able to straighten each foot easily by manipulating it gently with your fingers. If you cannot straighten a foot easily, discuss this with your doctor. In this situation, the bones may not be aligned perfectly, causing a problem known as **metatarsus adductus**. This problem is simple to correct if detected early in a newborn.

All infants have fat feet (not to be confused with *flat* feet). Unless there is an obvious bony deformity of the foot, with ankle bones protruding on the inside of the foot, you need not be concerned.

Toddlers

When children begin to walk, they keep their legs far apart and have their feet pointing out. This "duck walking" provides the most stable base for the new, unsteady walker.

Many toddlers appear to have bowed legs and later walk with their toes pointing in—"pigeon toes." Rarely, **toeing in** results because the leg is set into the hip at the wrong angle. With the child lying on his or her back, you should be able to turn the feet outward. If this is not possible, check with your doctor during your next visit. Toeing in can also be caused when one of the bones in the lower leg is twisted in excessively. As the child grows, the bone

naturally twists outward. You can detect excessive twisting by checking the child's ankle bones when he or she is sitting on a table. If the outer ankle bone is in front of the inner bone, toeing in is present.

Pigeon toes can also be caused by metatarsus adductus. Most children outgrow their pigeon toes by age four. A severe problem causing frequent tripping or any of the findings discussed in the previous paragraph require a discussion with your doctor.

Older Children

In an older child, you can check for flat feet by examining the child's shoes. A worn inner edge of the heels indicates possible flat feet. Children with severe flat feet may complain of foot pain and have no visible arch even if they stand on their toes. Most flat feet are more imagined than real.

Home Treatment

Most children will grow up to have straight feet and legs, and most variations are normal developmental occurrences. The best home treatment is to encourage physical activities, because muscles assist in the growing and straightening process. You need *not* spend large sums of money on shoes. The purpose of a shoe is to protect the bottom of the child's foot from scrapes and cuts. Except for the first few months of walking, when high-top shoes may facilitate the walking process, athletic shoes are a good choice. They are inexpensive (if you avoid designer labels), which is especially important for a rapidly growing foot, and won't cramp the toes.

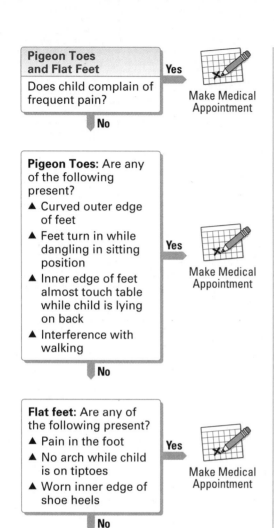

Pigeon Toes and Flat Feet

Does child complain of frequent pain?

Yes → Make Medical Appointment

No ↓

Pigeon Toes: Are any of the following present?

▲ Curved outer edge of feet
▲ Feet turn in while dangling in sitting position
▲ Inner edge of feet almost touch table while child is lying on back
▲ Interference with walking

Yes → Make Medical Appointment

No ↓

Flat feet: Are any of the following present?

▲ Pain in the foot
▲ No arch while child is on tiptoes
▲ Worn inner edge of shoe heels

Yes → Make Medical Appointment

No ↓

Use Home Treatment

What to Expect

The doctor will perform a thorough examination of the foot, ankle, knee, and hips and will observe the child's gait. If the doctor suspects a fixed foot deformity such as metatarsus adductus, he or she may order X rays. Treatment will depend on the child's age and the extent of the problem. Be reassured that perfectly straight feet and legs, though cosmetically more pleasing, do not offer any functional advantages. People with feet that are slightly turned in play tennis with greater ease, and those with feet slightly turned out have an easier time with fencing.

Foot problems. Pigeon toes (below) has several causes. You may be able to identify flat feet (bottom right) by first wetting your child's feet then standing him or her on a dry surface to leave an imprint.

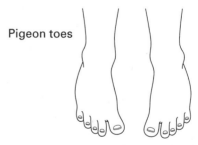

Pigeon toes

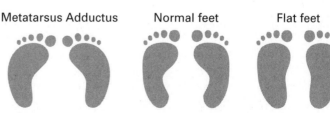

Metatarsus Adductus   Normal feet   Flat feet

Arm and Leg Lumps

Active children have countless ways of entangling, compressing, bruising, and sometimes shattering arms and legs. We are all accustomed to seeing a slight amount of swelling that accompanies a minor injury, but the presence of other symptoms can help indicate whether the problem is serious. When making decisions after an accident, always consider the severity of the impact. Also be sure to read Chapter B, "Common Injuries."

Whenever your child has difficulty moving an arm or leg or problems standing or walking, see the doctor immediately.

Severe pain, moderate pain lasting for more than a day, or a large amount of swelling may indicate more than a simple bruise and justify immediate medical attention.

Sometimes parents notice lumps that do not seem related to any injury. The most common cause of a lump in the thigh for infants is an **immunization**. Often you may not notice the lump for a day or two after the shot. Home treatment and time will usually alleviate this problem. On exceedingly rare occasions, an abscess may follow many days or weeks after any type of injection. See the doctor the same day you detect an abscess.

Children or parents often discover small, bean-shaped lumps in places such as the groin, the side of the elbow, behind the knee, or the armpit. These are **lymph nodes** that usually swell in the process of fighting infections. Look for a nearby stubbed toe or scratched finger. On rare occasions, lymph nodes swell because of more serious infections or other illnesses. A persistently swollen lymph node, as well as swelling accompanied by weight loss or other symptoms, requires a visit to the doctor. (See Swollen Glands, page 358.)

A small circular swelling on the back of the hand is usually due to a cyst known as a **ganglion**. Most resolve on their own, but persistence or pain should prompt a visit to the doctor.

Home Treatment

Simple bruises often feel better with something cool next to them. If pain is troublesome, you may wish to ask older children if they want acetaminophen or ibuprofen (page 218).

Warm compresses may help a leg that is swollen because of an immunization. Soak a washcloth in warm water and apply it several times a day to your infant's thigh. The lump should start getting smaller in three to five days, but a small hard spot may persist for weeks.

When dealing with lymph nodes, you must deal with the local infection. Soap and water is your first option. (See Swollen Glands, page 358.)

What to Expect

For traumatic problems, the doctor may perform a thorough exam and order X rays.

There is little your doctor can do to speed the healing of an immunization reaction. Prolonged or massive swelling after an injection may signal an abscess and require blood tests and even an X ray.

If the doctor is concerned about swollen lymph glands, he or she will probably investigate them by running skin and blood tests for a variety of common

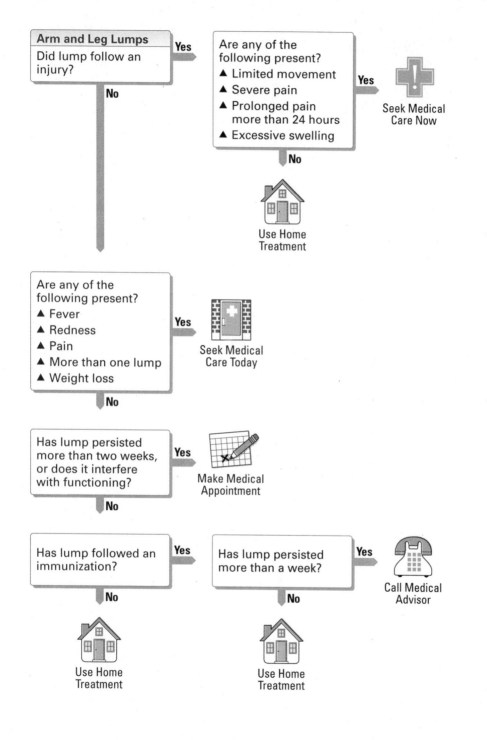

Arm and Leg Lumps

Did lump follow an injury? — **Yes** →

Are any of the following present?
▲ Limited movement
▲ Severe pain
▲ Prolonged pain more than 24 hours
▲ Excessive swelling

— **Yes** → Seek Medical Care Now

No ↓ Use Home Treatment

No ↓

Are any of the following present?
▲ Fever
▲ Redness
▲ Pain
▲ More than one lump
▲ Weight loss

— **Yes** → Seek Medical Care Today

No ↓

Has lump persisted more than two weeks, or does it interfere with functioning? — **Yes** → Make Medical Appointment

No ↓

Has lump followed an immunization? — **Yes** → Has lump persisted more than a week? — **Yes** → Call Medical Advisor

No ↓ Use Home Treatment

No ↓ Use Home Treatment

infections (strep, staph), less common infections (mononucleosis, toxoplasmosis, cat scratch disease), and unusual infections (tuberculosis). Doctors often prescribe antibiotics before all these tests are completed to see if a presumptive infection can be treated. Occasionally, they will put a needle in the lymph node to obtain material for testing. Ultimately, some nodes may be removed surgically.

Lower Back Pain

Lower back pain is uncommon before adolescence. If a young child complains of back pain and there is an accompanying fever or pain on urination, a urinary tract infection is often to blame. A fall on the tailbone is another fairly frequent cause of this symptom. **Infections of the vertebrae** are rare but more frequent in children than adults. Although children's bones are far more resilient than those of adults, **spinal injuries** do occur. Persistent pain or weakness in the lower extremities should alert you to this possibility. Weakness without pain is unusual. However, if it is clearly present, see the doctor.

Some developmental (congenital) disorders of the hip may present themselves first as back complaints. Often children with these disorders have a limp or other problems as well. Another cause of back complaints is a developmental **abnormality of the spine**. A spine that appears crooked in a side-to-side or back-to-front direction should be discussed with the doctor during a regularly scheduled visit.

Adolescents

Lower back pain in adolescents often results from muscular strain. The strain causes spasm of the supportive muscles alongside the spine. Any injury to the back may produce such spasm, resulting in severe pain and stiffness. Pain may be immediate or may occur some hours after the exertion or injury. Often the cause is not clear.

Muscular problems of the back due to exertion or lifting must heal naturally; give them time. The pain due to muscular back strain is usually in the lower back. If it extends beyond this area, a more serious problem may exist. Pain that travels down one leg (**sciatica**) suggests pressure on the nerves as they leave the spinal cord. Such complications require medical attention.

A backache may also be caused by the daily strain of supporting an obese body, by the rupture of small fat sacs, or by loose ligaments following rapid weight reduction. Obesity is not good for the back.

Lower back pain is common during the menstrual period. This is discussed further in Menstrual Problems, page 478.

Home Treatment

When a muscle strain is present, resting the injured part will help healing. The spasm of the muscle itself helps rest the part. When the pain first appears, having the child lie flat on his or her back for at least 24 hours may help. After this bed rest, the child can begin a gradual increase in activity, carefully avoiding reinjury.

Severe muscle spasm pain usually lasts for 48 to 72 hours and is followed by days or weeks of less severe pain. Complete recovery will generally take 6 weeks. Strenuous activity during that period can bring the problem back and delay complete recovery.

Slow improvement is the rule with back pain. But if there is no improvement within 48 hours, see the doctor.

After the back heals, an exercise program can help prevent reinjury. No drugs will hasten healing; they'll only reduce the symptoms. The child should sleep without a pillow on a very firm mattress, with a bed board under the mattress. Some individuals report being most comfortable on the floor. A folded towel beneath the lower back may increase comfort.

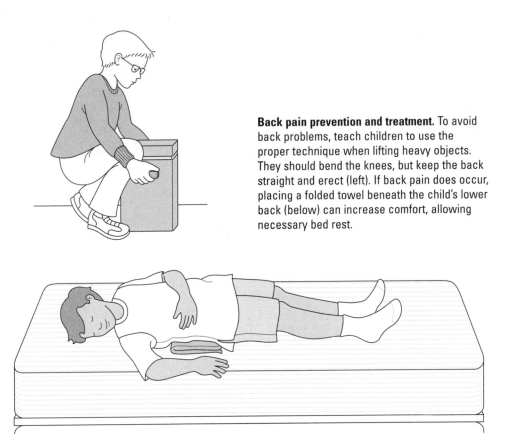

Back pain prevention and treatment. To avoid back problems, teach children to use the proper technique when lifting heavy objects. They should bend the knees, but keep the back straight and erect (left). If back pain does occur, placing a folded towel beneath the child's lower back (below) can increase comfort, allowing necessary bed rest.

Heat applied to the affected area will provide some relief. Acetaminophen or ibuprofen may be continued for as long as there is significant pain (page 218).

When the child is standing or sitting, at least one foot can be elevated and placed on an adjacent chair with the knee flexed. This position helps straighten the lower back and increase comfort.

What to Expect

The doctor will direct the physical examination toward determining whether the problem has its origins in the urinary tract, the skeleton, or the muscular system. The examination will center on the back, abdomen, arms, and legs, with special attention to testing the nerve function of the legs.

If the injury is the result of a fall or blow to the back, or if a limp is present, X rays are indicated; otherwise, they usually are not. X rays do not show injuries to muscles, only to bones.

If lower back strain is present, the doctor's advice will be similar to that described above. A urinary tract infection will require an antibiotic. Infections of the bones are very rare but quite serious. They can be diagnosed by X ray and will be

Lower Back Pain

Is pain associated with any of the following?

▲ Abdominal pain

▲ Nausea, vomiting, or diarrhea

▲ Pain, bleeding, or frequency of urination

▲ Menstrual period

▲ Flulike symptoms

Yes →

See:
Abdominal Pain, p. 465;
Recurrent Abdominal Pain, p. 468;
Nausea and Vomiting, p. 456;
Diarrhea, p. 459;
Urination Problems, p. 474;
Vaginal Discharge, p. 476;
Colds and Flu, p. 334

No ↓

Is any of the following present?

▲ Fever

▲ Pain traveling down one or both legs below the knee

▲ Weakness of the legs

Yes →

Seek Medical Care Today

No ↓

Use Home Treatment

treated with antibiotics and hospitalization. Developmental problems of the hip or spine may require special braces.

Muscle relaxants have not been found to be superior to heat and ibuprofen or aspirin for relief of pain due to muscle spasm.

Chest and Digestive Tract Problems

Chest Pain

Chest pain can come from the chest wall (including muscles, ligaments, ribs, and rib cartilage), lungs, outside covering of the heart (pericardium), gullet (esophagus), diaphragm, spine, skin, and organs in the upper part of the abdomen. Heart pain almost never occurs under 30 years of age.

Chest pain in children frequently results from severe **coughing**, which leads to a pain or burning sensation underneath the breastbone (sternum).

Chest pain is a very common problem in adolescents. Often it is difficult even for a doctor to determine the precise origin of the pain. In general, pains that are made worse by breathing, coughing, or movement of the chest are due to problems of the chest wall or lungs. You can check for **chest wall pain** by pressing a finger on the chest at the spot of discomfort and reproducing or aggravating the pain.

A shooting pain lasting a few seconds is common in healthy young people and means nothing. It is probably due to a trapped **gas bubble** in the stomach. A sensation of a "catch" at the end of a deep breath is also trivial and does not need attention. The hyperventilation syndrome (see Stress, Anxiety, and Depression, page 306) is a frequent cause of chest pain, particularly in adolescents. If there is dizziness or tingling in the fingers, suspect this problem.

Adolescent males often complain of chest pain when they experience tenderness in a swollen breast (see page 69). Adolescent females also may complain of chest pain when they are experiencing breast problems.

One of the serious problems that can present itself as chest pain is a **pneumothorax**. A pneumothorax is a problem in which the outside lining of the lung has ruptured and air begins to accumulate around the lung, compressing it. This problem often occurs in children with a history of asthma, but it can occur spontaneously without any prior lung problems. Breathing becomes progressively difficult. If chest pain is accompanied by shortness of breath, consult the doctor immediately.

When a family member suffers a heart attack, it can be a frightening experience for everyone. It is common at such a time for children to become concerned about their own hearts—to worry about minor chest problems and fear that they may also be having a heart attack. During other periods of family crisis, children may become anxious about minor chest pains they have had for some time. Take these complaints seriously. Reassurance is usually all that is required.

Finally, excessive hard exercise in someone not accustomed to prolonged exercise can produce chest pains. These pains are usually temporary and disappear with a few minutes of rest.

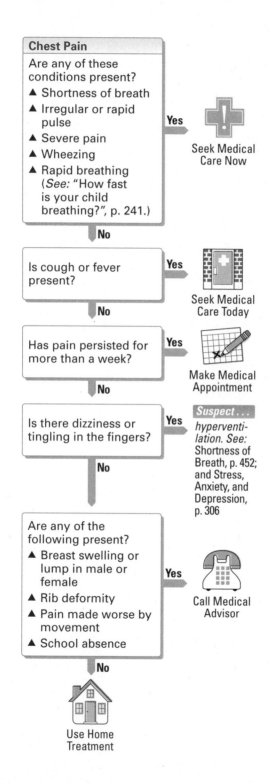

Chest Pain

Are any of these conditions present?
▲ Shortness of breath
▲ Irregular or rapid pulse
▲ Severe pain
▲ Wheezing
▲ Rapid breathing (*See:* "How fast is your child breathing?", p. 241.)

Yes → Seek Medical Care Now

No ↓

Is cough or fever present?

Yes → Seek Medical Care Today

No ↓

Has pain persisted for more than a week?

Yes → Make Medical Appointment

No ↓

Is there dizziness or tingling in the fingers?

Yes → *Suspect . . .* hyperventilation. *See:* Shortness of Breath, p. 452; and Stress, Anxiety, and Depression, p. 306

No ↓

Are any of the following present?
▲ Breast swelling or lump in male or female
▲ Rib deformity
▲ Pain made worse by movement
▲ School absence

Yes → Call Medical Advisor

No ↓

Use Home Treatment

Home Treatment

Pains arising from the chest wall can usually be managed at home with acetaminophen (page 218). Heat sometimes helps. For chest wall injuries, wrapping the chest loosely with an elastic bandage will limit the movement of the chest wall, which often aggravates the pain. If a persistent cough is responsible for the chest pain, time will heal this problem. In particularly severe chest pain due to coughs, honey or a cough suppressant with dextromethorphan may help. (See page 225.)

What to Expect

The doctor will take a thorough history and examine the chest wall, lungs, heart, and abdomen. Only if the doctor suspects a serious underlying problem such as pneumonia, pneumothorax, or inflammation of the heart will he or she order X rays or an electrocardiogram (EKG).

Shortness of Breath

When children run hard and long, they become short of breath. This is certainly normal. Medical use of the term "shortness of breath" does not include shortness of breath after such heavy exertion.

Shortness of breath can be due to several different problems. Your child may experience difficulty breathing in. This symptom is common in **croup** (page 352), where it is usually accompanied by a barking cough.

If a child is gasping for breath, drooling, or breathing with the head tilted forward, a serious obstruction of the airway passages is likely. Take the child to the doctor immediately.

If a child is having difficulty breathing out, the expiration will take longer than normal. Often difficulty breathing out is accompanied by **wheezing** (page 354) or may be due to **asthma** (pages 176–180). Wheezing cannot be heard unless you place your ear to your child's chest.

Rapid Breathing

The term "shortness of breath" is frequently used to mean rapid breathing. Respiratory rates in infants are usually high. Breathing rates of 50 to 60 breaths per minute are common. As infants grow older, the normal respiratory rate declines. By about one year of age, the respiratory rate is between 25 and 35 while resting. In an active but not exercising child, it may be as high as 45. It is therefore important to assess the breathing rate when the child is resting. Here are resting breathing rates that should cause concern:

▲ In children older than one year of age: 40 or more
▲ In children older than six: 30 or more

The most common causes of elevated respiratory rates are **fevers** (page 288) and **pneumonia**. One of the body's mechanisms for lowering temperature is to increase the respiratory rate. If you reduce the fever with acetaminophen (page 218) or cool baths and the child's respiratory rate is still elevated, you should be concerned about possible pneumonia.

Another cause for an elevated respiratory rate is an overdose of aspirin. If you suspect this, call the doctor.

More unusual causes of an elevated respiratory rate include diabetes and metabolic disturbances that may accompany severe diarrhea. These problems need the doctor's attention.

Home Treatment

Most causes of true shortness of breath require medical attention. Mist will usually relieve croup (page 352). Children with asthma will already be under medical supervision, and you should begin the usual regimen. For all other cases, see the doctor.

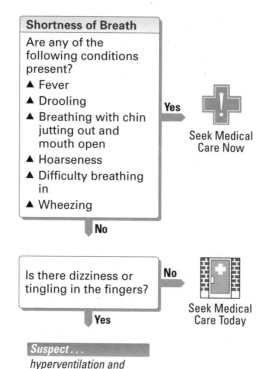

Shortness of Breath

Are any of the following conditions present?
▲ Fever
▲ Drooling
▲ Breathing with chin jutting out and mouth open
▲ Hoarseness
▲ Difficulty breathing in
▲ Wheezing

Yes ➤ Seek Medical Care Now

No

Is there dizziness or tingling in the fingers?

No ➤ Seek Medical Care Today

Yes

Suspect...
hyperventilation and call doctor today.
See also: Stress, Anxiety, and Depression, p. 306.

What to Expect

The doctor will take a thorough history and examine the lungs, heart, and upper airway passages. Depending on the nature of the problem, he or she may order chest and neck X rays. Severe obstruction of the airway will almost always require hospitalization. Pneumonia, asthma, and croup can usually be managed without hospitalization.

Palpitations

Pounding of the heart is brought on by strenuous exercise or intense emotion and is seldom associated with serious disease. Most of us have experienced what is known as "bent-bumper syndrome." After a near collision with another car, the heart seems almost to stop and then pounds with such force that you feel as though you're being punched in the chest. Simultaneously, the knees become wobbly and the palms sweaty. These events are due to a large discharge of adrenaline from the adrenal glands. Almost no one is concerned by such a pounding of the heart. But if there is no obvious exertion or frightening event, many people become worried.

Most people who complain of palpitations do not have heart disease, but are overly concerned about the possibility of such disease and thus overly sensitive to normal heart actions. Often this is because of heart disease in parents, other relatives, or friends.

Taking a Pulse

An irregular or very fast pulse may be more serious than heart pounding. There is a normal variation in the pulse with respiration (faster when breathing in, slower when breathing out). Even though the pulse may speed up or slow down, the normal pulse has a regular rhythm. Occasional extra heartbeats occur in nearly everyone. A consistently irregular pulse, however, is usually abnormal. You can feel the pulse on the inside of the wrist, in the neck, or over the heart itself. Ask the nurse to check your pulse-taking technique on your next visit to the doctor. Take your own pulse and those of your children, noting the variation with respiration.

The most common time for palpitations to occur is just before going to sleep. If the pulse rate is under 120, relax.

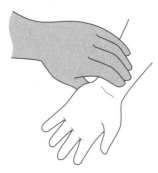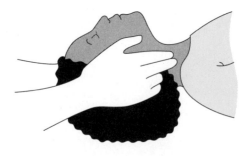

Pulse-taking. *Left:* This drawing shows the technique for taking a pulse from the inside of the wrist. (*Caution:* Do not use your thumb, which has its own pulse.) *Right:* This drawing shows the technique for taking a pulse from either side of the neck. (*Caution:* Do not take pulse from both sides of the neck at once.)

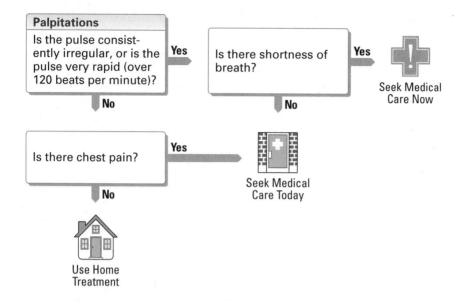

Palpitations

Is the pulse consistently irregular, or is the pulse very rapid (over 120 beats per minute)?

Yes → Is there shortness of breath? **Yes** → Seek Medical Care Now

No ↓   **No** ↓

Is there chest pain? **Yes** → Seek Medical Care Today

No ↓

Use Home Treatment

Causes

Hyperventilation may cause heart pounding and chest pain, but the heart rate will remain under 120 beats per minute. (See Stress, Anxiety, and Depression, page 306.)

In older children and adolescents, a resting heart rate over 120 beats per minute (without exercise) is a reason to check with the doctor. Young children may have a normal heart rate in that range, but they rarely complain of heart pounding. If your child does complain, check with your doctor. Keep in mind that the most frequent causes of rapid heartbeat (other than exercise) are anxiety and fever. The presence of **shortness of breath** (page 452) or **chest pain** (page 450) increases the chances of a significant problem.

Although most soft drinks have only a fraction of the amount of caffeine contained in coffee, excess intake can lead to palpitations.

Home Treatment

If a child seems stressed or anxious, focus on this feeling rather than on the possibilities of heart disease. If anxiety does not seem likely and the child has none of the other symptoms on the decision chart, discuss the problem with the doctor during your next visit.

What to Expect

Tell the doctor the exact rate of the pulse and whether the pulse rhythm was regular. Usually, the symptoms will have disappeared by the time you see the doctor, so your accuracy is important. The doctor will examine the heart and lungs. An EKG is unlikely to help if the problem is not present when it's being done. A chest X ray is seldom needed.

Nausea and Vomiting

Vomiting is one way that the body expels germs or other irritants. Unfortunately, it's a "drastic measure" that can be frightening and exhausting for children. Prolonged or excessive vomiting can cause more serious problems.

Dangers of Vomiting

A child who is vomiting and losing fluid in other ways, such as diarrhea or sweating, may suffer **dehydration**. Children become dehydrated more quickly than adults, and infants under six months of age can become dehydrated very quickly, especially in warm summer weather or while running a fever. Signs of dehydration include the following:

▲ Marked thirst, dry mouth
▲ Sunken eyes
▲ Dry skin that wrinkles easily (Gently pinch the skin on the stomach using all five fingers. If the skin does not spring back normally, dehydration has occurred.)
▲ No wet diaper for six hours
▲ Urine that is scant or deep yellow in color

If you see any of these signs in a small child, see the doctor immediately.

If vomiting is bloody, if it is accompanied by flecks of blood in the stool (feces), or if intermittent abdominal pain is present, an intestinal blockage is possible, and professional medical care is necessary.

Newborns

Most newborns and infants will spit up a small amount of food after feeding. Even with proper burping, you can expect small amounts of vomitus at this age. Persistent or violent vomiting and the failure to gain weight are signs that this may be more than simple spitting up. Vomiting green material may signify an obstruction requiring a surgical procedure. Fever is unusual in newborns. If it is present along with vomiting, see the doctor immediately.

Infants, Toddlers, and Older Children

Infants and toddlers will often vomit due to viral infections of the gastrointestinal tract. Nausea usually precedes or accompanies vomiting in children with mild gastrointestinal infections. With many gastrointestinal infections, diarrhea accompanies the vomiting. The younger the child, the more serious this combination can be. When abdominal pain is present, parents are often concerned about the possibility of appendicitis or other serious abdominal problems. These are discussed further under Abdominal Pain, page 465.

In younger children, don't overlook the possibility of accidental poisoning or medication intake. In older children, excess alcohol ingestion can cause vomiting.

Other Causes of Vomiting

Hepatitis may begin with nausea and vomiting. Often children with hepatitis have dark urine. Jaundice is not always present in hepatitis, but abdominal tenderness over the liver (the upper right quarter of the abdomen underneath the rib cage) usually is. If you suspect hepatitis, a visit to the doctor is important. Other members of the family can obtain gamma globulin shots, which will reduce the severity of the symptoms in the event that they come down with the disease.

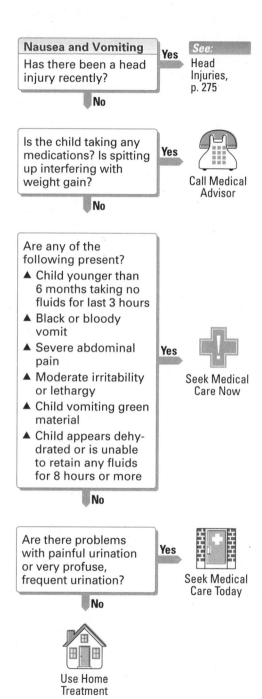

Nausea and Vomiting

Has there been a head injury recently? — **Yes** → *See:* Head Injuries, p. 275

No ↓

Is the child taking any medications? Is spitting up interfering with weight gain? — **Yes** → Call Medical Advisor

No ↓

Are any of the following present?

▲ Child younger than 6 months taking no fluids for last 3 hours

▲ Black or bloody vomit

▲ Severe abdominal pain

▲ Moderate irritability or lethargy

▲ Child vomiting green material

▲ Child appears dehydrated or is unable to retain any fluids for 8 hours or more

— **Yes** → Seek Medical Care Now

No ↓

Are there problems with painful urination or very profuse, frequent urination? — **Yes** → Seek Medical Care Today

No ↓

Use Home Treatment

Nausea and vomiting can accompany urinary tract infections. Fever (page 288), problems with urination, and occasionally abdominal or back pain also will be present. (See Urination Problems, page 474.)

A serious infection that produces vomiting, and fortunately is not very common, is **meningitis**. This infection of the covering of the brain and spinal cord will also produce either irritability or lethargy, and fever is almost always present. In young children, the soft spot (fontanel) will be bulging. Older children will have a stiff neck that prevents them from touching their chins to their chests. Meningitis is a medical emergency that must be attended to immediately.

Head injuries can cause vomiting and are discussed in further detail on page 275.

Vomiting often follows a cough and is known as post-tussive emesis (see page 349).

Excessive excitement or emotional stress also can cause vomiting in young children. Vomiting, when it accompanies a headache, may be a sign of migraine, discussed further in Headache, page 294.

Vomiting often occurs when no other symptoms are present, especially in children who have problems with **motion sickness**. Car sickness is aggravated by looking out the side windows of a moving vehicle, which forces the person to focus continually on objects rapidly moving past him or her. The eye movements required for this focusing bring about car sickness.

Many medications can cause nausea. Remember that if your child is taking medication, vomiting will interfere with the absorption of the medicine. Call the doctor.

Home Treatment

Avoid solid foods. Give frequent, small feedings of clear liquids instead. One tablespoon (15 ml) of clear fluid every few minutes will usually stay down. Often frozen Pedialyte popsicles will work if nothing else does.

As the child's condition improves, give him or her larger amounts of fluids and then bland foods. Sometimes sucking on hard candy or chewing ice chips helps. In younger children, you may wish to use a commercially available electrolyte solution (Pedialyte, Lytren). These solutions are effective in keeping children from becoming dehydrated but have very little caloric value.

After a period of 8 to 12 hours without vomiting, your child can begin to eat bland foods: bananas, rice, and applesauce for infants; these foods plus bread and soup for older children.

What to Expect

The doctor will focus the history and physical examination on the abdomen and on finding out whether the child is dehydrated. With girls, the doctor often will order a urinalysis. If a serious underlying condition is suspected, he or she will order blood tests and abdominal X rays.

For particularly severe vomiting, some doctors may prescribe trimethobenzamide (Tigan), promethazine (Phenergan), or prochlorperazine (Compazine) suppositories. These suppositories are not recommended for treating uncomplicated vomiting. Although useful in preventing vomiting in children who are taking anticancer medicines (known to cause vomiting), their effectiveness in controlling other types of vomiting is unknown. The side effects of these drugs include nervous system disturbances that may confuse a diagnostic evaluation.

If dehydration is a problem, intravenous fluids and hospitalization may be required. This is more usual for children under the age of two than for older children. Some doctors will give intravenous fluid therapy in their offices.

Diarrhea

Diarrhea is another common problem in children of all ages. Like constipation (page 300), it may be just a normal variation in bowel habits rather than a disease. Newborn infants who are exclusively breast-fed have more frequent and softer stools than bottle-fed infants do. Having more than a dozen of these soft stools a day is not uncommon. Despite the frequency, this is not diarrhea. Diarrhea in infants consists of a liquid, runny stool. In older children, two or three soft to runny stools a day may be considered a sign of diarrhea.

Diarrhea can be potentially dangerous, especially in young infants. Both water and body salts can be lost, leading to dehydration. It is always important to start giving your child the proper fluids when diarrhea begins.

Causes

The most common cause of diarrhea is viral gastroenteritis, or **stomach flu**. Often there are other symptoms, such as fever, runny nose, and fatigue. Like most viral infections, the problem should end in three to four days; rotavirus infection often lasts 5 to 6 days. The diarrhea is often accompanied by vomiting, which may aggravate the child's fluid loss. Because of this outpouring of fluid from both ends, it is crucial to maintain adequate hydration.

Diarrhea can also be caused by **bacterial infections**. The bacteria usually come from contaminated food or water and can be particularly severe in infants. Profuse, watery diarrhea, especially if it contains flecks of blood, should arouse your suspicion of a bacterial infection. The intestines respond to the presence of viruses and bacteria by increasing their movement. They are trying to get rid of the infection. This natural defense mechanism produces rapid, frequent bowel movements. There may be irritation of the lining of the intestines, and some of the cells that produce enzymes necessary to digest food may be temporarily damaged. Much of the ordinary digestive processes are hampered because the food does not remain in the intestines long enough to be digested.

Parasites such as Giardia are also common causes of diarrhea, and often occur in day care settings.

Antibiotics, by altering the normal bacterial pattern in the intestines, often cause diarrhea. If this seems to be the case, contact the prescribing doctor.

Milk allergy is often blamed for diarrhea in children, but it is seldom the cause. However, some children may have a limited amount of the enzyme (lactase) necessary for digesting milk. This may cause several symptoms, including diarrhea, bloating, and abdominal pain.

Chronic diarrhea is unusual in children, but when it occurs, it can be a serious problem. It requires professional medical care, especially when accompanied by weight loss.

Home Treatment

Management of diarrhea is primarily by fluid and dietary manipulation. All children have sufficient caloric reserves to withstand several days of no food intake. However, no child has sufficient *fluid* reserves to withstand several days of diarrhea without fluid intake.

Treatment of diarrhea begins with giving the child special liquids known as **oral electrolyte solutions**. Solutions available in supermarkets and pharmacies, such as Lytren and Pedialyte, are essential for infants because they replace fluid *and* the right amount of salt and sugar. Juices, flat sodas, or Gatorade may actually increase diarrhea in infants and young children because they have too much sugar. Avoid these products. Some juices (apple, pear) contain sorbitol, which increases diarrhea.

If the child seems to be tolerating the fluids, you can start feeding regular solid foods in small amounts. Avoid spicy foods.

Avoid giving the child too much milk. Milk contains a great deal of lactose, and because children often lose the enzyme lactase during a bout of diarrhea, milk cannot be digested properly. Avoid fats for several days, because they will not remain in the intestines long enough to be digested. Although there is no real evidence that the presence of undigested fats is harmful, they do make the bowel movement smell bad.

Infants can become dehydrated very quickly. Consult the decision chart for indications when to call the doctor. Don't hesitate to do so with young infants. If an older child is still having watery diarrhea after three days of clear liquid therapy, consult your doctor by phone. Often the recommendation will be to begin solid foods, because a continuous liquid diet also can eventually result in diarrhea.

There are no diarrhea medications that we consider safe and effective for use in children. The narcotic or narcotic-like preparations (paregoric, Parelixir, Lomotil) used by adults to control diarrhea should not be given to children.

Over-the-counter preparations that include kaolin and pectin will change the consistency of the stool from a liquid to a semisolid state, but they will not reduce the amount or frequency of the bowel movements. Although Pepto-Bismol has been shown to help moderate to severe dehydration when used with oral rehydration, the frequency of doses required is cumbersome and the medication changes stool frequency while stool volume is unchanged. We do not recommend it for children.

As soon as diarrhea begins, you may wish to protect the diaper area with petroleum jelly. If skin breakdown has occurred and sores are present, avoid ointments and try to keep the diaper area as dry as possible.

What to Expect

The doctor will take a thorough history and perform a physical examination with special attention to assessing dehydration. He or she will examine the abdomen. Frequently, the doctor will examine the stools under the microscope. Occasionally, he or she will take a culture. The physician may examine a urine specimen to assist in assessing dehydration. In cases of bacterial infection, he or she may prescribe an antibiotic. If so, give yogurt in between doses to encourage "healthy" intestinal bacteria, because the antibiotic will kill both helpful and harmful bacteria. Chronic diarrhea will require more extensive evaluation of the stools, blood tests, and often X rays of the intestinal tract.

Diarrhea

Is the child taking any medications? — **Yes** → Call Medical Advisor

No ↓

Is either of the following present?
▲ Blood in the stools (feces)
▲ Severe abdominal pain — **Yes** → Seek Medical Care Now

No ↓

Are any of the following present?
▲ Infant under 6 months has taken no food in 3 hours
▲ Infant under 12 months has had more than three watery stools in 24 hours
▲ Infant under 12 months has had more than seven loose stools and episodes of vomiting (either or both totaling more than seven) in 24 hours
▲ There has been no wet diaper in the past 6 hours — **Yes** → Seek Medical Care Now

No ↓

Does the child show these signs of dehydration?
▲ Decreased urination and tears
▲ Thirst
▲ Sunken eyes
▲ Drowsy or irritable behavior
▲ Dry lips — **Yes** → Seek Medical Care Now

No ↓

Has diarrhea persisted beyond five days without improvement? — **Yes** → Seek Medical Care Now

No ↓

Use Home Treatment

Colic

The word *colic* means "of the colon," but it is commonly used to mean a prolonged period of unexplained crying in infants. Typical crying patterns are discussed on page 79. Abdominal pain is probably not responsible for these bouts of crying.

The first episode of colic can be a disturbing experience. New babies seldom demonstrate symptoms of colic while in the hospital, for these simple reasons:

▲ Colic is very unusual within the first few days of life.
▲ Infants are often moved to the nursery if they are crying in the mother's room.

Once at home, the baby who has thus far seemed perfectly well behaved begins a pattern of screaming. This usually occurs in the evening when both parents are at home, and neither is able to supply an explanation. Is the baby having terrible pain? What can you do if the baby can't tell you where it hurts? Is this an emergency? Does the baby just want to be fed?

Often neither feeding, changing, nor cuddling the infant will provide comfort. Temporary relief may be found when the baby begins to suck on his or her fists or anything else available. Sometimes the child will eagerly accept a bottle, then violently reject it. Given this insatiable crying, panic may ensue, with frantic phone calls to the doctor or a frenzied trip to the emergency room. Sometimes before either of these courses of action has produced medical advice, the crying will stop, leaving the parents exhausted and baffled but thankful.

In most instances, the onset and resolution of this problem are not this dramatic. The baby simply has a crying spell that may last several hours, during which nothing seems to be of comfort.

Signs of Colic

Typical colic has a number of features that usually make it easy to recognize. It begins after the second week of life and peaks at about three months of age, ending shortly thereafter. For this reason, it is sometimes called "three-month" colic. Occurrences generally decrease rapidly after the age of three months. It is unusual for colic to begin after this age.

Colic usually occurs in the evening. Some people have postulated that the increased activity in the home during the evening hours may contribute to colic. Parents' tolerance of such activity also is far less in the evening, when they may be fatigued and a colicky baby can be of great concern.

The attack occasionally ends with a passage of gas or stool, and "gas" is often blamed for the problem. We feel that colic is caused by gas in some infants, but not the majority of them.

The baby will seem perfectly well before and after these attacks, and there should be no fever, vomiting, or diarrhea. Repeated episodes are the rule and may occur with great regularity at the same time each day.

Some people feel that colic is not related to abdominal pain but is merely part of the normal development of some children. Although all children cry, some seem to cry longer and are more difficult to console than others. Colic can be better appreciated by reading the section on crying (pages 79–80).

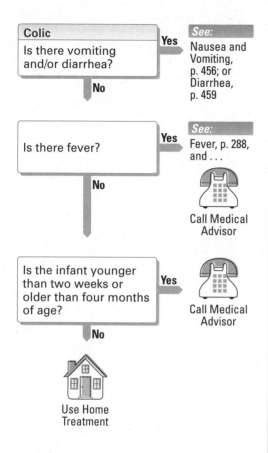

Colic

Is there vomiting and/or diarrhea?

Yes → *See:* Nausea and Vomiting, p. 456; or Diarrhea, p. 459

No ↓

Is there fever?

Yes → *See:* Fever, p. 288, and . . .

Call Medical Advisor

No ↓

Is the infant younger than two weeks or older than four months of age?

Yes → Call Medical Advisor

No ↓

Use Home Treatment

Home Treatment

Colic has been treated in many ways, all of which work some of the time, and none of which work all of the time. This leads us to believe that most of the time the problem cures itself and probably requires no treatment.

There is no reason to give the child any medication. Parents have found that cuddling, rocking, soothing music, walking with the baby, taking the baby for a car ride, wrapping the child snugly, soothing talk, a pacifier, and back rub are sometimes effective. Increasing the amount of time you hold your baby during quiet periods may be effective in reducing crying, although many truly "colicky" babies are characteristically inconsolable.

Many home remedies call for giving the child a small amount of an alcoholic beverage. We discourage relying on alcohol, or any other drug, for the relief of any but the most disturbing symptoms. Another popular home remedy is 1 to 2 ounces (30 to 60 ml) of warm, weak tea. Tea seems more likely to stimulate the bowel than to put it to rest, but it may occasionally provide relief.

In children who have insufficient lactase, switching to a soy formula or lactose-free formula may help. One study suggests a whey-casein hydrolysate formula may reduce symptoms. Breast-fed babies are not immune to colic, and trying a milk-free diet (though tough on a lactating mother) may help. Switching from one formula to another is another option, although the effectiveness of this cure is unknown. Because it is safe, it is worth a try. But don't forget to try going back to your original formula, which may be cheaper.

Finally, don't be afraid to leave your baby crying alone in the crib for a few minutes while you go to another room to rest your ears.

Colic is terribly frustrating for parents to deal with and is known to undermine confidence and cause depression in many parents. However, be assured that colic is *not* due to parental incompetence. You can take heart in knowing that your child will outgrow this stage in a few months.

If any one attack persists beyond four hours, give the doctor a call. If the attacks do not seem to be diminishing by four months of age, discuss them during a regular doctor visit.

We do not recommend any medication for colic, and we suggest that you avoid such medications, because their effectiveness has not been demonstrated.

What to Expect

If you see the doctor for a single long-lasting attack, he or she will perform a thorough physical examination to see if there is any reason for the crying other than colic. The doctor will pay particular attention to the ears, throat, chest, and abdomen.

If the visit is prompted by attacks that seem to be colic but are still occurring after four months of age, the doctor will take a careful history and perform a physical examination. Most often the diagnosis will be colic that is lasting longer than usual, and the doctor will recommend a policy of watching and waiting, perhaps with a dietary change. It is very rare for serious medical problems to be present.

Abdominal Pain

Abdominal pain is one of the most common concerns of parents, and the causes for it in children change with the age of the child. During the first few months of life, **colic** (page 462) is often believed to be abdominal pain, although this may not be the case. As children become older, they sometimes need to be reminded to have a bowel movement, which will relieve their abdominal pain.

Abdominal pain associated with vomiting and diarrhea is common with gastroenteritis, or **stomach flu**. These problems are of greater concern in infants (see Nausea and Vomiting, page 456, and Diarrhea, page 459) than in older children. Vomiting without diarrhea and especially without bowel movements is of concern because of the possibility of a blocked intestine. Obstruction can also produce severe intermittent pain and especially violent vomiting. All these signs signal the need for a trip to the doctor.

In older children, infections commonly produce abdominal pain, even though the infection itself may not be in the abdomen. Sore throats, ear infections, and excessive coughing from a cold can cause bellyaches. Pneumonia can also cause abdominal pain and is usually accompanied by rapid breathing and fever.

Hepatitis may cause abdominal pain (usually in the upper right corner of the abdomen) and is usually accompanied by nausea, vomiting, and sometimes jaundice. Household members can receive protection from the symptoms of hepatitis with gamma globulin shots.

Urinary tract infections can be accompanied by abdominal pain, along with discomfort or frequency in passing urine. (See Urination Problems, page 474.)

Appendicitis occurs less frequently than any of the problems discussed so far. Although appendicitis most commonly occurs in young adults, it can occur at any age. The diagnosis of appendicitis is especially hard to make in toddlers, who cannot describe the problem but may look very sick. Older children may begin by complaining of a pain in the center of the abdomen. In some children, this pain will move to the lower right part of the belly. Some children will have pain only in the lower right belly; about 20% will have pain elsewhere. Appendicitis is usually accompanied by fever and often by nausea and vomiting. Because of abdominal tenderness, children may rest with the right leg bent. Sometimes they will not bear weight on the right leg. The abdomen may be sensitive to the touch. If these symptoms are present, see the doctor. If you are uncertain, waiting a few hours will not substantially increase the risk of the appendix bursting. However, waiting a long time (more than 12 hours) will increase this risk.

Abdominal pain with unusual accompanying symptoms such as joint pain and a rash suggest rare illnesses such as rheumatic fever and Henoch-Shönlein-purpura, which require medical attention.

Ulcers are more common in adults, but they do occur in children. Vomiting of a dark material or blood signals ulcers as a possibility. Pain in the upper abdomen that recurs for many days needs to be checked by the doctor. If a severe injury has occurred, spleen or liver lacerations will require immediate attention.

Finally, do not overlook the possibility that your child may have swallowed some object, toxic substance, or medicine. Always be careful with medicines and dangerous products.

Home Treatment

Watchful waiting in the first few hours is the best approach. For diarrhea, see page 459. For nausea and vomiting, see page 456. Give the child small amounts of clear liquid. Do *not* give him or her aspirin, but you can treat discomfort caused by a fever with acetaminophen or ibuprofen (page 218). If pain and fever are the only problems, be sure to evaluate your child's appearance every few hours, and do not hesitate to call the doctor for further advice.

What to Expect

The doctor will take a thorough history and examine the ears, throat, chest, and abdomen. If the doctor suspects appendicitis, he or she will perform a rectal examination. Often the physician will order a blood test and a urinalysis. If the doctor suspects an intestinal obstruction, he or she will order X rays, although these are not helpful in most cases of abdominal pain.

Abdominal Pain

Are any of the following present?

▲ Black or bloody stools

▲ Severe pain

▲ Abdominal injury recently

▲ Rapid breathing (*See:* "How fast is your child breathing?", p. 241.)

Yes

Seek Medical Care Now

No

Are any of the following present?

▲ Vomiting without bowel movement

▲ Vomiting and intermittent pain

▲ Pain in one part of the abdomen

▲ Jaundice (yellowness of skin)

▲ Painful or bloody urination

▲ Sore throat

▲ Swollen glands

▲ Possible sickle-cell disease

▲ Possible drug or poison ingestion

▲ Rash and/or joint pain

Yes

Seek Medical Care Today

No

Is there nausea, vomiting, or diarrhea?

Yes *See:* Nausea and Vomiting, p. 456; or Diarrhea, p. 459

No

Has the pain lasted for more than six hours?

Yes *CALL DOCTOR NOW.*

No

Use Home Treatment

Recurrent Abdominal Pain

All children in the course of growing up will have a number of bouts of abdominal pain. As we have discussed under Abdominal Pain, page 465, these symptoms are often related to respiratory tract infections, coughing, urinary tract infections, or stomach flu. When we refer to recurrent abdominal pain, we are talking about repeated bouts of abdominal pain for which no explanation is obvious.

Somewhere between 10 and 20% of all children will complain of these recurrent problems. In several studies, serious medical problems were found to be the underlying cause of pain in fewer than 10% of these children. The most common underlying medical problems were in the urinary tract. Children with medical problems often complained of pain in one particular corner of the abdomen, as opposed to diffuse or vague central abdominal pain.

One possible cause of recurrent abdominal pain is the inability to digest the sugar (lactose) in milk. Some children lose this ability as they get older, and this can cause abdominal pain as well as swelling of the belly. Constipation is another common cause, while inflammatory bowel disease is unusual but serious.

Stress
The most common cause of abdominal pain in adults and children is stress. It is only natural for us to react to the environment in which we live. A bad day, the loss of a pet, or an argument with a friend creates stress in all of us. It is a common misconception that children's feelings are not as complex and sensitive as adults' feelings. Children become just as angry, anxious, and depressed as we do. Often if children are permitted to talk about these feelings, the symptoms—abdominal or other—may not be as severe.

Stress can sometimes cause serious medical problems such as ulcers. Although ulcers are less common in children than in adults, they do occur.

Being subjected to stress is part of growing up. However, if abdominal pain, or any other symptom, is interfering with the child's normal functioning in school, at home, or with friends, you should seek professional help.

Home Treatment
The home treatment for recurrent abdominal pain requires a commonsense approach. Care may include giving the child clear liquids, having him or her spend some time in a hot bath, and gently rubbing the child's belly. A child will often tell you what makes him or her feel better. In addition, you should try to find out the cause of the abdominal pain. Talking with your child about what is going on in school and what may be upsetting him or her can often be profitable. Children sometimes exploit abdominal pain to get attention or to get their own way. Your own judgment will guide you in these cases.

What to Expect
The doctor will spend the most time and attention taking the child's medical history. He or she will perform a thorough physical examination, including examination of the head, chest, abdomen, and genitalia, and order a urinalysis and most likely an examination of the stool. Often

Recurrent Abdominal Pain

Is abdominal pain causing any of the following?
- ▲ School absenteeism
- ▲ Disruption of family routines
- ▲ Problems with friends

Yes →

Make Medical Appointment

No ↓

Are any of the following present with recurring episodes?
- ▲ Fever
- ▲ Severe pain
- ▲ Pain localized other than around navel
- ▲ Nausea, vomiting, diarrhea

Yes →

Make Medical Appointment

No ↓

Have there been three or more bouts in the past year, or is child constipated?

Yes →

Call Medical Advisor

No ↓

Use Home Treatment

you can avoid an additional trip to the office by finding out beforehand whether or not a stool specimen will be required. X rays will be necessary in only a few circumstances; do not expect them as part of the routine evaluation.

Eating Difficulty

Toddlers often go through stubborn periods when other activities are more compelling than eating. At this stage, it is often helpful to offer finger foods at frequent intervals and fluids to keep them hydrated.

Older children may refuse to eat for longer periods. This may represent depression or may herald anorexia (see page 305). In these circumstances, consult the doctor.

Most children will lose their appetites during an illness, occasionally even during the most minor ones. When children feel bad, they often have neither the energy for nor an interest in eating. This is a feeling we all have experienced.

If an ill child appears interested in eating but experiences difficulty once the food is in his or her mouth, a sore throat or mouth sores may be the culprit. On rare occasions, the entrance to the child's windpipe (trachea) may become infected and so swollen that the child will refuse to eat and will often drool and hold his or her head forward to alleviate difficulty breathing. This is a clear-cut emergency.

Home Treatment

Most children can withstand a dramatic change in diet during a short illness. It is not necessary to consume all the basic food groups at every meal each day.

What is critical is that children receive a sufficient amount of liquids every day so that they will not become dehydrated. Cold juices seem to be time-honored favorites, but keep children with mouth sores away from lemonade or acidic juices such as orange or pineapple. Although sodas are not nutritionally commendable, during an illness any form of fluid or calories that may be acceptable to the child is okay. Sodas without caffeine are preferable. Commercially available electrolyte solutions, such as Pedialyte or Lytren, are helpful in decreasing the likelihood of dehydration, although they have little caloric value.

Most parents quickly learn that toddlers and younger children have variable appetites. Major struggles over food generally intensify into meal wars. Reasonable rules should be established—"If you're not hungry tonight, you still need to be at the dinner table for our family talk, but you don't have to eat"—and infractions must be dealt with immediately and appropriately—"You ignored our warning not to take your sister's dessert, so you will not be allowed to watch television tonight."

Once children are old enough to eat, they should not be "force-fed" unless that is part of a prescribed regimen for an eating disorder. Children who are picky eaters should have firm routines, few distractions during mealtimes, defined time periods for eating (about 20 minutes), and minimal snacking and fluids between meals. Avoid confrontations and negative comments.

What to Expect

After taking a history and performing a careful exam, your doctor may investigate certain infections with the appropriate lab tests, such as a throat culture. If the doctor suspects dehydration, he or she may order a urinalysis and/or a blood test. If the problem has been chronic, or if depression or anorexia is present, you should be

Eating Difficulty

Are any of the following present?
▲ Hoarseness
▲ Drooling and fever
▲ Difficulty breathing
▲ Decreased urination
▲ Won't swallow any liquids

Yes → Seek Medical Care Now

No ↓

Does your child have any of the following?
▲ Fever and sore throat
▲ Sore throat lasting more than a day
▲ Sore throat and other symptoms

Yes → Seek Medical Care Today

No ↓

Are there any mouth sores?

Yes → Call Medical Advisor

No ↓

Is child beginning to lose weight? (*See:* "Your Child's Weight," pp. 66–67, and Underweight, p. 304.)

Yes → Make Medical Appointment

No ↓

Use Home Treatment

prepared for a number of visits and the involvement of other professionals. Treatment of depression in childhood always involves counseling. Drug therapy is sometimes needed as well.

Rectal Problems (Bleeding and Itching)

Rectal complaints are seldom serious but can be annoying for children and frightening for parents.

Rectal Bleeding

Rectal bleeding is not a very common problem in children. It is most often seen during a diaper change when you notice a few streaks of blood, usually on the surface of the stool. In newborn infants, this is most often due to a tiny tear in the rectum (fissure). This tear will usually heal itself, as long as the stools are not hard. In older infants and children, rectal bleeding is usually due to **constipation** (page 300).

If abdominal pain accompanies rectal bleeding, this may be a sign of a blocked intestine or bacterial gastroenteritis. Both of these conditions require medical attention quickly. Painless bleeding may occur with polyps or a congenital abnormality known as Meckel's diverticulum.

Rectal Itching

Often a child will suddenly awaken crying with rectal pain in the early evening. There may be intense itching as well. This almost always means pinworms. Though these small worms are seldom seen, they are quite common. They live in the rectum, and the female emerges at night and secretes a sticky and irritating substance around the anus into which she lays her eggs. Occasionally, the worms move into the vagina, causing pain and itching in that area. The scratching can lead to vaginal infections in girls.

You can confirm the diagnosis of pinworms by checking for them with a flashlight several hours after the child's bedtime. They are about ¼ inch (6 mm) long and look like white threads. Although infestations of pinworms often resolve without medication, several prescription drugs can speed the process.

Bacterial infections can also cause rectal redness and itching. This is a consideration when pinworms are not seen.

Home Treatment

Rectal Bleeding

If rectal bleeding is due to constipation, the stool should be softened. This can be accomplished by including more fruit (especially prunes or prune juice), fiber (bran, celery, whole wheat bread), and fluids in the child's diet. Seldom are over-the-counter laxatives (Colace, Metamucil, Maltsupex) necessary.

Rectal Itching

Temporary relief of itching may be accomplished by giving the child acetaminophen or ibuprofen (page 218). If itching is present in girls, good hygiene and baths will help prevent vaginal infections.

What to Expect

Through an examination of the anus and rectum, the doctor can detect small tears and fissures. If polyps or a Meckel's diverticulum is suspected, expect an appropriate radiologic exam. Seldom are pinworms noticeable during the day. If you have seen them at night, the doctor may rely on your observation.

Often you may be asked to remove some of the pinworms with a piece of adhesive tape and bring them in for

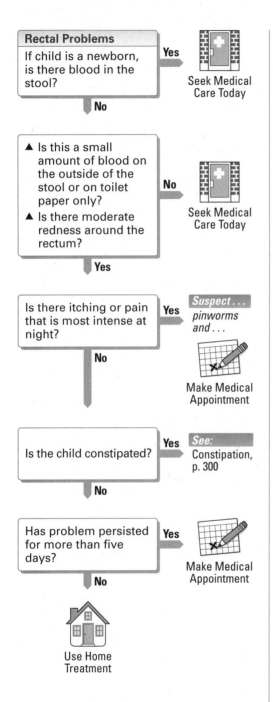

Rectal Problems

If child is a newborn, is there blood in the stool? — **Yes** → Seek Medical Care Today

No ↓

▲ Is this a small amount of blood on the outside of the stool or on toilet paper only?
▲ Is there moderate redness around the rectum? — **No** → Seek Medical Care Today

Yes ↓

Is there itching or pain that is most intense at night? — **Yes** → *Suspect...* pinworms *and...* Make Medical Appointment

No ↓

Is the child constipated? — **Yes** → *See:* Constipation, p. 300

No ↓

Has problem persisted for more than five days? — **Yes** → Make Medical Appointment

No ↓

Use Home Treatment

evaluation. After you have collected the pinworms, fold the tape over so that only the non-sticking surface is exposed. Even if you don't see the pinworms, tape applied to the area around the anus that is itching will collect the eggs, which the doctor can identify under the microscope.

Pinworms may be treated with one of several effective oral drugs. Treatment of the entire family is often necessary.

A moderate degree of redness around the rectum may signify a streptococcal infection, requiring antibiotics.

The Urinary Tract and the Genitals

Urination Problems

Painful, frequent, or bloody urination, usually indicating a bladder infection, is much more common in girls than in boys. In addition, many girls have episodes of frequent or burning urination in which there is no infection but only irritation of the end of the urethra. These episodes are characterized by frequent passage of small amounts of urine.

Chemical irritants such as bubble baths have been incriminated in these outside irritations of the urethra (**urethritis**). Both boys and girls are susceptible to urethral irritation from trauma, chronic itching from pinworms, or masturbation.

Some children will urinate very frequently but have no underlying problem. This condition is known as pollakiuria and diagnosis is often made after a urine test indicates the absence of diabetes and infection.

Boys seldom have episodes of painful urination, but those that occur are more likely to be related to an infection. In infants, a fever may be the only symptom of a **urinary tract infection**. Sometimes infections involve not only the lower urinary tract (urethra and bladder) but the kidneys as well. With a **kidney infection**, the child is likely to appear much sicker, the fever is significant, and there may be nausea and vomiting, abdominal pain, back pain, or true shaking chills.

The resumption of bed-wetting in a previously dry child may provide a clue to a urinary tract infection (see Bed-Wetting, page 298). If the child has a fever and the bed-wetting is not accompanied by any other stressful psychological event, suspect a urinary tract infection.

Sometimes a complaint of burning on urination is accompanied by a vaginal discharge in girls. In these instances, it is likely that the vaginal irritation has involved the urethra or urinary opening. If the doctor has investigated this problem before, follow the treatment recommended previously. This may include using vaginal suppositories or having the child soak in a bath with vinegar added.

Blood in Urine

Blood in the urine can indicate a problem with the bladder or kidneys, and you should always see the doctor. This can be a sign of an infection or a kidney stone, or it can be due to an injury. Red urine does not always signify blood. Beets can produce a pink urine color in some children.

Home Treatment

Home treatment is useful in relieving symptoms but not in eliminating an infection. All new episodes of urinary burning, frequency, pain, or blood require a doctor visit.

Drinking lots of liquids helps. Cranberry juice is better than some drinks, because it contains a chemical known as quinic acid, which is transformed in the body into another chemical having antibacterial properties. However, cranberry juice does *not* provide enough of these chemicals to make it a reliable therapy.

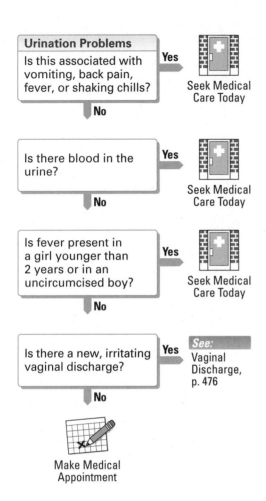

Urination Problems

Is this associated with vomiting, back pain, fever, or shaking chills? — **Yes** → Seek Medical Care Today

No ↓

Is there blood in the urine? — **Yes** → Seek Medical Care Today

No ↓

Is fever present in a girl younger than 2 years or in an uncircumcised boy? — **Yes** → Seek Medical Care Today

No ↓

Is there a new, irritating vaginal discharge? — **Yes** → See: Vaginal Discharge, p. 476

No ↓

Make Medical Appointment

It is *not* an adequate treatment for a bacterial infection.

Acetaminophen may help relieve pain. If a vaginal discharge is present, see Vaginal Discharge, page 476.

What to Expect

The doctor will perform a urinalysis and examine the back, abdomen, vaginal opening, and urinary opening or urethra. The urinalysis may indicate the need for a urine culture and/or antibiotics.

The doctor may prescribe Pyridium, a medication that is helpful in relieving urethral pain. If there is an infection, he or she may suggest X rays or sonogram of the urinary tract. Most doctors will suggest this for boys at any age and for girls younger than three years old after an initial infection, but this is controversial. Do not be surprised or discouraged if your child has a second urinary tract infection. Eighty percent of children with one infection will develop a second, but only a few will have long-term problems.

Vaginal Discharge

Doctors usually use the term *discharge* to mean something abnormal, and this can be confusing. Girls have vaginal secretions (discharges) that *are* normal, although the amount is much less than an adult's. Adult hormones increase the amount of secreted material. Children have naturally increased secretions in two situations.

The first is in the newborn baby during the first week of life. Often there is some vaginal discharge or bleeding during this time due to stimulation by the mother's adult hormones.

After the first two weeks, the child will have only a small amount of clear secretions until about one year before the onset of menstrual periods. At this time, girls begin to make their own adult hormones. The amount of the secretions increases, and they become thicker. These normal secretions are sometimes called "normal discharge." Some secretions are normal in mid-cycle after menstruation has begun.

Abnormal Discharges

Poor hygiene may contribute to vaginal discharges in girls. Scratching in the genital region often accompanies the rectal itching common with **pinworms** (see Rectal Problems, page 472) and can lead to a vaginal infection. Pinworms occasionally reach the vagina and cause itching directly as well.

Another cause of abnormal discharges in girls is a **yeast infection** (candida), just as in adults. Yeast infections are likely to occur when a child is taking an antibiotic.

Other causes of discharges in children are unusual in women. Just as children stick things in their ears and noses, they also may put objects in their vaginas. This may lead to a bacterial infection and a discharge with a particularly bad smell. (A forgotten tampon can cause the same reaction.) Sand and toilet paper particles can also lead to an infection and discharge. For this reason, we recommend that girls be taught to wipe with toilet tissue from front to back, rather than back to front. Sometimes the chemical irritation of bubble baths will begin an itch-scratch-infection cycle.

Occasionally, a discharge can result from gonorrhea or other **sexually transmitted diseases (STDs)**. These are always a result of sexual contact. Children are often too frightened to discuss these experiences with parents. In judging whether a venereal disease is possible, it is important not to jump to conclusions. This is an area in which your doctor can be of great help.

Home Treatment

Frequently, attention to the hygiene of the outside genital structures will be sufficient to clear up a discharge. Gentle washing with soap and water is helpful, as are warm baths. Eliminate bubble baths if they have been used.

If you suspect a foreign object in the vagina, it is possible to look for it yourself. Have your child lie with her chest on the ground or a table while she is on her knees. In a moment or two, the vaginal opening will relax enough for you to see inside (a flashlight will help).

Yeast does not grow well in an acid environment, and minor infections often respond to vinegar (3% acetic acid) sitz

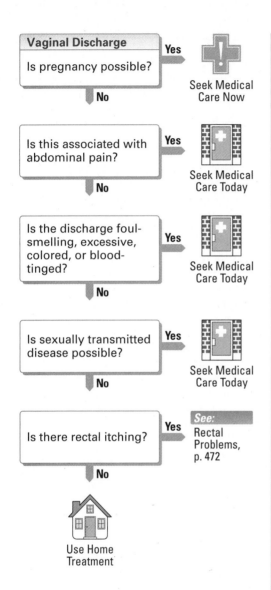

Vaginal Discharge

Is pregnancy possible? — **Yes** → Seek Medical Care Now

No ↓

Is this associated with abdominal pain? — **Yes** → Seek Medical Care Today

No ↓

Is the discharge foul-smelling, excessive, colored, or blood-tinged? — **Yes** → Seek Medical Care Today

No ↓

Is sexually transmitted disease possible? — **Yes** → Seek Medical Care Today

No ↓

Is there rectal itching? — **Yes** → *See:* Rectal Problems, p. 472

No ↓

Use Home Treatment

baths. Fill the tub with enough water to cover the child's bottom, then add 1 cup (240 ml) of white vinegar. Have the child soak for at least 15 minutes twice a day if possible. The baths will often clear up the problem, and you can avoid using vaginal suppositories. Clotrimazole cream is also effective and is now available over the counter. If the problem does not improve within five days, make an appointment with the doctor.

What to Expect

The doctor will examine the abdomen and outside of the vagina (vulva). He or she will look at the discharge under a microscope. Adolescents may require a pelvic examination. The doctor will usually avoid this if possible in younger children. The physician may order urine tests to check for infection. If the outside of the vagina is very irritated, he or she may prescribe an antifungal cream or ointment such as nystatin or miconazole. These antifungals are sometimes combined with steroids. If there is an infection inside the vagina, the doctor will make a presumptive diagnosis after performing a few immediate laboratory tests. He or she will recommend appropriate therapy, usually with an oral antibiotic, until a definitive laboratory diagnosis is possible.

Menstrual Problems

There are a number of "problems" involving menstruation that are really normal. However, they often concern parents and their daughters and can lead to unnecessary anxiety and avoidable trips to the doctor.

New parents are sometimes shocked to find blood coming from the vagina in the first two weeks of life. This bleeding is due to stimulation of the baby's uterus by the mother's hormones during pregnancy. When a baby is born, she is no longer exposed to these hormones, and what amounts to a small menstrual period follows. This is essentially the same series of events that will cause her own periods later in life when she produces her own adult hormones. Do not be concerned about some vaginal bleeding in the first two weeks of life.

Menstruation Patterns

The normal time for the first menstrual period is quite variable. We have chosen the ages of 9 and 16 as the limits for this range; some people feel that it should be extended to between ages 8 and 18. Although there is probably no problem, we feel that a visit to the doctor is indicated if a girl's periods begin before age 9 or have not begun by age 16.

After periods begin, a girl's cycles are seldom regular for the first two years. The amount of flow also tends to vary widely, and these variations usually last for the first several years. During this time, consult the doctor if periods are extremely heavy, frequent, or prolonged, or if they have stopped altogether for more than four months.

Young women who have had several years of regular periods will often experience missed periods. An emotionally upsetting experience may cause missed periods. Rapid weight loss during a crash diet or a severe illness also can cause missed periods. Certainly, pregnancy must be considered in a sexually active adolescent who is not practicing birth control. If the girl's periods have previously been regular and one is missed, pregnancy is a possibility.

Tension or Pain

Approximately 15% of all women complain about some form of premenstrual tension. Included in this category are headaches, irritability, abdominal bloating, breast tenderness, and thirst. These changes are most likely due to the fluid shifts in the body brought about by changes in the hormone cycle.

Approximately 5% of women experience **dysmenorrhea**, or severe pain during menstruation. These symptoms most often begin during the first few years of the menstrual cycle. These crampy, lower abdominal and back pains usually begin shortly before the onset of the period and last for about 24 hours. Occasionally, the pain may begin two days before the period and may last up to a total of about four days. Fewer than 5% of the women with this problem have any abnormality of their reproductive systems.

Home Treatment

If the problem is irregularity alone, no treatment is necessary other than reassuring your daughter that this is normal for

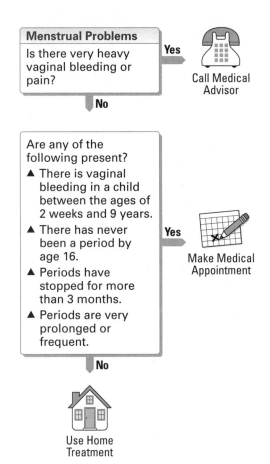

Menstrual Problems

Is there very heavy vaginal bleeding or pain? — **Yes** → **Call Medical Advisor**

No ↓

Are any of the following present?

▲ There is vaginal bleeding in a child between the ages of 2 weeks and 9 years.

▲ There has never been a period by age 16.

▲ Periods have stopped for more than 3 months.

▲ Periods are very prolonged or frequent.

— **Yes** → **Make Medical Appointment**

No ↓

Use Home Treatment

What to Expect

The physical examination may include a pelvic examination. A Pap smear and a pregnancy test may be needed on occasion. If the girl is 16 years old or older and has never had a period, the doctor may order blood tests and a urinalysis. These tests also may be done if periods started but have now stopped.

In some situations, the doctor may prescribe hormones (by mouth or injection) to try to trigger a period. Doctors should never prescribe hormones unless a pregnancy test is negative. For extremely heavy, prolonged, or frequent periods, blood tests to evaluate endocrine problems may be in order. If the problem is one of painful and heavy periods, the doctor may prescribe hormones (most often birth control pills). Because of the risks of birth control pills, we feel that adolescents should decide whether the symptoms they are experiencing are sufficiently incapacitating to warrant the use of potentially hazardous drugs. Most dysmenorrhea can be successfully treated with a group of medications known as prostaglandin inhibitors (for example, Motrin).

Evaluation of periods beginning in children under the age of nine is usually quite extensive and will include evaluation of hormones (pituitary, thyroid, and ovarian) and X rays. The doctor will take a thorough history and perform a physical examination, and he or she will ask questions to determine whether the child may have taken some of her mother's birth control pills or other hormones.

the first few years and even after. An occasional heavy period may be helped by bed rest to decrease the amount of flow. Using a heating pad on the abdomen and a pain reliever such as ibuprofen may relieve menstrual cramps.

If menstrual symptoms are accompanied by a feeling of bloating, salt restriction for several days before the expected period may be helpful. For severe pain, a prostaglandin inhibitor such as naproxen (Alleve) may help.

Problems with the Penis

Skin oils and secretions tend to accumulate underneath the foreskin of an uncircumcised penis. This accumulation may cause irritation and lead to infection (balanitis). With a severe infection, the foreskin may swell and prevent the passage of urine.

To avoid these problems, parents can begin a program of foreskin hygiene. The foreskin in very young infants cannot be pulled back, but by the end of the first year, the underlying glans should be visible. Parents can begin to gently pull the foreskin back and carefully wash the area as part of every boy's bath. Retraction should never be forceful and can begin in late infancy. Once-a-week retraction is sufficient. Do not worry if the foreskin is not fully retractable by age four or five years, because this is common in many boys. Return the foreskin to its normal position after washing. As the child becomes older, this should become part of his bath routine as well.

Sometimes the foreskin is so tight (phimosis) that it cannot be pulled back. This problem requires the help of the doctor. If the foreskin is retracted and cannot be returned to its former position, the blood supply to the end of the penis may be impaired. This problem also requires the prompt attention of the doctor.

Discharges from the urinary opening of the penis are rare before adolescence, but at any age they require a visit to the doctor. Sometimes an infection under the foreskin will produce enough pus so that there appears to be a discharge. If this is the case, the infection is bad enough to consult your doctor. For minor irritation underneath the foreskin, use home treatment.

Another common problem is getting the skin of the penis caught in a zipper. This most often occurs when parents are in a hurry to zip up a younger child. Little boys seldom zip fast enough to cause this problem themselves.

Home Treatment

Careful cleaning of the area under the foreskin is essential. This is most easily accomplished with a soft washcloth dipped in warm water. Remember to put the foreskin back in its normal position after washing. Soaking in a warm tub is also useful with foreskin problems.

What to Expect

If the foreskin is pulled back and restricting blood flow to the end of the penis, treatment usually consists of cold compresses and medications. Rarely, a minor surgical procedure will be necessary to relieve the constriction. If the foreskin is so tight that it cannot be pulled back in an older boy, it may be stretched. You will be instructed in a method of stretching the foreskin. This is a gradual process and requires some time. Circumcision is almost never necessary in dealing with foreskin problems.

If a discharge is present, the doctor will examine it under the microscope. He or she will most likely take a culture. Boys have been known to put foreign objects inside their penises. This can cause an infection. Most discharges do not indicate gonorrhea, but gonorrhea and other STDs can occur at any age. These infections will be treated with antibiotics.

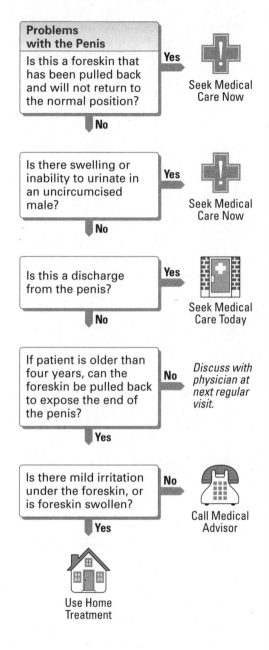

**Problems
with the Penis**

Is this a foreskin that has been pulled back and will not return to the normal position?

Yes → Seek Medical Care Now

No ↓

Is there swelling or inability to urinate in an uncircumcised male?

Yes → Seek Medical Care Now

No ↓

Is this a discharge from the penis?

Yes → Seek Medical Care Today

No ↓

If patient is older than four years, can the foreskin be pulled back to expose the end of the penis?

No → *Discuss with physician at next regular visit.*

Yes ↓

Is there mild irritation under the foreskin, or is foreskin swollen?

No → Call Medical Advisor

Yes ↓

Use Home Treatment

Swollen Scrotum

Many parents are surprised at the large size of their newborn baby boy's genitals, especially the scrotal sac that contains the testes. The size is actually accounted for by an accumulation of fluid in a sac, called a **hydrocele**. This common condition usually resolves on its own in the first six to nine months of life.

Another common problem that can cause the scrotum to swell at any time in a child's life is a **hernia**. A small opening in the muscles of the abdomen allows a portion of the child's intestine to slide into the scrotum. Once the muscle opening is present, the intestine may slide in and out of the scrotum, so that the swelling is present one minute and gone the next. The problem usually occurs on one side, although some children also will develop a hernia on the opposite side. Because it is possible for the intestine to become either twisted or permanently entrapped in the scrotum, it is necessary to repair the hernia surgically.

Adolescents may find painless masses in their scrota (a varicocele is a swollen and tangled group of veins). All painless masses should be evaluated by a physician. A firm mass may be cancer. Nonfirm conditions are common; they are not emergencies but do require medical management.

Pain

Pain in the scrotum is of serious concern. Injury to the scrotum can be painful, but if pain persists for more than several hours or is accompanied by swelling, see the doctor. If there has been no trauma, your child may be experiencing either a twisting of the testicle (testicular torsion) or an infection of the stalk of the testicle (epididymitis). Both of these conditions need immediate attention.

Home Treatment

There are no specific actions for you to take at home. Hydroceles in newborns will resolve on their own. All other problems need professional care.

What to Expect

Your doctor will probably use a flashlight when examining the scrotum. It is sometimes possible to distinguish the way fluid lights up compared to more solid structures such as the intestine. In older children, the doctor will order a urinalysis, possibly accompanied by a blood count if he or she suspects an infection. If a serious twisting problem is suspected, blood flow to the testicle may be measured by a Doppler technique or by a special X ray (radionuclide scan). If the doctor finds an infection, he or she will prescribe an antibiotic.

Surgery is required immediately for twisted testes and eventually to repair a hernia.

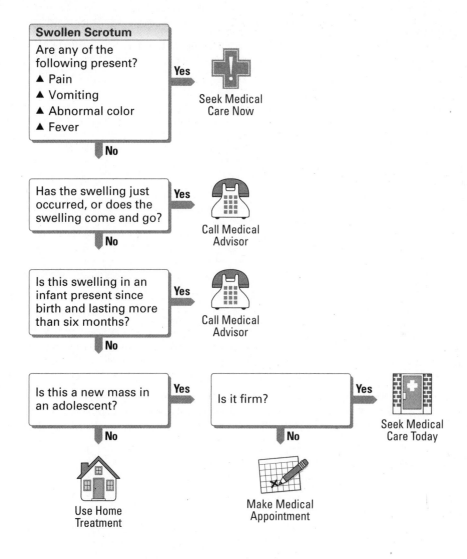

Swollen Scrotum

Are any of the following present?
▲ Pain
▲ Vomiting
▲ Abnormal color
▲ Fever

Yes → Seek Medical Care Now

No ↓

Has the swelling just occurred, or does the swelling come and go?

Yes → Call Medical Advisor

No ↓

Is this swelling in an infant present since birth and lasting more than six months?

Yes → Call Medical Advisor

No ↓

Is this a new mass in an adolescent?

Yes → Is it firm?

Yes → Seek Medical Care Today

No ↓   **No** ↓

Use Home Treatment   Make Medical Appointment

Adolescent Sexuality

Preventing Unwanted Consequences

The many surveys on adolescent sexuality give slightly different results because of their different methods, but the basic message is the same: The majority of youths today will have a sexual experience in their teens, with 7% having an initial experience before age 13. Nearly half (48%) of high school students had ever had sexual intercourse in 2007. Teenage sexual experience extends across all major segments of our population. Among high school students, 67% of African Americans, 42% of whites, and 51% of Hispanics report having had sexual intercourse. Some trends have improved: 54% of high school students acknowledged having had intercourse in 1991 while 47% acknowledged the same in 2003; also safer sex is increasing with 46% reporting condom use at last intercourse in 1991 compared with 61% in 2007. However, each year there are nearly 10 million new STD infections in 15 to 24 year olds.

Sexually Transmitted Diseases (STDs)
When an adolescent becomes sexually active, he or she is at risk for a variety of STDs, including the following:

▲ AIDS
▲ Syphilis
▲ Gonorrhea
▲ Herpes
▲ Chlamydia
▲ Human papillomavirus (genital warts)
▲ Trichomonas
▲ Lymphogranuloma venereum
▲ Pelvic inflammatory disease
▲ Lice
▲ Scabies
▲ Monilia
▲ Hepatitis
▲ Chancroid

All the above are preventable.

Some adolescents face higher risks for these problems, due to early maturation, other risk-taking behaviors besides sex, and the use of alcohol or other drugs. Developmentally, many adolescents are not good planners, and some have difficulty understanding real risks. Adolescent women are more vulnerable to certain diseases because of biological factors relating to the cervix. However, it is behavior more than biology that leads to serious health consequences.

Compared with the United States, many other Western countries have lower rates of STDs among their teenagers. Clearly, the cost of treating these diseases, added to the cost of teen pregnancies, is one factor in rising U.S. health care bills. No country in the world spends more than the United States on medical care, and reforming the U.S. health care system requires reversing such trends.

The growing list of serious sexual diseases makes it imperative that your adolescent discuss the full range of contraceptive and disease prevention options with his or her doctor. A variety of techniques prevent pregnancy, but only a few of those protect against STDs. As a parent, your role is to foster open communication and responsible decision making and to help your adolescent make good use of the health care system. The following information may be helpful to you and your child, but your child and his or her physician should make the ultimate decision about contraception.

Contraception

The most effective method of contraception and STD prevention is, of course, not to have sexual intercourse. There are psychological, social, and developmental arguments against having early intercourse as well.

Other than abstinence, only condoms (best used in combination with a spermicide) can prevent infection. Your adolescent should discuss with his or her doctor the full range of contraceptive and disease prevention options. Following is a brief discussion of currently available methods. Table 10 (pages 486–487) lists pregnancy rates for the various contraceptive methods and for no protection at all. Intrauterine devices (IUDs) are not recommended for teens.

Factors in the Choice

Contraception methods vary in risk to the user, in effectiveness, and in convenience. Methods that are most effective unfortunately tend to have the highest risks. Methods that pose little risk, such as diaphragms and condoms, are somewhat less effective for contraception. Some of the lack of effectiveness is due to inconvenience or aesthetic considerations, causing people to use them improperly or not at all. The amount of preparation a method requires is especially important to teenagers. Sexual encounters at these ages often occur at erratic intervals and are unplanned. Some adolescents (and adults) lack a strong motivation toward planning and control, especially when lovemaking begins.

Several methods of birth control are particularly likely to fail and are not recommended.

▲ Coitus interruptus, the withdrawal of the penis just before ejaculation, is not totally effective even when practiced faithfully, and it can be emotionally difficult.
▲ Douching immediately after intercourse has the same drawbacks as coitus interruptus.
▲ The rhythm method requires fairly regular menstrual cycles, which are often lacking in adolescence, and is often ineffective.

In reality, the only advantage of these three methods is their lack of side effects and, for some, their religious acceptability.

Methods of Contraception

Condoms have a good deal to recommend them. If used correctly, they are 97% effective. They are now available in both polyurethane and latex. There are no side effects, they are inexpensive and widely available, and they give protection against STDs, especially if used with a spermicide containing nonoxynol-9. They don't work if they are in the wallet or on the drugstore shelf during intercourse, and that's where they often are.

Spermicides, or chemicals that kill sperm, are available for vaginal application in the form of foams, gels, creams, and suppositories. Used alone, they are a poor contraceptive choice. There are essentially

Table 10: Birth Control Guide

Method	Number of Pregnancies Expected per 100 Women	How to Use It	Some Risks
Implantable rod	1	One-time procedure; nothing to do or remember	Acne Weight gain Cysts of the ovaries Mood changes Depression Hair loss Headache Upset stomach Dizziness Sore breasts
Oral contraceptives (Combined pill) "The Pill"	5	Must swallow a pill every day	Dizziness, Nausea Changes in your cycle (period) Changes in mood Weight gain High blood pressure Blood clots Heart attack Strokes
Oral contraceptives (Progestin-only) "The Pill"	5	Must swallow a pill every day	Irregular bleeding Weight gain Breast tenderness
Oral contraceptives Extended/Continuous Use "The Pill"	5	Must swallow a pill every day	Risks are similar to other oral contraceptives Bleeding Spotting between periods
Patch	5	Must wear a patch every day	Exposure to higher average levels of estrogen than most oral contraceptives
Vaginal contraceptive ring	5	Must leave ring in every day for 3 weeks	Vaginal discharge Swelling of the vagina Irritation Similar to oral contraceptives
Male condom Except for abstinence, latex condoms are the best protection against HIV/AIDS and other STIs	11–16	Must use every time you have sex; requires partner's cooperation	Allergic reactions

Method	Number of Pregnancies Expected per 100 Women	How to Use It	Some Risks
Diaphragm with spermicide	15	Must use every time you have sex	Irritation Allergic reactions Urinary tract infection Toxic shock
Sponge with spermicide	16–32	Must use every time you have sex	Irritation Allergic reactions Hard time removing Toxic shock
Cervical cap with spermicide	17–23	Must use every time you have sex	Irritation Allergic reactions Abnormal Pap test Toxic shock
Female condom May give some protection against STIs	20	Must use every time you have sex	Irritation Allergic reactions
Spermicide	30	Must use every time you have sex	Irritation Allergic reactions Urinary tract infection
Emergency contraceptives "Morning After Pill" It should not be used as a regular form of birth control	15	Must use within 72 hours of unprotected sex	Nausea Vomiting Abdominal pain Fatigue Headache

Adapted from FDA Office of Women's Health "Birth Control Guide," 2007; www.fda.gov/womens

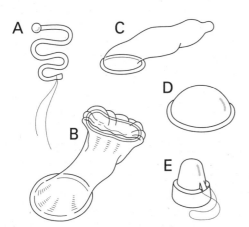

Contraceptive devices. (A) intrauterine device, or IUD (this figure shows a Lippes Loop; other types are available); (B) female condom; (C) male condom; (D) diaphragm; (E) cervical cap.

no side effects, but these methods are effective for only about one hour after insertion, and you must follow their instructions for use *exactly* if they are to be fully effective. Their cost may represent a significant expense for an adolescent.

The combination of a condom and a spermicide such as nonoxynol-9 is nearly as effective as the birth control pill for contraception and has the added benefit of preventing some sexual diseases. This is a highly recommended form of prevention for teenagers, especially for those with infrequent intercourse who may find daily pills less desirable and expensive.

Other barrier methods include the diaphragm, cervical cap, and female condom.

A diaphragm with spermicidal jelly is a compromise that is acceptable to some people. It is effective in preventing pregnancy, though not as effective as birth control pills. Protection lasts for 12 hours or so after insertion. A diaphragm requires that intercourse be anticipated; this can be a problem. The woman must wear the diaphragm for several hours following intercourse. Rare occurrences of toxic shock syndrome have been associated with diaphragm use in situations where the diaphragm was not removed after 24 hours. Diaphragms must be individually fitted. Women who are allergic to latex products cannot use them. There are no other side effects or complications of diaphragms, and we highly recommend them.

Cervical caps are similar to diaphragms in the way they are used. The basic difference is that the cervical cap has a smaller diameter than the diaphragm, and it fits snugly over the cervix. It must be inserted before intercourse and remain over the cervix for six to eight hours after intercourse. The cervical cap is com-

parable to the diaphragm in its effectiveness, and some women may find it more comfortable. Very infrequently, a woman may have difficulty removing the cervical cap. Another rare problem with the cervical cap is the development of cervical discomfort and/or abrasions in women who are using one that does not fit properly. The cervical cap must be fitted by a professional who has been thoroughly trained in the proper techniques. The cautions about toxic shock syndrome included in the discussion of diaphragms also apply here.

Birth control pills are the most frequent choice for contraception because they are the most effective means of preventing pregnancy, if taken properly, and because they do not require any thought at the time of intercourse. Obviously, their use requires a doctor's prescription (usually the doctor will perform an examination as well), and the patient must remember to take the pill daily. If the pills are taken regularly, protection against pregnancy is almost 100%.

The risks of birth control pills can be significant depending on a woman's medical history and/or family history of specific diseases. They may cause blood clots, which have been fatal on occasion. They may cause or contribute to high blood pressure. There are many less dangerous side effects: weight gain, nausea, fluid retention, migraines, vaginal bleeding, and yeast infections of the vagina. Some of the side effects can be eliminated by changing to a pill with a different ratio of hormones.

Most birth control pills contain combinations of two hormones: progestin and estrogen. The "mini-pill" is a progestin-only pill. It is nearly as effective as regular

Table 11: Risk of Pregnancy, Contraceptives, and Other Dangers

	Chances of Death in a Year
Motorcycling	1 in 1,000
Playing football	1 in 25,000
Pregnancy continuing beyond 20 weeks	1 in 10,000
Automobile driving	1 in 5,900
Oral contraceptive	
Nonsmoker less than 35 years old	1 in 200,000
Smoker less than 35, 25 or more cigarettes/day	1 in 5,300
Intrauterine device (IUD)	1 in 100,000
Barrier methods (diaphragm, condom, or spermicide)	
Death resulting from use	None
Death resulting from 10 percent becoming pregnant	1 in 100,000
Legal abortion	
Less than 9 weeks	1 in 262,800
9–12 weeks	1 in 100,100
13–15 weeks	1 in 34,400
More than 15 weeks	1 in 10,200

Source: Robert A. Hatcher, James Trussell, Felicia Stewart, et al., *Contraceptive Technology*, 18th Revised Edition. (New York: Ardent Media, Inc., 2005.) Reprinted by permission.

birth control pills, but often accompanied by irregular bleeding or lack of menstrual periods. This creates the need for periodic pregnancy testing to see if the user is pregnant. The mini-pill is especially useful for adolescents with certain chronic diseases (diabetes, sickle-cell) and for others who need to avoid estrogen.

Hormonal injections such as Depo-Provera, a progesterone injection given every three months, is growing in popularity, but the accompanying weight gain often discourages teens.

A vaginal contraceptive ring (Nuva-Ring), a soft device containing contraceptive hormones, is inserted in the vagina every 28 days and removed after 21 days. It is very effective but must be combined with a barrier method to prevent STDs.

The transdermal contraceptive patch delivers hormones through the skin. It is convenient and 99% effective. It must be changed weekly and is not recommended for obese teens. While "perfect use" is easier than with daily pills, the patch can be seen on the teenager's skin and can cause skin irritation. Also, condoms need to be used to protect against STDs.

Since 1997, oral contraceptives have been approved for emergency contraception or "morning after" pills. Several types are available. One type contains a combination of estrogen and progestin (Previn), while the other type, Plan B, contains progestin only. In addition, specific doses of more than a dozen commonly used standard oral contraceptives can be used for emergency contraception.

Plan B is available without a prescription in pharmacies for 18 year olds; younger girls will need a prescription or have it dispensed at a clinic. The American Academy of Pediatrics supports the availability of emergency contraception without a prescription.

Safety and Reliability

How safe are contraceptive methods? It is impossible to predict a specific risk for a particular patient. The best information available boils down to this: The risk of any of these two methods is less than the risk of not using them if a young woman's sexual activity may be anything more than very occasional. Table 11 (page 489) demonstrates the relative risks of various contraceptive methods and other activities.

Where to get reliable advice about sex and contraception is sometimes a problem. Teenagers should be able to get advice in an atmosphere that is nonjudgmental and supportive. All family doctors and pediatricians should maintain confidentiality, and most provide sound and supportive advice. However, many young people feel embarrassed discussing sexuality with their childhood physicians. Public health clinics are alternatives. Planned Parenthood clinics provide competent sex advice in general and contraceptive advice in particular, as well as the medical services necessary for all forms of contraception. Emergency rooms and walk-in clinics are not good places to obtain this type of help.

Additional Reading

A Pocket Guide to Managing Contraception, 2005–2007 ed., R. A. Hatcher, M. Zieman, et al. (Tiger, Georgia: Bridging the Gap Foundation, 2005).

Part V

Family Records

Name: _____

Birth Information

Date _____ Weight _____ Mother's age _____ Length of pregnancy _____
Complications _____

Medical History   Date   Illness

Hospitalizations   _____   _____

Other medical problems   _____   _____
  (Include serious illness or injury,   _____   _____
  hearing or vision problem,
  positive TB test, etc.)   _____   _____

Allergies

Medicines _____
Other _____

Family Medical History

Allergy/Asthma _____ High blood pressure _____

Heart disease _____ Tuberculosis _____

Diabetes _____ Other _____

Immunizations

The recommended age or age range for each immunization appears in **bold**. Write your child's immunization date in the space provided. (See also Figure 9.1, on page 173.)

Birth	**4 months**	**6–18 months**	**18–24 months**
Hep B _____	DTaP _____	Hep B _____	Hep A _____
1–4 months	HIB _____	IPV _____	**4–6 years**
Hep B _____	IPV _____	**12–15 months**	DTaP _____
2 months	PCV _____	HIB _____	MMR _____
DTaP _____	Rota _____	PCV _____	IPV _____
HIB _____	**6 months**	MMR _____	Varicella _____
IPV _____	DTaP _____	Hep A _____	**11–12 years**
PCV _____	HIB _____	**12–18 months**	Tdap _____
Rota _____	PCV _____	Varicella _____	**11–18 years**
	Rota _____	**15–18 months**	Men _____
		DTaP _____	

DTaP = Diphtheria, tetanus (lockjaw), and pertussis/acellular pertussis (whooping cough); **DT** = Diphtheria and tetanus (lockjaw); **MMR** = Measles, mumps, and rubella; **Hep B** = Hepatitis B; **IPV** = Inactivated poliovirus vaccine; **Hep A** = Hepatitis A; **PCV** = Pneumococcus; **HIB** = *Hemophilus influenzae* B vaccine; **Men** = Meningococcus; **Rota** = Rotavirus; **Varicella** = Chicken pox.
NOTE: Diphtheria and tetanus immunization is recommended every 10 years for life, with an additional tetanus booster for contaminated wounds more than 5 years after the last booster.

Name: _____

Birth Information

Date _____ Weight _____ Mother's age _____ Length of pregnancy _____

Complications _____

Medical History

	Date	Illness
Hospitalizations	_____	_____
Other medical problems (Include serious illness or injury, hearing or vision problem, positive TB test, etc.)	_____ _____ _____	_____ _____ _____

Allergies

Medicines _____

Other _____

Family Medical History

Allergy/Asthma _____   High blood pressure _____

Heart disease _____   Tuberculosis _____

Diabetes _____   Other _____

Immunizations

The recommended age or age range for each immunization appears in **bold**. Write your child's immunization date in the space provided. (See also Figure 9.1, on page 173.)

Birth
Hep B _____

1–4 months
Hep B _____

2 months
DTaP _____
HIB _____
IPV _____
PCV _____
Rota _____

4 months
DTaP _____
HIB _____
IPV _____
PCV _____
Rota _____

6 months
DTaP _____
HIB _____
PCV _____
Rota _____

6–18 months
Hep B _____
IPV _____

12–15 months
HIB _____
PCV _____
MMR _____
Hep A _____

12–18 months
Varicella _____

15–18 months
DTaP _____

18–24 months
Hep A _____

4–6 years
DTaP _____
MMR _____
IPV _____
Varicella _____

11–12 years
Tdap _____

11–18 years
Men _____

DTaP = Diphtheria, tetanus (lockjaw), and pertussis/acellular pertussis (whooping cough);
DT = Diphtheria and tetanus (lockjaw); **MMR** = Measles, mumps, and rubella; **Hep B** = Hepatitis B;
IPV = Inactivated poliovirus vaccine; **Hep A** = Hepatitis A; **PCV** = Pneumococcus; **HIB** = *Hemophilus influenzae* B vaccine; **Men** = Meningococcus; **Rota** = Rotavirus; **Varicella** = Chicken pox.
NOTE: Diphtheria and tetanus immunization is recommended every 10 years for life, with an additional tetanus booster for contaminated wounds more than 5 years after the last booster.

Name: _____

Birth Information

Date _____ Weight _____ Mother's age _____ Length of pregnancy _____

Complications _____

Medical History	Date	Illness
Hospitalizations	_____	_____
Other medical problems (Include serious illness or injury, hearing or vision problem, positive TB test, etc.)	_____ _____ _____	_____ _____ _____

Allergies

Medicines _____

Other _____

Family Medical History

Allergy/Asthma _____ High blood pressure _____

Heart disease _____ Tuberculosis _____

Diabetes _____ Other _____

Immunizations

The recommended age or age range for each immunization appears in **bold**. Write your child's immunization date in the space provided. (See also Figure 9.1, on page 173.)

Birth
Hep B _____

1–4 months
Hep B _____

2 months
DTaP _____
HIB _____
IPV _____
PCV _____
Rota _____

4 months
DTaP _____
HIB _____
IPV _____
PCV _____
Rota _____

6 months
DTaP _____
HIB _____
PCV _____
Rota _____

6–18 months
Hep B _____
IPV _____

12–15 months
HIB _____
PCV _____
MMR _____
Hep A _____

12–18 months
Varicella _____

15–18 months
DTaP _____

18–24 months
Hep A _____

4–6 years
DTaP _____
MMR _____
IPV _____
Varicella _____

11–12 years
Tdap _____

11–18 years
Men _____

DTaP = Diphtheria, tetanus (lockjaw), and pertussis/acellular pertussis (whooping cough);
DT = Diphtheria and tetanus (lockjaw); **MMR** = Measles, mumps, and rubella; **Hep B** = Hepatitis B;
IPV = Inactivated poliovirus vaccine; **Hep A** = Hepatitis A; **PCV** = Pneumococcus; **HIB** = *Hemophilus influenzae* B vaccine; **Men** = Meningococcus; **Rota** = Rotavirus; **Varicella** = Chicken pox.
NOTE: Diphtheria and tetanus immunization is recommended every 10 years for life, with an additional tetanus booster for contaminated wounds more than 5 years after the last booster.

Growth Charts

These charts will help you keep a record of your child's growth; three are for girls and three for boys. (Find the latest growth charts on-line at www.cdc.gov/growthcharts.)

On the first four charts, you can plot your child's height (or length) and weight at various ages. The line for height and the one for weight will be plotted on two different scales on the same chart. Weight and height are shown on the left and right margins of the chart.

To plot your child's height:

1. Find the vertical line for his or her age at the bottom of the chart.

2. Find the horizontal line for the child's height on the side of the chart.

3. Mark the point where the two lines cross.

4. The next time you measure your child, mark the new age and height position on the chart.

5. Connect the points. The line will show your child's growth.

To plot weight:

1. Find the line for the child's age at the bottom of the chart.

2. Find the horizontal line for the child's weight on the side of the chart.

3. Mark the point where the two lines cross.

4. Proceed as for the height part of the chart.

The curved lines with numbers represent "percentile" of normal children. For example, if your boy weighs 31 pounds (14 kg) at 27 months, he is in the 75th percentile. This means that about 75% of normal boys weigh less than he does and about 25% weigh more.

To plot body mass index (BMI):

1. Calculate your child's BMI by taking weight in pounds, dividing by height in inches, dividing by height in inches a second time, and then multiplying by 703. Or use the special BMI calculator at http://nhlbisupport.com/bmi.

2. Find your child's age on the bottom of the chart.

3. Find your child's calculated BMI from the scale on the chart's right side.

4. Mark the point where the two lines cross.

Birth to 36 months: Girls
Length-for-age and Weight-for-age percentiles

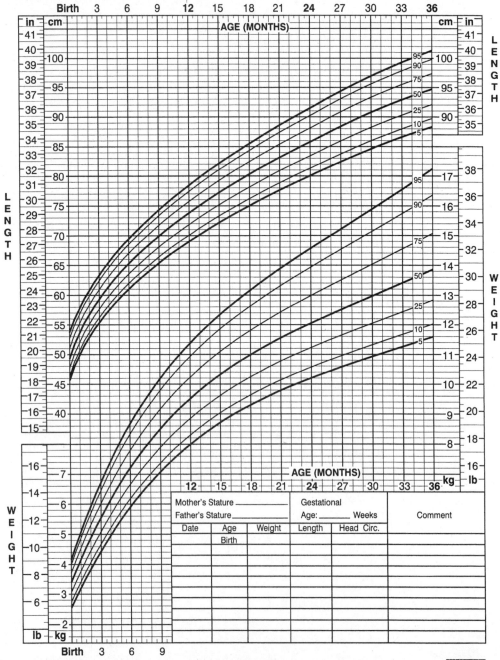

Published May 30, 2000 (modified 4/20/01).
SOURCE: Developed by the National Center for Health Statistics in collaboration with
the National Center for Chronic Disease Prevention and Health Promotion (2000).
http://www.cdc.gov/growthcharts

SAFER · HEALTHIER · PEOPLE™

2 to 20 years: Girls
Stature-for-age and Weight-for-age percentiles

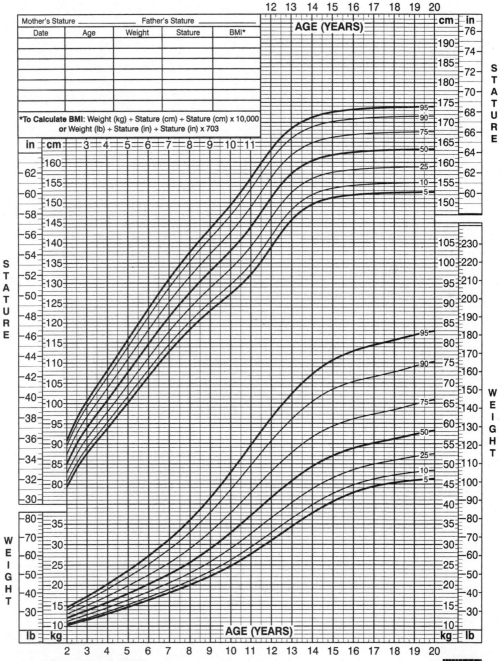

Published May 30, 2000 (modified 11/21/00).
SOURCE: Developed by the National Center for Health Statistics in collaboration with
   the National Center for Chronic Disease Prevention and Health Promotion (2000).
   http://www.cdc.gov/growthcharts

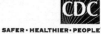

SAFER · HEALTHIER · PEOPLE™

Birth to 36 months: Boys
Length-for-age and Weight-for-age percentiles

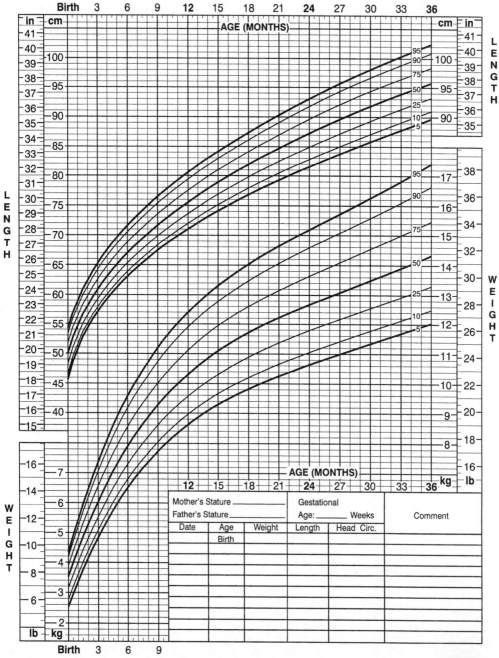

Published May 30, 2000 (modified 4/20/01).
SOURCE: Developed by the National Center for Health Statistics in collaboration with
the National Center for Chronic Disease Prevention and Health Promotion (2000).
http://www.cdc.gov/growthcharts

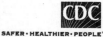

SAFER · HEALTHIER · PEOPLE™

2 to 20 years: Boys
Stature-for-age and Weight-for-age percentiles

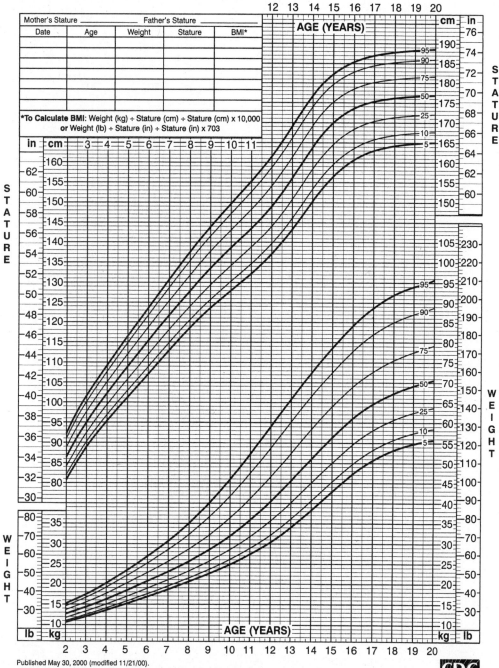

Mother's Stature _____ Father's Stature _____

Date	Age	Weight	Stature	BMI*

*To Calculate BMI: Weight (kg) ÷ Stature (cm) ÷ Stature (cm) x 10,000
or Weight (lb) ÷ Stature (in) ÷ Stature (in) x 703

AGE (YEARS)

Published May 30, 2000 (modified 11/21/00).
SOURCE: Developed by the National Center for Health Statistics in collaboration with
the National Center for Chronic Disease Prevention and Health Promotion (2000).
http://www.cdc.gov/growthcharts

SAFER · HEALTHIER · PEOPLE™

2 to 20 years: Girls
Body mass index-for-age percentiles

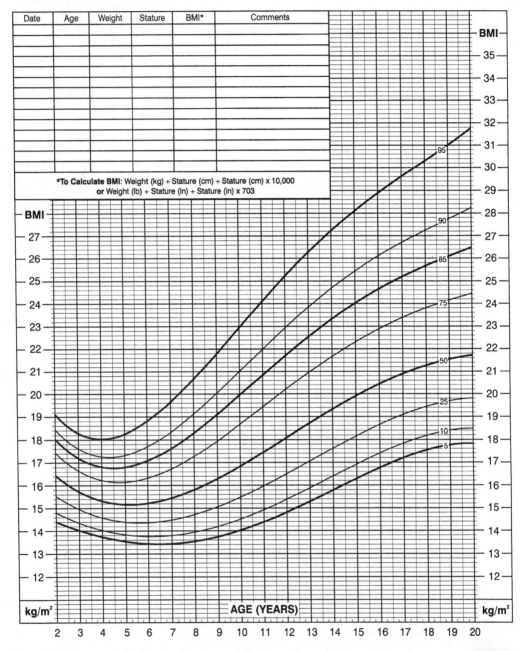

Date	Age	Weight	Stature	BMI*	Comments

*To Calculate BMI: Weight (kg) ÷ Stature (cm) ÷ Stature (cm) x 10,000
or Weight (lb) ÷ Stature (in) ÷ Stature (in) x 703

AGE (YEARS)

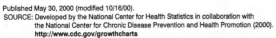

Published May 30, 2000 (modified 10/16/00).
SOURCE: Developed by the National Center for Health Statistics in collaboration with
the National Center for Chronic Disease Prevention and Health Promotion (2000).
http://www.cdc.gov/growthcharts

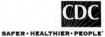

SAFER · HEALTHIER · PEOPLE'

2 to 20 years: Boys
Body mass index-for-age percentiles

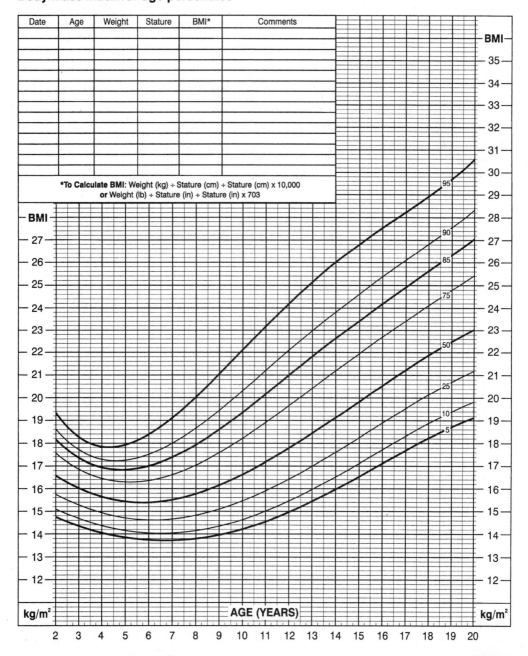

Date	Age	Weight	Stature	BMI*	Comments

*To Calculate BMI: Weight (kg) ÷ Stature (cm) ÷ Stature (cm) x 10,000
or Weight (lb) ÷ Stature (in) ÷ Stature (in) x 703

Published May 30, 2000 (modified 10/16/00).
SOURCE: Developed by the National Center for Health Statistics in collaboration with
the National Center for Chronic Disease Prevention and Health Promotion (2000).
http://www.cdc.gov/growthcharts

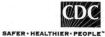

SAFER · HEALTHIER · PEOPLE™

Please fill out the following about how your child usually is. Please try to answer every question. If the behavior is rare (e.g., you've seen it once or twice), please answer as if the child does not do it.

1. Does your child enjoy being swung, bounced on your knee, etc.?	YES	NO
2. Does your child take an interest in other children?	YES	NO
3. Does your child like climbing on things, such as up stairs?	YES	NO
4. Does your child enjoy playing peek-a-boo/hide-and-seek?	YES	NO
5. Does your child ever pretend, for example, to talk on the phone or take care of a doll or pretend other things?	YES	NO
6. Does your child ever use his/her index finger to point, to ask for something?	YES	NO
7. Does your child ever use his/her index finger to point, to indicate interest in something?	YES	NO
8. Can your child play properly with small toys (e.g., cars or blocks) without just mouthing, fiddling, or dropping them?	YES	NO
9. Does your child ever bring objects to you (parent) to show you something?	YES	NO
10. Does your child look you in the eye for more than a second or two?	YES	NO
11. Does your child ever seem oversensitive to noise? (e.g., plugging ears)	YES	NO
12. Does your child smile in response to your face or your smile?	YES	NO
13. Does your child imitate you? (e.g., you make a face—will your child imitate it?)	YES	NO
14. Does your child respond to his/her name when you call?	YES	NO
15. If you point at a toy across the room, does your child look at it?	YES	NO
16. Does your child walk?	YES	NO
17. Does your child look at things you are looking at?	YES	NO
18. Does your child make unusual finger movements near his/her face?	YES	NO
19. Does your child try to attract your attention to his/her own activity?	YES	NO
20. Have you ever wondered if your child is deaf?	YES	NO
21. Does your child understand what people say?	YES	NO
22. Does your child sometimes stare at nothing or wander with no purpose?	YES	NO
23. Does your child look at your face to check your reaction when faced with something unfamiliar?	YES	NO

Tick if parent gives answer indicated below. Child fails screening test if two or more critical (in **bold**) items are ticked or if three or more items ticked in total.

1.	Does your child enjoy being swung, bounced on your knee, etc.?	NO	☐
2.	Does your child take an interest in other children?	**NO**	☐
3.	Does your child like climbing on things, such as up stairs?	NO	☐
4.	Does your child enjoy playing peek-a-boo/hide-and-seek?	NO	☐
5.	Does your child ever pretend, for example, to talk on the phone or take care of a doll or pretend other things?	NO	☐
6.	Does your child ever use his/her index finger to point, to ask for something?	NO	☐
7.	Does your child ever use his/her index finger to point, to indicate interest in something?	NO	☐
8.	Can your child play properly with small toys (e.g., cars or blocks) without just mouthing, fiddling, or dropping them?	NO	☐
9.	Does your child ever bring objects to you (parent) to show you something?	**NO**	☐
10.	Does your child look you in the eye for more than a second or two?	NO	☐
11.	Does your child ever seem oversensitive to noise? (e.g., plugging ears)	YES	☐
12.	Does your child smile in response to your face or your smile?	NO	☐
13.	Does your child imitate you? (e.g., you make a face—will your child imitate it?)	**NO**	☐
14.	Does your child respond to his/her name when you call?	**NO**	☐
15.	If you point at a toy across the room, does your child look at it?	**NO**	☐
16.	Does your child walk?	NO	☐
17.	Does your child look at things you are looking at?	NO	☐
18.	Does your child make unusual finger movements near his/her face?	YES	☐
19.	Does your child try to attract your attention to his/her own activity?	NO	☐
20.	Have you ever wondered if your child is deaf?	YES	☐
21.	Does your child understand what people say?	NO	☐
22.	Does your child sometimes stare at nothing or wander with no purpose?	YES	☐
23.	Does your child look at your face to check your reaction when faced with something unfamiliar?	NO	☐

Children who fail more than 3 items total or 2 critical items (particularly if these scores remain elevated after the follow-up interview) should be referred for diagnostic evaluation by a specialist trained to evaluate ASD in very young children. In addition, children for whom there are physician, parent, or other professional's concerns about ASD should be referred for evaluation, given that it is unlikely for any screening instrument to have 100% sensitivity.

Index

For advice on a common medical problem, look up the primary symptom in this index. Numbers in **boldface** indicate the pages where you can find the most information on each subject. These are usually the pages with decision charts and advice on home treatment and when to see a doctor.

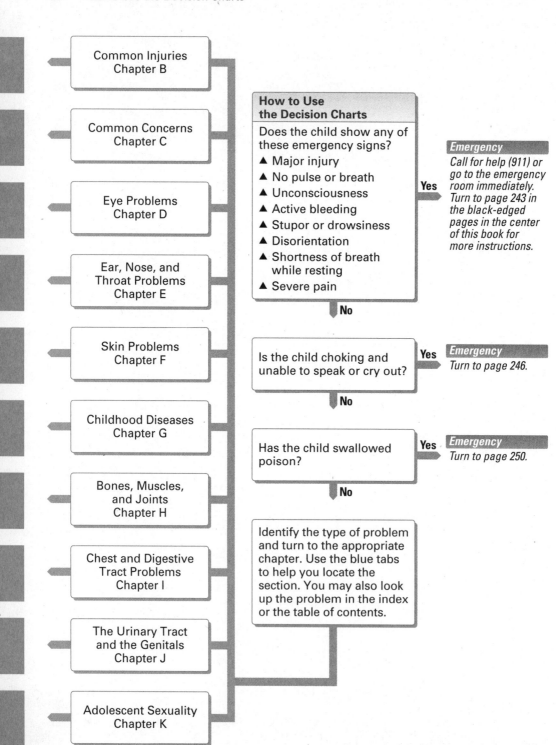

Common Injuries
Chapter B

Common Concerns
Chapter C

Eye Problems
Chapter D

Ear, Nose, and
Throat Problems
Chapter E

Skin Problems
Chapter F

Childhood Diseases
Chapter G

Bones, Muscles,
and Joints
Chapter H

Chest and Digestive
Tract Problems
Chapter I

The Urinary Tract
and the Genitals
Chapter J

Adolescent Sexuality
Chapter K

**How to Use
the Decision Charts**

Does the child show any of
these emergency signs?
▲ Major injury
▲ No pulse or breath
▲ Unconsciousness
▲ Active bleeding
▲ Stupor or drowsiness
▲ Disorientation
▲ Shortness of breath
   while resting
▲ Severe pain

Yes

Emergency
*Call for help (911) or
go to the emergency
room immediately.
Turn to page 243 in
the black-edged
pages in the center
of this book for
more instructions.*

No

Is the child choking and
unable to speak or cry out?

Yes

Emergency
Turn to page 246.

No

Has the child swallowed
poison?

Yes

Emergency
Turn to page 250.

No

Identify the type of problem
and turn to the appropriate
chapter. Use the blue tabs
to help you locate the
section. You may also look
up the problem in the index
or the table of contents.